SICKNESS AND THE STATE

SICKNESS AND THE STATE

SICKNESS AND THE STATE
Health and Illness in Colonial
Malaya, 1870–1940

LENORE MANDERSON

*Australian Centre for International
and Tropical Health and Nutrition
The University of Queensland*

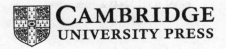
CAMBRIDGE
UNIVERSITY PRESS

PUBLISHED BY THE PRESS SYNDICATE OF THE UNIVERSITY OF CAMBRIDGE
The Pitt Building, Trumpington Street, Cambridge, United Kingdom

CAMBRIDGE UNIVERSITY PRESS
The Edinburgh Building, Cambridge CB2 2RU, UK
40 West 20th Street, New York NY 10011–4211, USA
477 Williamstown Road, Port Melbourne, VIC 3207, Australia
Ruiz de Alarcón 13, 28014 Madrid, Spain
Dock House, The Waterfront, Cape Town 8001, South Africa

http://www.cambridge.org

First published 1996
First paperback edition 2002

A catalogue record for this book is available from the British Library

National Library of Australia cataloguing in Publication data
Manderson, Lenore.
Sickness and the state: health and illness in colonial
Malaya, 1870–1940.
Bibliography.
Includes index.
1. Public health – Malaysia – Malaya – History.   2. Public
health – Social aspects – Malaysia – Malaya – History.
3. Medical care – Malaysia – Malaya – History.
4. Malaya – Colonization.   I. Title.
362.109595

Library of Congress Cataloguing in Publication data
Manderson, Lenore.
Sickness and the state: health and illness in colonial Malaya,
1870–1940 / Lenore Manderson.
p.   cm.
Includes bibliographical references and index.
1. Medical policy – Malaysia – Malaya – History.   2. Social medicine –
Malaysia – Malaya – History.   3. Public health – Malaysia – Malaya –
History.   4. Malaya – Colonization.   I. Title.
RA388.M4M36   1996
362.1′09595′1–dc20   95-42786

ISBN 0 521 56008 X hardback
ISBN 0 521 52448 2 paperback

Contents

Figures

Tables

Spelling and Abbreviations

I have used the contemporary English spelling of most places mentioned in this work, since these are the names of the politico–geographic entities of the colonial state, hence Penang not Pulau Pinang, Malacca not Melaka. Other spelling used for place names in the Indonesian Archipelago and for Malay terms follows the conventional orthography of the period, thus Acheh rather than Aceh or Atjeh, for example.

Abbreviations used in the text, notes, references:

FMS	Federated Malay States
GB	Great Britain
IMR	Institute of Medical Research
LSHTM	London School of Hygiene and Tropical Medicine
SS	Straits Settlements

Sources

BAKed	British Adviser to Kedah
BAKel	British Adviser to Kelantan
BATr	British Adviser to Trengganu
CO	Files of the Colonial Office
FMS	Federated Malay States
GB	Great Britian
GRO	General Register Office
Mss Indian Ocean	Colonial Records Project, Indian Ocean Manuscripts
Sel. Sec.	Files of the Selangor Secretariat
SSR	Straits Settlements Records
ZHCI	Great Britain, Colonial Office, Accounts and Papers, ZHCI

See also Archival Sources, p. 308, for locations

Publications

AJE	*American Journal of Epidemiology*
ATMP	*Annals of Tropical Medicine and Parasitology*
BDJ	*British Dental Journal*
BHM	*Bulletin of the History of Medicine*
BIMR	*Bulletin of the Institute of Medical Research*
BJA	*British Journal of Anaesthesia*
BMJ	*British Medical Journal*
CMP	*Culture, Medicine and Psychiatry*
EDCC	*Economic Development and Cultural Change*
FMSAR	*Federated Malay States, Colonial Reports, Annual Report*
HTR	*Health Transition Review*
IJHS	*International Journal of Health Services*
JAS	*Journal of Asian Studies*
JBS	*Journal of Biosocial Science*
JMBRAS	*Journal of the Malay Branch of the Royal Asiatic Society*
JMBMA	*Journal of the Malayan Branch, British Medical Association*
JMH	*Journal of Modern History*
JRSA	*Journal of the Royal Society of Arts*
JSP	*Journal of Social Policy*
MH	*Medical History*
MJA	*Medical Journal of Australia*
MJM	*Medical Journal of Malaysia*
MMJ	*Malayan Medical Journal*
MMJES	*Malayan Medical Journal and Estate Sanitation*
SKAR	*State of Kelantan Annual Report*
SSAR	*Straits Settlements Annual Departmental Report*
SSI	*Social Science Information*
SHM	*Social History of Medicine*
SMJ	*Singapore Medical Journal*
SSM	*Social Science and Medicine*
SSS	*Social Studies in Science*
ST	*Straits Times*

Preface

When I commenced work on this book, a good decade ago, little had been

When I commenced work on this book, a good decade ago, little had been published outside medical journals dealing with health and medicine in Malaysia, either for the colonial period or since independence. Even in recent years as interdisciplinary interest in the field has expanded – spawning anthropological, sociological, historical demographic and social historical studies – a small corpus of writing only has been concerned with death and disease, health and medicine under colonialism.[1] There remains a vacuum in historical epidemiology and the documentation and analysis of changes in morbidity and mortality, the development of health and medical services, the nature of decision-making, and the implementation of subsequent programs, the ideological and pragmatic considerations which determined these programs, and their effects on people's health. The voluminous literature on education and schooling for the colonial period stands in marked contrast to this apparent disinterest in or shying away from issues of health and medicine.

Medical administrative innovations under British colonial rule related to and followed from economic developments, and occurred in response to the perceived political and economic effects of ill health. To date, however, we lack a history of medicine or health services for the colonial period which would provide an overview within a political, economic and social context, which might explore the effects on health of colonialism. We lack too documentation of the ways in which people responded to the broad changes that colonialism brought: changes to the environment and ecology of the Peninsula, the distribution and prevalence of infection, the means of production, subsistence and well-being, and the means provided for the treatment of injuries and illness.

Lack of attention by social scientists to matters of health and medicine reflects in part the professional territoriality and epistemological

tensions that have existed within the field and remain characteristic of
the interdisplinary projects seeking to better understand the interface
of biology, culture, and society.[2] The practice of medicine was – over a
century – to be increasingly confined to a small group of professionals,
even in areas traditionally beyond their concern and interest (for
instance, childbirth). So too the records of medical practice and policy
were to become and remain within their territory, generally uncritical
assessments which emphasised the supremacy of biomedicine and the
desirability of its structures and institutions. In the context of this work
the lack of critical analysis pertaining to colonial Malaya is most significant. However, it is important to note that until the past decade or so
little had been written anywhere which located the provision of health
and medical services in a political and economic context or which
examined them in terms of public policy formulation and practice.[3]
Rather, medical history for the most part was concerned with the history
of the great men (and rarely women), with the establishment of medical
and related welfare institutions, and with clinical advances. Few medical
histories until recently have shown much interest in patient perspectives
or the population as a whole,[4] or in biomedicine as a cultural system.
Finally, in histories of health care in colonial societies, there has been
little interest in traditional medicine and its interrelationship with
biomedicine.

The first article on health care in colonial Malaya appeared early, in
1913, and related to the establishment of the Tan Tock Seng Hospital in
Singapore.[5] Fifty years later, with few intermittent publications, H. C.
Chai published a chapter on health and medical research in the
Federated Malay States (FMS).[6] From 1972 to 1977, Y. K. Lee published
a series of articles on public health and medicine in the Straits
Settlements in the nineteenth century;[7] and Ross in 1980 published a
paper on medicine in Penang, drawing on the letters of Dr Francis King,
the East India Company surgeon posted to the island from 1857 to
1865.[8] Excepting Chai's work, these articles focused on institutions or
programs. Lee, for example, details the establishment of pauper and
general hospitals and lunatic asylums, programs to reduce the incidence
of smallpox and cholera, the development of medical education,
forensic medicine, the use of anaesthesia, and the establishment of the
municipal health department, but without exposition of the logic that
underlined the processes and determined the nature of the
developments. Yet these steps in nineteenth-century medicine were far
more than simple humanitarian or public health innovations following
from the penetration and establishment of colonial rule.[9]

These early histories of colonial medicine have their counterparts in
other colonial settings. Baker's history of medicine in Malawi, Bayoumi

for the Sudan, Beck for German East Africa, Herrmann for British
Honduras, provide accounts of the appointment of medical staff and the
establishment of hospitals and clinics in the context of colonialism and
its economies, providing some of the groundwork on the basis of which
we can now interpret the relationship of medicine to colonialism.[10]
Baker, for instance, notes that by the 1930s expatriate planters in
Nyasaland (present-day Malawi) had begun to see the economic advantages of a healthy workforce, and hence medical services to rural areas
increased, despite continued European privilege.[11] Elsewhere, political
considerations directly influenced the extension of medical services.
Bopegamage, for example, documents the role of the British Indian
Army, following the Indian Mutiny in 1857, in initiating public health
and medical services: treatment of malaria, innoculation against typhoid
fever, sterilisation of water with chlorine, provision of piped water and
underground drainage in urban areas, and general improvement of
communications.[12] To some extent British Malaya followed this model:
the prime focus of medical care was the European population; medicine
was most often curative rather than preventive; indigenous populations
were usually (although not in Malaya) left to the Christian missions.[13]

In this book, I aim to begin to fill out the picture in Malaya. I begin
with a description of the nature of empire, then review political economic approaches to colonial medicine, together with an exegesis of
recent discussions of health and empire, colonial capitalism and disease.
The introduction also sets the scene in terms of political geography,
describing the colonies of the Straits Settlements and Malay States, and
discussing issues associated with administrative arrangements, demographic structure, and economic development. It also describes contemporary (1870 onwards) understandings of the etiology of disease, the
purported effects of the environment on health outcomes, and the ways
in which such vulnerability was understood to be mediated by race. I
illustrate too the complex health and healing systems of the region, into
which biomedicine was introduced.

I bring to my use of the term 'colonial capitalism' not only an understanding of the way in which specific political and economic conditions
shaped and gave meaning to material life in Malaya, but also the fact that
in this context, biology, ecology, the circumstances of material life and
knowledge interacted and produced health and illness. I include therefore not only the specific conditions and circumstances of capitalist
penetration and relations of production, and the disruptions that
colonialism created in terms of social and material life, but also colonial
perceptions of territory and space, order and control, and ideas of
moral authority and cultural difference that saturated state policies
and programs.

This use of political economy provides a framework within which to view an eclectic and disparate range of epidemiological, demographic, and historical data. The approach provides a mechanism for the interrogation of state initiatives in the areas of health and medicine, forcing us to question the nature, direction, structure, and outcomes of health interventions in terms both of their epidemiological impact and their ability to serve the interests of the state. In addition to my use of political economy, I am concerned also with the significance of the introduction of biomedicine as a cultural system, in terms of practice, institution and belief,[14] and with the role of gender within the state and with respect to health and illness, as in all aspects of social life.

To take these points, briefly, in turn. Edward Said, following the early work of Eric Stokes, draws attention to the significance of nineteenth-century English philosophy in legitimating colonialism – in Stokes' example, British dominion of India. Said argues that the entire history of nineteenth-century European thought is predicated on presumptions of them/us, inferior/superior, upper/lower, hence also ruler/ruled.[15] This apparently crude binarism underpinned much nineteenth and early twentieth-century colonial discourse in Malaya (and in the Colonial Office in London), and provided the intellectual arguments to justify the colonial enterprise; it introduced 'superior' cultural trappings (ideas and beliefs, methods and technologies, structures and institutions) to 'primitive' peoples, and established systems of Western science through schools and medical services. The development of a hospital system, the provision of British doctors and assistant doctors and apothecaries trained in biomedicine, and the availability of a pharmacopoeia derived from this (without acknowledging the debts owed to other systems with prior presence in Malaya) established, in the context of the colonial polity, the primacy of Western science, and the need to maintain a political system to ensure the continuing advantages of its technical offerings. Tropical medicine was 'invented' in this light.

I have implied, above, the importance of gender in understanding health and illness. I do not propose here to demonstrate the ways in which many histories, gender-blind, have represented the realities of men as if they were all people, nor to spell out why gender matters. But colonial Malayan history provides a nice case study of gender at work: the structure of the colonial population, the distribution of power, the sexual divisions of labour and the concomitant varying risks of infection, and access to medical care, are all as much matters of gender as they are of class and race. Less easily documented are the variations in meaning, knowledge and treatment between women and men, and by ethnicity, although as I describe later, state understandings of the sexual distribution of disease and salience of various ailments is relatively straightforward. Colonial

understandings of gender and the colonial construction of sex and
sexuality pervade the epidemiology of disease and its interventions whilst
informing also colonial demography. In official accounts, men not
women suffer from malaria and beri-beri, cholera and tuberculosis, not
because women were protected from such infections but because the
sexual division of labour and the demographic disequilibrium of the sexes
created a series of hierarchies that affected exposure, infection, illness
and its treatment. Ideas about women and their health derive from the
segregation of women and men, and women from each other; and
women's sexual roles divide into recreational and procreational roles that
subsume colonial women, their biology, functions and behaviour. Whilst
in general health services collapsed the categories of woman and
reproduction (women's health was of interest only in the context of
reproductive health),[16] in Malaya the population of women was bifurcated
into essentialist categories – mother and whore – and their health needs
defined in terms of antenatal care for the former, venereal disease for the
latter. For mothers, women's health services concentrated on ensuring
their ability to reproduce. For sex workers, the focus was on preventing
others from being infected by them; these women were vectors rather
than victims of disease.

The distribution of disease by race and sex, and changes over time due
to economic and demographic changes, is documented in Chapter 2.
Colonial Malaya was characterised in the late nineteenth century by
rapid changes in morbidity, mortality and demographic structure. Whilst
there was a dramatic decline in the incidence of some epidemic infectious diseases through simple controls (for example, smallpox through
vaccination), for other diseases the etiology was more complex, treatment was unavailable or offered varied success, and control was problematic. Health statistics are unreliable, but even so, it is apparent that
health status was equivocal for many, and the incidence of a number of
endemic ailments, including diarrhoeal diseases, respiratory infections
and malaria, continued to take a major toll of the population. Although
the infant mortality rate as well as adult mortality declined from the early
twentieth century, several major factors contributed to this and
morbidity statistics for the period to 1940 suggest that improved health
was sometimes illusory.

For many Malays colonial capitalism resulted in changes in the mode
of production from peasant subsistence farming and fishing to wage
labour. However most labour was provided by immigrant Indian and
Chinese men. Chapter 3 is concerned with understandings of illness and
race, and the way in which this was played out in the context of
particular diseases. It considers the incidence of various ailments as
influenced by material circumstances of everyday life, and dominant

beliefs and actions consequent upon the etiology of illness, diagnostic categories, and available treatments. Economic changes resulted in disruptions to the environment, affecting particularly the epidemiology of malaria and resulting in changes in food supply, in turn affecting the nutritional status of peasants and fisherfolk as well as agricultural labourers. In addition, specific conditions which prevailed in parts of Malaya resulted in the prevalence of particular diseases: beri-beri among Chinese miners was the most notable and best documented. The chapter discusses government interventions in malaria and beri-beri, the impact of which was harshest among immigrant workers, as pursued for estate works in Chapter 5; these public health programs were accorded high priority in an effort to minimise the cost (and exploit the potentiality) of the colonial economy.

In Chapter 4, the focus shifts from the country to city. For evidential reasons I focus on Kuala Lumpur and Singapore, where health risks and outcomes were calqued onto the social geography of the towns, reflecting colonial social and racial categories. Hygiene and sanitation were poor, visibly so with open sewers, drains, and refuse in the streets. Dry and wet waste disposal presented one problem to public health officials, so too did the pace of urbanisation. Towns expanded rapidly, resulting in overcrowding and spread of disease. Coffee houses, bars and brothels, markets, food stalls and dairies, and residential cubicles were all sites of contagion; this chapter describes the management of urban space that was based on this understanding.

Chapters 5 and 6 concentrate on two populations that might be considered exemplary or indexical of the colonial setting. In Chapter 5, the setting is rural, the workers estate labourers; the chapter details the organisation of labour, health conditions on estates and the health status of the labourers, and the provision of medical care, potable water and sanitation. Poor health from infectious disease was compounded by conditions of deprivation and cruelty. Malaria was a major risk to estate workers and death rates at the turn of the century were especially high. Malaria control measures were implemented variously on the estates, with continual tension between state and capital, as represented by the malaria control boards and town councils on the one hand, and estate owners on the other – one seeking to reduce mortality and the other to expend as little as possible on a labour force which it regarded as replaceable.

Chapter 6 focuses on working women: the commercial sex workers of the colonies. The colonial economy relied on immigrant labour, mostly men. Around the turn of the century the sex ratio was some 12 men to 1 woman, a significant number of whom were involved in prostitution. Most lived and worked in oppressive conditions, in substandard and overcrowded housing, their mobility limited, their money strictly controlled. From the late nineteenth century their health needs were partly met by private medical clubs and lock hospitals, driven by a wider interest to control venereal disease. Shifts in morality and political pressure from outside the colony led to government movements to 'rescue' the women by encouraging them into commercial sewing, domestic service, or marriage and, as a result of growing international pressure in the 1920s, by steps taken to close down the brothels.

State accommodation and regulation of prostitution reveals one aspect of its understanding of gender. Midwifery and child welfare, as discussed in Chapter 7, provides a further vehicle for the engendering of colonial subjects. State interest in mothers and children, infant mortality, child welfare and the control of midwifery date from the early twentieth century. Female medical officers ('lady doctors') provided a means of surveillance of mothers, midwives were trained and registered, and infant welfare clinics were established so that babies could be weighed and measured. Babies who performed poorly were proof of maternal incompetence, and the ability of native and immigrant women to be 'good' mothers was constantly in question. A growing concern that initiatives with adults be consolidated led to the development of curricula for young women (future mothers), and this chapter explores the development and content of the curriculum and the perceived role of women as gatekeepers of their families' health.

The concluding chapter documents the shifts in logic that occurred towards the end of the British empire. Growing sensitivities at criticism of the health and wellbeing of subject people in British colonies (from the USA as well as from international organisations and agencies), led to considerable reflection within the Colonial Office about colonialism and the moral responsibility of the state. Enquiries in the 1930s and the development of post-war plans for the colonies reflect a growing concern with a 'moral economy' of colonialism. The foreshadowed end of colonialism pushed government awareness of the need for 'social' development, and for social services that addressed the inequalities created by economic development. It is on this note that the book closes.

If the work were to begin now – in the 1990s – it might be difficult to start from archival sources and to remain so embedded in those records that the work could proceed without matching alternative documentation, the provision of moderating voices of those Chinese, Indians and Malays who left textual records through the 'vernacular' press, for example, or through oral history interviews with those who might still recall the end days of the empire. But this is a work commenced a

decade earlier, and the excavations of archives in Malaysia, Singapore
and the United Kingdom proved far more complex and compelling
than might have been imagined; the source material is eclectic and
voluminous. This work brings together part of that data, and presents a
starting point for a continuing project that seeks to better understand
the diverse and pervasive impact of colonial rule on a society, a
biosphere, a people, and their everyday life.

Much of the research for this book was undertaken whilst I was a
Research Fellow with the Department of Southeast Asian and Pacific
History, in the Research School of Pacific Studies, the Australian
National University, although the theoretical and thematic interests of
the book reflect also the very disparate environments of the School of
Sociology, the University of New South Wales, and the Tropical Health
Program of the Faculty of Medicine, the University of Queensland.
Financial support was provided from a grant from the Australian
Research Council;[17] the Faculty of Arts, the University of New South
Wales; the Research School of Pacific Studies, the Australian National
University; and the Tropical Health Program, the University of Queens-
land. In addition, I benefited from the hospitality and colleagiality of the
University of Oxford as a Visitor to the Department of Biological
Anthropology in 1984, and to the Wellcome Unit for the History of
Medicine in 1992. The Wellcome Unit especially provided me with a
lively intellectual environment and a tranquil haven from routine
academic life that enabled me to make the first good draft of this book.

The book draws on diverse holdings. In London, I used the libraries of
the London School of Hygiene and Tropical Medicine, the Wellcome
Institute, the Royal Commonwealth Society, and the Foreign and
Commonwealth Office, in addition to the Public Records Office in Kew
and its India Office holdings in South London. In Oxford I used the
Rhodes House Library and the library of the Wellcome Unit for the
History of Medicine; in Singapore the National Archives of Singapore
and the library of the National University of Singapore; in Kuala
Lumpur the libraries of the University of Malaysia and the Institute of
Medical Research, together with Arkib Negara Malaysia. In Canberra, I
worked primarily in the National Library of Australia. I have used the
libraries of the Australian National University, the University of Oxford,
the University of New South Wales and the University of Queensland for
supplementary material.

Institutions I can name; individuals are more difficult. I have scored
up many personal debts over the lengthy period when I worked, intermittently, on this book, and I risk omitting or undervaluing the role of
some were I to name those who might now first come to mind. Four
exceptions are in order: Leanne Kerr, Alyson Stibbard and Kiruba

Rajanayagam for their research assistance in Australia and Jenny Cooper for her superb word processing skills. To others, I acknowledge simply my true gratitude for the roles that they have played in this work: those who provided me with computing and clerical assistance, and those colleagues, friends and kin whose keen wit pointed me in the direction of new ideas, information and interpretations. I carry full responsibility for this work, of course.

The conception of this book predates my children; they were born while the research for it was most concentrated; they went to school in high winter in England as I drafted the manuscript; they spent a summer without me as it underwent refinement. They have been tolerant of my moods and generous of my absences for this project as of all other aspects of my working life, and I remain, always, indebted to them and in wonder of them. Pat Galvin has lived with the ideas of this book, and its material evidence, for years. I am deeply grateful to him for his interest, generosity, support, care and sacrifices.

The book is dedicated to my mother, whose compassion and lifetime interest in health and medicine inspired me, and in memory of my father, whose own life was profoundly affected by colonialism and racism, and his flights from both.

LENORE MANDERSON
Brisbane

CHAPTER 1

Introduction:
Imposing the empire

The expansion of British colonial jurisdiction facilitated, from the mid-nineteenth century, the development of extractive industries and plantations on the Malay Peninsula and its offshore islands. This expansion required increased control over both people and resources, resulting first in the enumeration and registration of land, goods and people. From 1857, with the transfer of government of the Straits Settlements from the East India Company to the Colonial Office, and from 1874 with the extension of direct rule over the Malay States, the bureaucracy extended its surveillance. By the end of the century, it had established the mechanisms to maintain and extend demographic and epidemiological surveillance, as well as economic and political control, of British Malaya (see Figure 1.1).[1]

The data gathered on migration, births, deaths, and morbidity were without doubt underestimates and therefore disguised the burden of sickness on select populations, even of those whose lives were most closely tied to the workings of colonial capitalism and who were subject to its closest scrutiny. Even so, the statistics expressed summarily in terms of hospital beds and inpatient days, stools examined, parasites counted, injections administered, and cases recorded, treated, cured or lost, provide some account of illness, suffering and death under colonialism.

The human experiences that lie behind these numbers – beliefs and perceptions of health and illness, patterns of diagnosis, treatment and care, and the nature of suffering, for example – are captured only occasionally in fragmentary allusive notes on the margins of the departmental files of colonial officials. Memoranda, reports and scientific papers often provide such bare accounts of the experiences of sickness and death, however, that any mention of social, cultural or personal context captures our attention, forcing us to look beyond the text for a

1

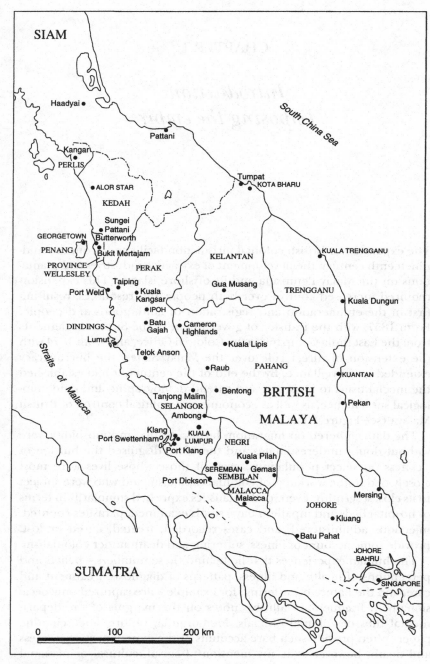

Figure 1.1 Map of British Malaya, 1920.

more complete account. On the other hand, organisational aspects of colonial health services, including the establishment, maintenance and activities of hospitals, clinics and dispensaries, the public health measures taken to reduce transmission of infection and disease, and the work of medical departments, councils, boards and committees, are well documented and give the historian a substantial body of information from which to work. Similarly data on population trends, morbidity and mortality, with anecdotal commentaries on sickness and death, provide the building blocks to reconstruct a social and epidemiological past. Births, deaths, outbreaks of infection, injuries and accidents are all ways of characterising the patterns of health and illness and finding meaning in apparently singular experiences. Behind these figures we must imagine the lived experience: picture a funeral and a family locked in grief; a mother fleeing to a dispensary or a traditional healer with a sick child in arms; a labourer lying, shaking and sweating on a sleeping platform in a labourers' lines; a young and frightened woman, emprisoned in a brothel and alone in childbirth.

The task of reconstructing the social history of sickness is not entirely a task of the imagination, for both contemporary descriptions of material life and the official epidemiological record allow us to conjure up these events.[2] The empirical data available for colonial Malaya is rich and varied. As already noted, routine reports of government departments, agencies, committees and councils; reports of and submissions presented to enquiries and commissions; unpublished papers of medical officers, district officers, sanitary inspectors and civil engineers; police and coroner's reports;[3] parliamentary papers; unpublished institutional records; journal articles on colonial and tropical medical matters; and newspaper accounts, memoirs, travel diaries and other papers contribute to an extraordinarily eclectic archive.

From these records, despite their omissions and biases, we can begin to reconstruct life and death in British Malaya. Since the collection of statistics and other information was part of a broader colonial project, the data inevitably privileges the accounts and views of the colonial authors, who, through their particular reading of social distance, argue for the logic of European penetration and its subsequent policies and practices.[4] Colonial subjects had least chance to speak for themselves in any context, including any in which to document their experiences. Malays living beyond colonial boundaries, in spaces and economies of little interest to settlers and the state, were largely invisible or treated as such, incorporeal spectators of imperial endeavours. Others, co-opted as labourers, producers or service providers, even so were rendered silent, as if children, under the paternalism of colonialism, and their experience entered into social knowledge largely as it was mediated by others.

Despite this, the written accounts offer the basis for a continuing project, one that might turn to a more diverse range of written and oral sources of individuals and groups subject to colonialism as well as those who enforced it. This book is a beginning.

British Malaya was a benevolent regime, and blatant oppression was unusual. Still, illness and deaths occurred which for many were shaped by the inequities, powerlessness and poverty produced by the structures of colonialism, resulting in small resistances, labour strikes, and insurgency.[5] Dramatic acts, whilst present prior to the establishment of colonial rule, sometimes took on new meaning – and were certainly managed in different ways – with the extension of state control; theft, murder, rape, suicide, and alcohol and opium abuse were all part of the underside of and (partly) were produced by colonialism.[6] Committees of inquiry were established in response to such resistance. In documenting the conditions of labour and living, they revealed the extensiveness of emiseration and poverty among the Malay peasantry as well as immigrant labourers, the hardship endured by those employed on tin mines and rubber estates, and the crowded squalor of urban slums. In the conditions that prevailed in both urban and rural Malaya, the corporeal costs of colonial rule included those of nutritional deficiency diseases, such as beri-beri, increased transmission of endemic diseases such as malaria, and the spread of communicable and often fatal infections including tuberculosis, pneumonia, and venereal and diarrhoeal diseases.

Framing the period

In writing of the 'Age of Empire', Eric Hobsbawm draws the empire to a close in 1914, as major changes in economy and society were foreshadowed by the outbreak of the First World War.[7] Although war was played out in a colonial as well as European theatre, its staging was primarily Africa. In Malaya, the war did not result in disjuncture, and here the natural 'end of empire' is with the Pacific War, when Japanese occupation disrupted colonial rule and gave a small group of reformists and revolutionaries a new language of resistance.

By concluding at around 1940, the periodisation of this book is conventional, employing the same chronological frame as many other histories of Malaya. It follows a chronology not dissimilar to other histories of colonial medicine, too. The notion of empire, governing a period that extends to the outbreak of the Second World War, has proved heuristically useful as well as historiographically convenient for a number of writers. MacLeod, for instance, characterises the period from 1815 to the Second World War as 'the "classic" period of nineteenth century colonialism'.[8] The history of medicine during this period enables a focused exploration of 'the twinned relations of political and professional power'. Medicine is exposed as participating in the expansion and consolidation of political rule through its service to political, commercial and military arms of empire, leading to campaigns to conquer diseases that threatened the integrity and economic potentiality of the state, and to the systematic delivery of sanitary, health care and medical services.[9] In MacLeod's account, medicine is clearly an arm of empire. This was the perspective of Fanon too, when he drew attention to the symbolic and structural role of the doctor, 'always ... belonging to the dominant society ... a link in the colonialist network'.[10] The mix of metaphor of medicine and the military in imperial contexts, given this, is an appropriate one, for medicine served and sustained the troops that coerced imperial rule, while it waged its own campaigns against new, tropical biospheres – landscapes, insects, and microbes.

The time frame of this book – from the nineteenth century to the outbreak of the Pacific War – has its own logic. In the late nineteenth century, the population of British Malaya expanded rapidly to meet demands for labour. Population needs were met through immigration rather than natural increase, since the need for workers was immediate as new land was opened up, as the economy expanded, and as each new cohort of immigrants was culled by parasitic infection and death. Conflicting and paradoxical understandings of the processes of colonialism and the role of the colonists shaped the institutions of the state, including its medical and health services. The late nineteenth century was a period marked by conflicting sentiments of racism and humanitarianism, reflected in the contradictory yet complimentary exploitation of labour and establishment of a colonial welfare state.[11]

At the outbreak of the Pacific War, this story had moved into a time of self-reflection and change, as officials of the Colonial Office in London and their representatives in the colonies expressed increasing concern that the price of colonialism – for those subject to colonial rule – had been too high. In consequence, the days of the empire were numbered. The impact of plantation agriculture and mining on the lives and life chances of its workers, and the relations of authority and control determined by colonialism, were in question, and staff in the Cabinet Office in the intrawar years spent considerable effort developing appropriate mechanisms for post-war independence. By the end of the period covered by this book, therefore, the empire was all but over.

The creation of tropical medicine

Late nineteenth-century thought was influenced, Said has argued, by utilitarian philosophy which legitimised imperial domination and

governance.[12] At the same time, the evolutionary ideas of Herbert
Spencer and Charles Darwin, among others, were influential in providing the footings of a (loosely articulated) philosophy of colonisation
which legitimised relations of power and authority. Darwinian ideas were
sometimes crudely translated into naive misunderstandings of race,
biology, social development and social organisation. They provided
legitimacy to the institutions and structures that enabled the systems of
extraction and appropriation, however, while they rationalised colonisation in terms of its 'civilising' functions, including those in relation to
health, medicine, sanitation and hygiene.[13] Recast in terms of moral
obligation and social and economic development, evolutionary theory
provided the explanatory model for (the excesses of) colonial capitalism. According to this account, Malays, Chinese, Indians and 'others'
were subject to a beneficent paternalist regime and fared differentially
under it because they were lazy, indolent, stupid, ignorant, dirty or
greedy. Even those contemporary accounts most sensitive to the oppres-
sions of colonialism replicated these views. At worst, colonial subjects
were likened to beasts of burden, 'draught bullock ... equally helpless
among (their) new environment',[14] worthy only of the labour that they
might contribute to build up the wealth of the empire. At best, they were
represented as children, waiting for patronage and tutelage. The texts
show little sympathy for the lives of their subjects, although many are
sensitive, in terms of nineteenth-century economic rationalism and
Taylorism, to the human costs of colonial development. This was consistently so, hence C. A. Wiggins' justification of public health expenditure in 1919, that 'apart from the humanitarian aspect of the question,
there can be no doubt that money, judiciously and carefully spent on
sanitary measures would, ere long, bring its reward in the shape of
revenue'.[15]

It would be inappropriate to judge too harshly the participants in this
system, certainly those who sought to temper the effects of colonisation
and to mediate the differences between colonists and colonised. The
majority of European officials and others working in British Malaya were
products of their own time, unquestioning of their superiority and moral
rights, and impressed by their obligations and the broader ethical
responsibilities of colonialism. The time, as already noted, was that of
social Darwinism; it was a time of Victorian confidence, of innocent
enthusiasm for science, technology and the products of expanding
manufacturing industry.[16]

Prior to the industrial revolution, biomedicine was in its infancy and
little was known of the cause of many of the 'tropical' diseases that
limited European expansion. Then, medical care was a task practised by
a variety of professionals, midwives, apothecaries, barbers and surgeons.

As Headrick points out, certain technologies were available and used to prevent or treat disease; the prophylactic and therapeutic use of quinine, originally in the form of cinchona bark but commercially manufactured from 1827, is a case in point.[17] But by the 1890s, major advances in science had occurred, and biomedicine had gained strength. Medical claims to power and authority were bolstered by scientific discoveries and the development of new knowledge and skills, doctors enjoyed increased professional standing, and their authority over individuals and medical services expanded.[18] Major advances in microbiology, parasitology, and vaccine development occurred. Considerable advances were made in understanding the transmission and distribution of malaria, cholera, leprosy, plague, yellow fever, and dysentery. The scientific endeavour that resulted in these discoveries was intensely competitive and nationalistic, and in this context health research and 'tropical medicine', and its institutionalisation, took on a particular edge; the relationship between science and the state – as represented by tropical medicine and empire – was made clear.[19]

The successes of science, too, were a nice example of evolution, fitting well with the broader colonial project; this is wonderfully captured by three tableaux in the entrance hall of the Wellcome Bureau of Scientific Research in London, intended to portray medical progress: an African medicine-man at work, a mediaeval alchemist in his cell, and a modern laboratory bench.[20]

Influenced by general theories of evolution and race and by notions of the superiority of British political organisation, technology, industry and science, British attitudes towards colonised peoples were consistently paternalistic and often racist. This extended to discussions of medical conditions, the etiology and epidemiology of disease, and sickness behaviour within the colonies. During the period of early colonialism, most doctors had little understanding of disease causation, and they were as likely as their patients to subscribe to a variation of miasmic theory, whereby the environment was considered to be a critical factor in the incidence and transmission of disease. This understanding was tempered somewhat by ideas of immunity, not as an acquired resistance following exposure to pathogens (although this idea was circulating by the late nineteenth century), but as an artefact of race and heredity. Accordingly, as Harrison and Anderson both document, people were best suited to the environment of their ancestral realm, as reflected by the 'natural' resistance of 'natives' (or immigrants from similar climates) to 'tropical diseases', and particularly the vulnerability of white men in the tropics.[21] This belief was modified somewhat by other behavioralist theories: leprosy and diseases of the skin, for example, were linked to frequent bathing, believed to weaken the skin.[22] Episodes of illness including fevers were treated by purging, blood letting and salivation to rid the body of invading and accumulated 'poison'; European patients were sent to hill stations for a change of air and the completion of the cure.[23] These views were revised with advances in bacteriology, and notions of native innate immunity subtly shifted to notions of acquired immunity and the role of native as carrier. In the early twentieth century, the appropriate measures to be taken to reduce the toll of the tropics on Europeans, as described later in this volume, were to moderate native behaviours and habits, with an emphasis on sanitation, hygiene and diet: excretion, ingestion, pure water, fresh air. Hence, poor health – now construed as the result of 'native ignorance', lack of hygiene and sanitation, 'superstition' and 'primitiveness' – led to the development of public health programs as well as hospital-based curative services.[24] At the same time, the continuing high morbidity rates and the risk of disease and death to British settlers and immigrant workers and soldiers, whose continuing health was essential for the consolidation of the empire, led to the development of a research program directed specifically to the health problems of the colonies.

The empire's interest in tropical medicine dates from the late nineteenth century, when scientific discovery and a nascent new confidence that science, or rather biomedicine, could control illness coincided with the high point of imperial expansion. Such confidence was fueled, as outlined above, by a number of significant advances in the biology and epidemiology of disease. Jenner's work in virology, and the development of a vaccine against smallpox, occurred relatively early – in the 1790s – but thereafter scientific research gained momentum, encouraged by the successful work by Koch on tuberculosis and Pasteur on rabies, the development of other live vaccines, and the discovery in 1880 by Alphonse Laveran that the *Plasmodium* parasite, invading the blood stream, caused malaria. The subsequent identification by Patrick Manson of *Plasmodium falciparum* which caused the heaviest toll on life, and in 1897, the discovery by Ronald Ross, Giovanni Grassi and Amico Bignami that the *Anopheles* mosquito was the vector, encouraged further interest in tropical medical research, as the collision of interests between science on the one hand and nation–empire on the other was clear to the major players on the scene: France, Belgium, the Netherlands, Italy and the United Kingdom.[25]

In the United Kingdom, Joseph Chamberlain, Secretary of State for the Colonies from 1895, was particularly interested in the implications of new developments in parasitology and bacteriology for the colonies, given that the incidence and toll of disease was a major impediment to continued economic expansion. His concern with health status, as it affected colonial pecuniary success, led to the appointment of Manson as the first medical adviser to the Colonial Office in 1897. From 1899 until his retirement in 1912, Manson was founding director of the London School of Hygiene and Tropical Medicine, established to provide appropriate training for colonial medical officers, to undertake basic and applied research, and to provide the Colonial Office with technical advice and services, which included the anthropology as well as the biology of tropical disease.[26] Informed by belief that the future of imperialism lay with the microscope,[27] the school was run as a research institute, influenced by developments in biological sciences. It exemplified in many respects the privileging of laboratory science over field research, and biomedicine over public health.[28]

Ross was appointed also in 1899 as founding lecturer of the Liverpool School of Tropical Medicine.[29] This school maintained close ties with the professional and business community that had been instrumental in its establishment, promoting itself as 'an investment in colonial trade' and economic development. Hence Ross' commitment to vector control and the practical application of his research, and his bitterness, although not in the Malayan case, that environmental procedures such as vector control strategies were applied 'in a patchy and piecemeal way amidst much vacillation and discord'.[30] Industrial and mercantile interests maintained the impetus to continue the London and Liverpool schools, and later to establish the Ross Institute to 'keep industry in touch with science, to make the tropics healthy and to expand the markets of the world'.[31]

In 1901, on the recommendation of Swettenham, then High Commissioner of the Federated Malay States (FMS), the Pathology Institute opened in Kuala Lumpur, as death and disease from tropical infections appeared to be increasing throughout the empire.[32] This was not the first research and training institute established in the colonies: a Pasteur Institute had opened in Saigon in 1891, and a number of other institutes and smaller laboratories had been established with support from Paris in Tunisia, Senegal, Turkey, Brazil and Algeria.[33] Dutch interests in tropical medicine developed along parallel lines.[34] In each case the establishment of a research institute offered national scientists a field station to pursue their interests in diseases directly affecting the colonial enterprise, and to carry laboratory developments into the field. Through the involvement of local staff, other than in a menial capacity, they also shaped colonial science,[35] although even where institutes were concerned with local recruitment, training and technology transfer, a fundamental divide pertained that reinforced the function of the institution: applied research in the colonial peripheries, pure science at the centre.[36]

The opening of the Pathology Institute in Kuala Lumpur, which was renamed the Institute of Medical Research the following year, occurred in the context of scientific imperialism and international scientific competitiveness. Locally it was precipitated by high mortality rates from malaria and beri-beri and, according to Chai,[37] by a change in colonial rule from a policy of laissez-faire to one of welfare and efficiency. Its achievements included establishing the etiology of beri-beri. Its malaria control program was the first to implement Ross' proposals for broad-based environmental controls and the extension of these measures throughout the country was hailed as 'the greatest sanitary achievement ever accomplished in the British Empire'[38] and 'an epic in the history of modern preventive sanitation'.[39]

A number of public health measures occurred at around the same time, including the development of maternal and infant health services and primary health care. These early initiatives in medical research, hospital and auxiliary clinical services reflected nascent state concern regarding the political and economic effects of ill health. For example, Chamberlain, Medical Adviser to the Colonial Office in the late 1890s, noted that 'malaria, black-water fever, yellow fever, and other afflictions brought death, sickness and debility, at an appalling rate, to the Empire's officials and traders, as to the hapless natives. Sudden burials, repeated invalidings, and chronic enfeeblement made regular administration difficult and continuous policy impossible'.[40] Tropical medicine, born of the collusion of science and colonialism, developed as a speciality to reduce the incidence of these afflictions.

Tropical medicine was a cultural construct, the scientific stepchild of colonial domination and control.[41] Recognition of the political economy of disease was not unique to late twentieth-century discourse, however, and the doyens of tropical medicine were in no way deluded that pathogens were uniquely transformed by geography. Hence Sir Andrew Balfour argued in 1928 that most diseases, including malaria, beri-beri, dengue fever, plague, leprosy and schistosomiasis, were 'not strictly diseases of the tropics although, partly on account of their etiology, partly because of their association with unhygienic conditions, they now-a-days prevail to a much greater extent in hot countries than elsewhere'.[42]

The political economy of colonial medicine

The above discussion suggests the utility of a conventional political economic account of health and illness to capture the logic of the provision of medical services and health care for those whose welfare was essential to sustaining the colonial enterprise, neatly tying the centre and periphery – tin mine and canning factory, rubber estate and car. But such an account needs to note too that in British Malaya class, gender, race and geography patterned the nature of illness, the kinds of care that were available, and the access to such care. The effect of ill health on the relative success of colonial ventures influenced the timing of interventions and the structure and activities of control programs. However, most of the health programs in Malaya (and social welfare and education programs) were implemented soon after they were introduced in the centre, and reflected not government understanding of colonial needs, but rather contemporary changing ideas and practices in public health occurring within the United Kingdom. Environmental health and sanitation programs, home visiting and infant welfare work started in the Straits Settlements a few years after their implementation in Britain. These programs, and the philosophies that informed them, were determined by and reflected relations of power and authority that existed within the colony, but also reflected class relations in the centre. In Malaya, for example, infant welfare programs were implemented to enable the reproduction of labour to continue to meet the workforce needs of colonial estates and mines; in Britain, they ensured the reproduction of the working class to meet state strategic and military needs and, again, the labour needs of manufacturing industries that were fed by the raw materials of the empire.[43]

The political economy of health and medical services within colonial settings was made complex, however, by other agendas. There is, as Denoon argues, a separate logic of colonialism that brings about changes beyond those required to meet the demands of capital.[44] Colonial policies were directed not only by capitalist interests, and colonialism and capitalism did not always operate in tandem, although often the differences between state and commercial sectors were institutional and tactical rather than due to contradictory goals. Denoon suggests that in Papua New Guinea, for example, social and political rather than economic imperatives of colonialism drove medical policy. In particular, the survival of the colonists, and the reproduction of colonial government and its class of elite officers, was 'an absolute priority'.[45] It is tempting in recounting the subjugation of individuals under colonial capitalism to overlook the wider patterns and context of conditions of everyday life and the developments that occurred. The excesses of many of the colonies – for example, the brutal appropriation of labour on sugar estates in nineteenth-century Java or the Philippines, or on the plantations of Indochina – were relatively although not entirely absent in Malaya.[46] Yet colonialism in British Malaya was no less characterised by poverty, misery, exploitation and violence. In colonial Malaya, as elsewhere, life was often unpleasant, rough, dangerous and brief. But so it was in czarist Russia, Dickens' London, the American south, or feudal Italy. Conditions in the nineteenth century were generally harsh for those other than gentry, both in the expanding centres of capital and in their peripheries. In Malaya, life was in many respects exemplary rather than exceptional.

These comments reflect my concern to contextualise health status, health care services and programs within a framework that explores the interplay of global forces and local circumstances. The health status of a people is determined both by local exigencies – biological, environmental, economic, social and cultural – and by state and wider relations; and the introduction of political economic theory into the history of medicine, in order to pursue this interplay of polity and biology, has resulted in fundamental shifts in the way in which medical history has been written. The works of Vicente Navarro and his colleagues provide the most eloquent descriptions of these processes and documentation of the way in which relations of production have produced illness.[47]

Many of the earlier histories of medicine, including those in imperial settings, described the establishment and extension of curative and preventive health services, and the history of the conquest of disease, as if these occurred outside or were quarantined from politics. Beck's study of medicine in colonial East Africa is a case in point,[48] and provides a useful contrast to the discussions concerning colonialism and medicine in Malaya. Although her work is based on the premise that medical care in a colony cannot be examined or understood without reference to 'political, social, economic, and cultural problems',[49] the relevance of such 'problems' to the delivery of health and medical services is never fully articulated.

As in other colonies, in East Africa (Kenya, Uganda, Tanganyika) medical care was provided firstly, 'understandably so',[50] for the European population, particularly soldiers and administrative staff, then for the Indians imported to build the railroad and promote trade. Until after the First World War the British had little interest in the indigenous population of these territories; deaths of Africans during the war years were regarded as near inevitable given the lack of roads, shortage of quinine, absence of sanitation and the meagre diet of the troops. In Beck's account the deaths of 46,618 of the 350,000 Africans involved in the campaign was 'part of the cost of winning the war' since the provision of porter transport was essential, and 'it [was] almost sheer good luck that the Colonial Office was able to coast along [during the war] *without a major catastrophe*'.[51] Until the 1920s, most health care was delivered to Africans, with liberal doses of Christianity, by missionaries.[52] Only later were measures taken to control epidemics (malaria, plague, and trypanosomiasis) that were most threatening also to Europeans, and to 'promote the prevention, limitation, or suppression of infectious, communicable or preventable diseases' and 'the economic and cultural improvement of the native population'.[53]

The lack of reflection in this work is echoed in other recent scholarship. A collection dealing with the Dutch East Indies, for example, uses colonial archives to sketch the topography of disease and institutional responses: the structures and staff of military, general civilian and plantation medical services; the development of medical education; the priorities – the very definitions and boundaries – of tropical medical research; and the focus on particular 'tropical' diseases.[54] Yet there is a twist. In many colonies, preventive medicine and public health enjoyed far greater profile on the periphery than the centre. In the Dutch East Indies this was already very much so in the nineteenth century, and whilst the political and cultural environment of disease was largely overlooked by contemporary practitioners and policy makers and by subsequent historians, the complex interaction of human population, pathogen and environment was well recognised at the time. This was the case for smallpox in India, as Arnold describes, where local practices and practitioners, institutions and sensibilities – the cultural acceptability and established practices of variolation (innoculation for smallpox), caste restrictions, and so on – made compliance with vaccination problematic.[55] Further, epidemiologists around the turn of the century were cognisant of associations between poverty, hygiene, sanitation, and health outcome, and at times they were self-conscious of the label of 'tropical' medicine lest the term implied adherence to a belief in the role of telluric and meteorological miasma in the etiology and distribution of disease.[56]

Tropical medical history, floating from any geographic moorings, has featured in a tradition of a history of medicine focusing on heroic effort and the defeat of pathogens, with the twentieth century represented as an age of triumph of science over environment.[57] This perception of progress informed contemporary medical accounts of disease control, and it is perhaps not coincidental that interest in the political economy of medicine and, later, the social construction of tropical medicine, occurred as the confidence of medical scientists in their control over nature faltered.[58] The growth of interest in the social, political and economic context of health and disease occurred as historians turned their attention from metropolitan centre to imperial periphery. Although a few works (Beck's is one) of the history of colonial medicine predate this, it is (now) impossible to tell the story without attention to the manipulation of services, patients and knowledge by the political economic forces that created, in the first instance, the empire and its outposts. While colonial participants, perhaps not surprisingly, were relatively insensitive to the politics of their own history-telling and their versions of the triumph of medicine and science, it is difficult to ignore these forces now, in light of post-colonial critiques, when the substance of the history is the bodies of the oppressed.[59]

Fanon's critique of colonialism, first published in 1961, provides a starting point for many of the recent critical analyses of imperial medicine.[60] While Fanon is concerned with the economics of oppression, he extends our understanding of the political significance of colonial medicine in his insistence that its institutions and apparatus not simply served but were also part of a wider system of oppression – the doctor, the administrator, and the constable were identical embodiments of the imposed polity. As Fanon argues, Western medicine was introduced into colonial societies as part of the introduction of Western cultural values.[61] Encounters with Western medicine – its doctors, its institutions, its *materia medica* – were for colonised subjects always an encounter with the colonising society; their acceptance of its services implied a complicity with the ideology and polity that enabled it. This was the point. Public health education and other public health measures (house visitors, vaccinations, travelling dispensaries, maternal and child health clinics) were all part of a front line of imperialism that strove to dominate by care and cure; medicine, as MacLeod (after Fanon) maintains, was an agency of – or an agent for – Western expansion.[62]

Fanon's work has been influential in directing recent analyses of the ideological and material dimensions of colonial medicine, which take account of the location of medicine, as institution and as ideology, within contemporary political and social thought.[63] Along these lines, Arnold, and MacLeod and Lewis – following Headrick[64] – argue that European medicine and public health served as 'tools of Empire', symbolically and practically, as an instrument by which means the European presence and its supporting labour force were maintained, and as an 'imperializing cultural force' wherein professional and political tensions among colonisers and between colonisers and subject peoples were played out.

Location

The historiography of medicine and empire is geographically biased, focused primarily on Africa. In contrast, there have been relatively few publications for Asia or the Pacific which document the patterning of disease and institutional responses or which illustrate the imbrication of medicine, state and society, the relationships of production and reproduction, and the politics of sickness and health.[65] This is despite the strategic significance of the region with respect to trade, colonialism and colonial medicine.[66]

Disease was a major obstacle to European expansion, and 'the conquest of sickness was a basic condition for colonial expansion and development'.[67] In British Malaya, the first medical care was provided following the arrival of ship surgeons of the East India Company. With the establishment of naval bases and trade posts in Penang (in 1786), Singapore (in 1819) and Malacca (in 1824), military doctors provided medical care to colonial administrators and other colonists as well as to troops. In 1826, with the incorporation of the Straits Settlements with Penang as the capital, a medical department was established under the professional and administrative head, the Senior Surgeon, with assistant surgeons supported by a few apothecaries located in Penang, Malacca, and Singapore. In 1835 the headquarters of the department were transferred from Penang to Singapore and facilities were slowly upgraded and extended. Local men, usually Eurasians, were recruited as bonded apprentices to train as hospital dressers and sub-assistant surgeons to English professionals seconded from India or, in the late nineteenth century, direct from England.[68] In 1905 the Straits Settlements and Federated Malay States Government Medical School (later the King Edward VIII Medical School) opened to train physicians locally.

A hospital providing basic medical and surgical services was therefore operating in Georgetown, Penang, from the time of the establishment of British political and military presence on the island. Similarly, the first hospital was operating in Singapore from 1819, primarily to treat minor complaints of troops and to refer more serious cases to Penang. The Singapore hospital was administered until December 1822 as a military hospital, although it was referred to as a General Hospital and provided separate facilities (and graded provisions) for European soldiers, sepoys (Indian troops) and native paupers. The pauper ward became the Pauper Hospital, relocated on a number of occasions, providing primary care to vagrants, beggars and other poor people until Tan Tock Seng Hospital was established in 1844.[69] Paupers were also treated at the General Hospitals in Malacca and Penang, with these services supported by public contributions as well as taxes.[70]

Health services were administered centrally in the Straits Settlements. In the FMS all public health and clinical services were delivered on a state basis until 1911, when the government established a federal health department in Kuala Lumpur. The first hospital in the FMS was opened in Taiping in 1878, a second in Kuala Lumpur soon after. Salaried practitioners served the military and civil European community first, then other urban dwellers; Chinese associations and individual philanthropists played an important role in the delivery of health care to the non-European population, at times in cooperation with the colonial administration. In both the settlements and the FMS, medical services operated primarily out of town-based clinics, with the primary objective to protect the health of Europeans associated with the administrative, military and mercantile arms and the colony, then, secondly, to maintain

the health of the local (or imported) labour force employed within the
colonial economy.[71] Those marginal to the colonial economy had little
access to medical services:

> From an early date there were hospitals of the East India Company in
> Singapore, Malacca and Penang: the Surgeons of the Company had medical
> charge of the garrisons and the government officials and their families, and
> they treated the local inhabitants who were disposed to enter the civil or
> pauper hospitals: yet we see the medical science of the West as an exotic plant,
> flourishing only in the Straits ports, contributing little to the public health
> and scarcely touching the traditional medicine of the Asian peoples ...
> Organised medicine in Malaya, as in Europe, has spread from the towns. The
> first hospitals were built for the needs of the urban populations. The surgeons
> of the East India Company, and later the doctors of the Colonial Medical
> Service, were stationed where the medical needs arising from modern
> economic development were most pressing. They served mainly the immi-
> grant populations, the Europeans and Asians in and around the towns,
> plantations and mines. The conservative Malays have witnessed these changes
> without enthusiasm.[72]

The colonial medical service adopted a two-pronged approach. Clinical
treatment was provided by hospitals and 'outdoor dispensaries'; the
prevention of the spread of epidemics was addressed through the development of public health programs. This involved epidemiological
surveillance of the population residing beyond the hubs of colonial
capitalism, including Malay peasant farmers and fisherfolk who were
often excluded from direct involvement in colonial enterprises. Their
general health status was not at issue, however, and their very isolation
from centres of residence, administration and production provided to an
extent a *cordon sanitaire*. Despite the extension of preventive and curative
services – Perak, for instance, in 1896 established floating dispensaries to
deliver medical care to the Malay villages (*kampungs*) – in most cases
relatively few Malays, Indians, or Chinese had access to state health
facilities. Contemporary explanations of the disparity of their use
emphasised native reluctance to present for treatment and to comply with
biomedical treatment regimes, whilst minimising the differential distribution of services. At the same time, while the government recognised
the economic significance of 'tropical disease', it failed to take account
of the extent to which colonisation had created health problems.

Incorporating gender

Although nineteenth-century health conditions were poor everywhere,
Turshen points out that by the end of the century they had improved
considerably in Europe and had at the same time worsened on the

periphery as a consequence of colonial policies and strategies.[73] In Africa, colonialism undermined the economic basis of society through the annexation of land, the recruitment and movement of labour and the establishment of the plantation sector and monocultures, with a consequent decline of subsistence food production, changes in farming technology, the displacement of women in production, low wages, poor living conditions, taxation, and uneven development.[74]

Turshen's arguments of the effect of changes in production, as well as the transfer of an inappropriate model of medical services to African colonies, extends to considerations of gender and class, and the particular impact on women's health of colonial capitalism. She argues that in addition to unequal access to medical care, women's authority in agriculture and within the household pre-colonially enabled them to control their own and their children's health and nutrition. This was compromised by social and economic transformations following the establishment of colonial rule.[75] As an example, she refers to the role of women in production in Kilimanjaro. From the 1920s much of women's subsistence agricultural land was appropriated by men for coffee production, and households became increasingly dependent on purchased foods; later men moved into wage labour and women were left with the responsibility of both coffee and food crops. The returns were insufficient to provide for family needs, resulting in increased recruitment of women as wage labour. Changes in the organisation of their work affected their ability to prepare and distribute food; hence impacting directly on their children's health and nutritional status.[76] Although her argument draws primarily on African experience, conditions in Asia were little different. Ione Fett's work on changes in patterns of land ownership in Negri Sembilan points to trends along these lines for Malay women.[77]

The intersections of class, ethnicity, gender and culture hence influenced health through changes in basic social and economic conditions – access to money, decision-making and authority, food and nutrition – as well as individual exposure to disease and the availability, accessibility and utility of health care. Ideas about health status, the nature and focus of health services, the disproportionate allocation of resources between town and country, elite and worker, and so on, are all shaped by these fundamental divisions among individuals. Individual health has an economic value, and whilst the concern for human welfare might provide the rhetoric for the instigation of health care programs, funds tended to be made available along rather more pragmatic lines: colonial Malaya illustrates the ways in which these were made explicit by colonial officials. A healthy body of a labourer had a value, reflected in the wage, greater than that of an unhealthy one, and health services were established and operated precisely to maintain health in order to meet the

labour needs of the economy. Women were seen particularly as
reproducers, with primary or sole responsibility for the domestic sphere;
and the devolution of the responsibility of family health and daily as well
as biological reproduction effectively cut the cost of health in the
colonies.[78] But it was not simply that women would undertake the basic
surveillance, monitoring, and treatment of their own, their children's,
and their husbands' health; state intrusions into women's lives, through
the education system, ensured more fundamental changes in ideas and
understandings of health and illness that increased dependence on the
state and its medical services. Here is the irony in colonial logic. The
creation of dependency on its technical and professional services – on
its hospitals, doctors, and drugs – rendered the system indispensable.

The health and welfare of colonising and colonised populations in
peripheral states were of concern to and debated in the centre, and over
time a variety of institutions and mechanisms were developed in response to these issues. In the concluding chapter of this book, I return
to this theme to consider, in the light of reports of increasing poverty
within the colonies, the growing awareness of the state of the relationship between health and development. Here, in this introduction, the
point is simply that health was not a state that existed independently of
colonial policy. Health policies and programs – decisions about the
balance of curative and preventive services, for example, the nature of
clinical medicine services, the extension of water, sanitation and 'scavenging' services – were developed in the context of certain empirical
realities and practical exigencies. Shifts in emphasis and developments
in medical services and public health in the colonial periphery reflected
central concerns and ideas, and biomedical science, medical services
and public health programs reflected European ideas about the
pathogenicity of the tropical environment, the transmission of disease
and appropriate measures for control.

The social canvas of colonial Malaya

There are many ways to approach the history of health and medicine in
colonial Malaya. For each time and place, competing stories create new
ways of capturing the convergence of ideas, individuals, and pathogens.
Over the period that is covered by this book, colonial Malaya was divided
into three broad systems that facilitated colonial administrative procedure and reflected the different agreements of suzerainty and
autonomy between the British and the Malay rulers. These (incorporated into British Malaya from 1857 to 1921) were twelve geopolitical
units, pre-existing Malay states and merchant port settlements,
maintaining their own identity, local jurisdiction and governance. The

settlements (Singapore, Penang and Malacca), the Federated Malay States (FMS, Selangor, Perak, Negri Sembilan and Pahang), and the Unfederated Malay States (UFMS, Kelantan, Trengganu, Perlis, Kedah and Johore) included also other smaller significant subdistricts (the Dindings and Province Wellesley, for example), many places which had evaporated (or rather, lost political and hence statistical salience) by the end of the period.

Colonial Malaya brought together different polities within a system of graded authority shared by British civil servants and Malay sultans. It brought together two different social, economic and cultural systems. Subsistence agriculture and fishing co-existed with mining and plantation agriculture whose markets were European, not Malayan, traditional modes of production flexed and adapted with increasing monetisation. Land was registered, sold, alienated, planted with new crops; railways and roads cut through primary jungle that had been home only to *orang asli* gatherer-hunters. Towns grew: frontier towns providing food and services to the miners, planters, traders and bankers; larger towns serving the administrative, political, commercial and financial needs of the expanding economies of these states. They were centres with an extraordinary intermingling of peoples from Southeast, East and South Asia and from Europe: Sikhs, Tamils, Punjabis, Javanese, Minangkabau, Portuguese from Goa, Thais, Filipinos, Hakka, Hailam, Cantonese, Teochew, Japanese, Jews, Russians, Englishmen, Scots, Arabs, Malays from the Peninsula and Riau, and more. Groups carved out enclaves in the cities where native foodstuffs, clothing, devotional paraphernalia and native medicines were readily available. Houses were built haphazardly, too slowly for the expanding populations; with crowding and without clean water or sanitation, infectious disease was rampant. In the mines and on the estates, workers from single language groups or home regions crammed together in crude dormitories, isolated groups of fortune seekers or simple poor peasants trapped in inhospitable environments. The Europeans who gained most from the colonies lived in isolated grand houses and more modest dwellings, assisted by Malay gardeners, Chinese cooks and 'houseboys', and Indian dhobies; their beds warmed by a local mistress (or houseboy): adventurers largely, often employees of English companies or officers of the empire posted to the colonies and hopeful of a final more prestigious post; or opportunists, grabbing the chance of money and power. Many were poorly educated and few had any insight, understanding or interest in the people they employed. Their arrogance was often the brave face of fear: the Malays, Indians and Chinese in their employ challenged their notion of order, and they clung to ideas of national right and racial superiority to justify the system that gave them privilege and prestige.

Priests from Christianity, Buddhism, Islam, Judaism and Hinduism provided pastoral support for at least some people. Ayurvedic, Unanic, Chinese, Thai and Western medical practitioners, representing competing professional traditions, together with Malay *bomoh* (medical practitioners) and *bidan* (midwives), masseurs, pharmacists, patent drug sellers, bone-setters and quacks competed to meet the physical and mental health needs of this diverse population pre-colonially and following the establishment of British rule. Hart suggests that Muslim traders and missionaries, who visited and established settlements in the region from the seventh century, introduced humoral pathology from the time of first contact.[79] Documentation from the late nineteenth and early twentieth century, as well as more recent evaluations of these sources and other texts, all point to the historical depth of Malay ties with Unanic practitioners and those from other medical systems, and the probable adaptation of those systems in their interface with indigenous medical beliefs;[80] in addition, Chinese medical practitioners and Ayurvedic practitioners met the health needs of their compatriots in the trading ports of the Peninsula.[81]

Colonial biomedical services therefore were introduced into a landscape where there was already a wide variety of healing specialists serving community needs and hospitals, clinics, travelling dispensaries, and British trained private practitioners were only part of a much richer and diverse system. Civil servants and medical officers posted to the colonies, most notably Skeat and Gimlette, provided testimony of the extensive armamentarium of Malay *bomoh* and *pawang* (healers with supernatural powers)[82] whose theories and practices derived from a mix of indigenous knowledge and beliefs with humoral medical theory. Individual Malays sought care from an appropriate specialist to alleviate their physical or mental suffering, and Golomb's extraordinary list of healers in Patani in the early 1980s gives us some idea of the wealth of expertise that would have been available fifty or a hundred years earlier.[83] Traditional healers were, in addition, responsible through the supervision and administration of village rites and ceremonies for village health and welfare. Bone-setters, masseurs, specialists in internal medicine, urinary tract infections, and reproductive health, herbalists and others met the needs of people both within their own locale and further afield, prescribing herbs, rubefacients, inhalations, dietary change and rest in addition to prayers and specialist incantations. These men and women turned to healing through dreams, meditation and inspiration, or travelled often far from their *kampungs* for religious and healing apprenticeships.[84] Some may have been charlatans and others lucky, but some were highly skilled, their therapeutic protocols based on their understanding of an elaborate body of theory and an extensive variety of indigenous and imported plants and their complex pharmacology.

Contemporary colonial observers described Malay medicine as 'essentially pagan' – 'a blend of ancient folk-lore, Hindu mythology and Moslem orthodoxy enriched by an Arabic pharmacopoeia' – and were tolerant but condescending towards its practice. Unlike the case in India, there was not in Malaya great interchange and borrowing of ideas,[85] nor a belief that local practitioners were best placed to deal with diseases of the tropics.[86] Biomedicine's lack of interest in local healing practice relates to the timing of the establishment of the British presence in Malaya; physicians and surgeons arrived when scientific advances had already captured the medical imagination, and they were supremely confident of its superiority. Even so, whilst some indigenous health professionals – particularly midwives – were consistently characterised as wilful, negligent and stupid, they and others were used as a resource in public health activities; this occurred sporadically throughout the period. For example, J. W. Field, Director of the Institute of Medical Research, in 1951 wrote of Malay healers in the following terms:

> The *pawang* who specialised in the healing art is the *bomor*, the village medicine man, often a simple herbalist and a 'lovable old fellow' who may dispense *kampung* remedies or set a simple fortune, or advise on matters of birth or death, accident or illness: who knows the folk-lore of disease and may chide or coax evil spirits as occasion seems to demand ... In the campaign against disease the *bomor* is less a rival than a potential ally. Dr Wolfe tells, for example, of the great assistance given by the *bomors* in the recent small-pox outbreak in Trengganu. They are near to the hearts of the conservative peasants, and their ancient role in *kampung* society yields only in those directions which the West has clearly more to offer in the form accessible and acceptable to the villager. By a happy gesture to Malay tradition the river boats launched in 1926 by the Medical Department as travelling dispensaries on the Pahang and Perak rivers, were named the *Pawang* and *Bomor*.[87]

In addition to these local practitioners there were other professionals who had been educated within other modalities. As already noted, Thai, Chinese, Ayurvedic and Unanic medicine operated in Malaya, each offering its own complex and systematic nosology of disease, diagnostic procedures, therapeutic regimes and drugs based on highly refined understandings of physiology and pathology.[88] We do not know the numbers nor the geographic distribution for all of these, but Chinese medical practice was extensive in the Straits Settlements. Yeoh gives 1867 as the date of the first Chinese medical institution in Singapore which, as a result of subsidisation by the Thong Chai Medical Institution, provided free consultations, advice and prescriptions for its patients.[89] From 1884 to 1991, it served the needs of nearly 40,000 patients, and the growing demand for Chinese medicine saw, in the early twentieth century, the establishment of other outpatient clinics and Chinese hospitals. These in turn were supplemented by Chinese pharmacists or medicine shops; a census in 1883 undertaken by the colonial government recorded 139 pharmacies in the Straits Settlements.[90] Other Chinese medical practitioners operated from temples, clan associations and their homes. Chinese practitioners were arguably most active in the Straits Settlements and in urban centres in states such as Perak and Selangor where Chinese labourers were concentrated. Ayurvedic practitioners were concentrated in those towns where Tamils and other Indians were most numerous; Thai practitioners were primarily located in the border states, with Malays, Thais living in those states, and others travelling to Patani and beyond to take full advantage of Thai medicine.

European suspicion of traditional medicine dates from the nineteenth century and continued, with the *Malayan Medical Journal* responding to the establishment of an Ayurvedic clinic in Kuala Lumpur in 1926 with dire warnings of chaos.[91] In general, however, the colonial government, certainly to the turn of the century, was tolerant of these practices since, as Yeoh argues,[92] they obviated the responsibility of health and welfare provision to the communities they served. Moreover, some were relatively open-minded with respect to their potential, arguing that the numbers of practitioners and the size of their practices depended not on government policy but rather on more complicated social and geographic circumstances. On Chinese medicine Field was to write:

> When the Chinese is sick he is likely to go first to the herbalist who dispenses in his drug shop from ancient formulae a vast array of remedies from animals, and from the leaves, flowers, roots, bark and seeds of a legion of shrubs, trees and fungi, ... dried scorpion, insect excrement, tiger bones ... (t)here is much of undoubted value in Chinese traditional medicine.[93]

In contrast, Ayurvedic practice appeared to have the least established presence in the colonies and was least available to potential patients:

> Ayurvedic medicine, unlike the traditional systems of Malays and Chinese, has no roots in Malaya. There are Ayurvedic dispensaries in the towns but the social milieu of the Indian has not favoured the blossoming of the Hindu system. The Indians on the plantations are cared for in the hospital provided by the rubber estate; the Indian clerical classes have open to them the resources of the Government hospitals. The Hindu system, while given no official support, is not opposed but left to find its own level.[94]

But Malay *bomoh*, Chinese pharmacists and acupuncturists, and Ayurvedic doctors were only part of a more extensive network of healers and modalities, and others from all communities provided an informal

fringe to these professional practices. Geomancers, astrologists, clairvoy-
ants and numerologists guided people in their everyday decision-
making, selected auspicious days for weddings and circumcision
ceremonies, advised on funerary rites and mourning procedure,
protected families and villages from vast and varying casts of spirits,
ghosts and fairies, and exorcised, nursed, prayed and cared for the sick
and troubled. It was easy to discount their services then, as now, since
they had little impact on biological infection, but they provided the core
of familiar health care and were the specialists to whom many turned in
times of physical as well as mental or emotional crisis. *The Annual
Medical and Sanitary Report* for Trengganu in 1935, in describing local
spirit beliefs and the role of spirits in the etiology of infection, provides
one example of the lack of fit between these beliefs and available state
medical services, hence the continuing need for a variety of practitioners, sorcerers and healers:

> Spirits and other malign influences are still held by a large section of the
> Trengganu people to play a great part in disease and of the 218 deaths due to
> 'other causes' ... 4 were ascribed to 'kelintasan' and 4 to 'badi'. Kelintasan is
> believed to be caused by the spirits of the forest or other places who resent
> the interruption of a traveller or wood cutter into some special preserve of
> theirs; it usually befalls a man journeying in the heat of the day in some lonely
> spot. It is accompanied by loss of speech and paralysis; in fact it is sudden
> death caused by a stroke and is found in middle-aged and old people. 'Badi'
> are ghostly influences haunting the scene of the slaughter of human beings,
> of animals such as tiger and elephant, and of certain birds while apparently
> even trees may have this power of retaliation. Of the 41 cases, all but 6 were
> under 2 months of age and the oldest was 2 years. 'Jugi' appears to be the
> same as 'badi' when only an attempt to kill has been made.[95]

We must imagine, therefore, that Malaya of the nineteenth and early
twentieth century included a wide range of formal and informal healers
and druggists. Some lived in villages and provided help as needed – a
bidan would provide service to a woman through pregnancy, birth and
confinement but thereafter, her obligation would cease; other *pawang* or
bomoh might be consulted once only or on numerous occasions over a
period of time. Some had consulting rooms in towns or cities, not unlike
the surgeries and dispensaries of the Western doctors with whom they
competed; some had shop fronts to advertise their specialities, with lists
of diseases treated and photographs of symptoms. Pictures of haemor-
rhoids in Chinese medical shop windows in the 'Chinatowns' of contemporary Singapore and Kuala Lumpur are remnants of this past; so are
the promises printed on the labels of brand-name rubefacients such as
Tiger Balm, Kwan Loong and similar medicated oils and embrocations
of their healing power for headache, colds, catarrh, rheumatism, urinary

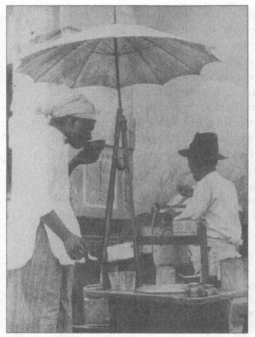
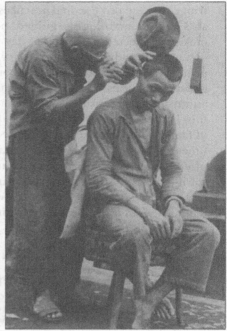

Figure 1.2 Food and beverage hawker in Singapore, c. 1910. Printed with permission from the Royal Commonwealth Society, London. Files of the British Association of Malaya, BAM/1 – Singapore.

Figure 1.3 Health care in the streets of Singapore, c. 1910. Printed with permission from the Royal Commonwealth Society, London. Files of the British Association of Malaya, BAM/1 – Singapore.

infections, low 'vital energy' and arthritis. Other healers had smaller and less lucrative practices and operated from roadside stalls, selling advice and medicine to those with faith and in need. People moved among these practitioners as required, combining therapies, seeking second and third opinions, presenting elsewhere when a treatment failed to relieve or cure, and '(n)o doubt in many instances the coolie instead of coming to the hospital went and obtained advice and physic from the many medicine shops now opened in various parts of the state'.[96]

Introduced into this landscape, Western medicine was simply another option. Government, for its part, tried to control the practice of non-Western healing through legislation, while promoting Western health and medical services. Medicinal wines, such as those that included a mix of wine and cocaine, were to be sold only through chemists, for example; but other 'rubbish', such as 'wines and meat extracts, Chinese decoctions of fruits and frog skins in alcohol, etc.', were sold through liquor stores and subject to liquor legislation.[97] Most drugs, herbs and medication, however, and the practitioners who prescribed them, were outside government control. In addition, patent medicines from British and other European pharmaceutical companies flooded the market from the late nineteenth century and made no less wild claims to prevent and cure. Holloway Pills in the 1880s, for instance, were advertised as preventing and curing 'diseases originating in bad blood and depraved humours'. One advertisement – drawing on humoral medical theory that placed the pills in the same modality as Chinese and Ayurvedic treatments, while at the same time alluding to current ideas of climate and immunity – described the pills as a 'cooling medicine [which] has the happiest effect when the blood is overheated and a tendency to inflammatory acting is set up in the system … [the pills] cleanse and perfectly regulate the circulation, and beget a feeling of comfort in hot climates and high temperatures'.[98] These and other tonics and medicines, advertised to the 1940s, promised cures for diverse ailments: diseases of the blood, stomach, liver, kidneys, women's 'nerves', neuralgia, rheumatism, gout and 'nervous affections when storms or atmospheric disturbances prevail'.[99]

Here was true medical pluralism, a complex mix of different practitioners and therapists to serve the varying needs of sick, injured, or disturbed people. The health care system and medical services of the colonial settlers were relatively haphazard and operated best to serve the curative needs of the military and other civilian British officials, and there was little need to tamper with the alternative systems. Those who could moved among them all.

From the vantage point of any of these people, the events of time and place looked different. A railway labourer, a shopkeeper, a hospital assistant, a rice farmer, a school teacher, or a medical officer: they were each positioned and positioned themselves differently one from the other with respect to the dominant political structures and the colonial economy: they exploited or were exploited in different ways; they lived differently in accordance with different sets of beliefs and behaviours; they were exposed and vulnerable to different infections; their explanations of sickness, appropriate management and outcome diverged. The challenge of a broad history such as that attempted in this book, weaving between intellectual, institutional, political, social and medical histories, is to capture these differences in perspective and experience, at least to some extent.

Text strips experience of its sensual complexity. Yet corporeality and ideology are juxtaposed; the flesh and its senses, like items of material culture and the fabric of the physical environment, ground the anonymity of history as it moves to the study of process and the theoretical renderings of its play. Beyond the opaque distance of planning and policy, beyond the broad economic and political processes here represented in terms of colonial capitalism, and beyond the teasing contradictory sets of ideas and beliefs, there is a sensual field: the sights, sounds and smells of everyday life. On the labour lines, the competing smells of stale rice and alcohol, curry, stagnant water, vomit, raw sewage; soft sounds of men singing and the harsher tones of quarrelling, quiet dusk cut by the noise of children playing or an infant screaming for a meal, whispers of bitterness or desire of a couple curled into a cot a foot from their sleeping neighbour. In the brothels: kitchen drains clogged with tea leaves and grey dishwashing water; a woman taking time off work to eat and chat; the pungent smell of garlic and frying oil cut by the stale odour of urine and dried sperm; confused sounds of sex and tears, lust and abuse. In the *kampungs*: chilli and fish paste in a *kuali* as a woman makes *belacan* for an evening meal, a cock crowing, men squatting to exchange the news of day, a voice across the field, the imam's call to pray cutting through the village peace. Or a hospital: here sharp sweet smells of disinfectant competing with the stench of ulcers, gangrenous sores, rotting lepromatous feet, and sour diarrhoeal fluids.

These sights and sounds and smells fade. Their absence underlines the difficulty of capturing the reality of everyday life in a time that is now imagined. But they are the backdrop to the explorations of sickness and the state that follow.

CHAPTER 2

State statistics and corporeal reality: Problems of epidemiology and evidence

Domestic violence and retaliation, ending in the hospitalisation or burial of individuals, were among the causes which brought the local population as well as recent immigrants (British officers, merchants and Indian troops) to British hospitals. The context of the injuries, the lives and deaths of individuals, are lost in the broad sweep of demographic history, however, and if we had the statistical data to allow us to write about morbidity and mortality in this early colonial period, we would simply note a small percentage of deaths due to homicide and murder and a small proportion of hospital admissions due to injury and assault. But the brief accounts raise a number of questions on the context of violence, illness, injury and death: the cause of the quarrel, for example, the extent of violence within the population, or the role of the colonial state in maintaining order. Further, statistical accounts – infant mortality rates, case fatality rates, life expectancy – silence the undocumented, ordinary and unremarkable lives and deaths of the men, women and children of the colonies. Changes in the demographic structure of the colonies, their political and economic organisation, living conditions and the workforce, including both the nature and conditions of work, were reflected in changes in patterns of morbidity and mortality, the perceptions of these changes by individuals, and their responses to specific instances of morbidity. Health and illness are socially embedded phenomena, and the description and analysis of these, of diagnostic procedure and therapeutic practice, all reflect the singular circumstances of time and place. Deaths too occur in social context.

From the late nineteenth century to 1940, infectious diseases declined dramatically as a consequence of simple control measures. Variolation, using minute amounts of infective material to control smallpox, was introduced in the late eighteenth century, and the later development, production and use of vaccines against smallpox had major impact on the Malay and immigrant populations and provide one tangible benefit of colonialism.[1] In the 1920s, the British enjoyed similar success in treating yaws with injections of salvarsan; the incidence of hookworm and other intestinal parasites were reduced through improved sanitation and mass treatment with anti-helminths (carbon tetrachloride); scientific discoveries led also to the means to reduce certain preventable diseases such as beri-beri.[2] Control was problematic, however, for diseases more complex in terms of etiology, epidemiology and prevention, and the decline in their incidence was far less dramatic even where there were concerted state efforts to improve treatment and decrease transmission. This was the case with diarrhoeal diseases, respiratory infections and malaria.

Epidemiological and demographic data suggest that the people's health status was rather more equivocal than contemporary commentators would have liked, although conditions did not deteriorate generally, as occurred from 1890 elsewhere in the empire. In Malaya, adult, infant and maternal mortality all declined from the early twentieth century but improvements in health were not universal, variations in the incidence of disease were not strictly due to seasonal fluctuations or changes in registration and record keeping, and advances in the control of some diseases were offset by the increased incidence of others and by growing evidence, in the 1930s, of poor nutrition. Improved services had variable impact and were, as will be discussed, rather more successful for curative than preventive purposes.

The peopling of colonial Malaya

Voluntary migrants were attracted to the settlements as the East India Company established its presence and as the ports grew in importance as centres of commerce; the transfer of their jurisdiction to the British colonial government, and the consequent expansion of commercial crops and extractive industries, was facilitated by the organised recruitment of indentured workers from China and India.[3] They were brought to a region which, despite a long history of diplomatic, cultural and mercantile links with other states in Asia and beyond, was still comprised of sultanates relatively sparsely populated by Malay subsistence agriculturalists and fisherfolk, most of whom, through colonial intent, remained marginal to the colonial enterprise. Most Chinese and Indian immigrants were men, although women workers (perhaps 10 percent of the total number of workers) were recruited too and some elderly dependents and children also migrated. However, immigrants were written of as if all were adult men, and the diseases that were most prevalent among them were treated as if they were the only health problems. These diseases, such as malaria, commonly related to economic and occupational circumstance: they occurred with the colonisation of land, the conversion of primary forest to sugar and rubber plantations and smallholdings, with the expansion of tin mining, the building of railways and roads, and the establishment of new towns.[4] Health policy developed in reaction to the deaths that occurred in this process, as a result of exposure to vectors (particularly to *Anophelene* mosquitos, the vector of malaria), lack of potable water, and lack of variety of foodstuffs.[5] The health of the indigenous Malay population was not at issue until into the twentieth century, as health officials drew attention to their poor health status also.

Strategically located on the sea trade routes that linked south and east Asia, the ports of the Malay Peninsula had always been host to different people. Trade, seasonal agricultural work and kinship ties were maintained between Sumatra and other islands of the Indonesian archipelago and the Peninsula, and many people from these islands migrated to and settled in Malaya: Sumatrans in Penang, Selangor, Malacca and Negri Sembilan, Bugis in Johore and Selangor, and Javanese in the southern and western parts of the Peninsula.[6] Muslims from Arabia and northern India came to the region, trading and studying in such centres as Acheh (north Sumatra) and Kota Bharu (Kelantan), and marrying peninsular and island Malays. Portuguese adventurers, traders, priests, soldiers and government officials settled in Malacca in 1511, the Dutch – in the form of the Dutch East India Company (Vereenigte Oost-Indische Compagnie, VOC) – from 1641. Forced migration occurred too for a number of reasons: *kerah* and debt-bondage, due to civil war, led to outmigration from Selangor and Pahang; political changes resulted in the emigration of Malays from Kedah during the period of Thai suzerainty to 1842; famine in Kelantan in the late nineteenth century led to the immigration of Kelantanese to west coast Malay states. Various natural disasters, including floods and crop failures, provided further push factors for local migration and resettlement, resulting in contemporary and later accounts of numbers of 'sick and starving beggars and vagrants'.[7] Local migration between Kelantan and Patani, and among the peninsular states, continued into the twentieth century. The immigration of Malays and other Indonesians as well as Chinese, Indians, and others from Asia and beyond, and circular migration within the region, made mapping the population a complex and approximate task, and population figures are therefore problematic.

The establishment of the British presence encouraged the voluntary migration of Chinese miners and merchants, but it was only after the transfer to Colonial Office control that economic activities and labour requirements expanded significantly. These were met systematically through the organised immigration of Chinese and Indian labourers, although an early *sinkeh* system was in operation by the mid-nineteenth century with an estimated two or three thousand Chinese entering Penang and Province Wellesley annually.[8] They were joined by other voluntary migrants – punters, labourers, traders, adventurers, and miscreants – from Asia and Europe.

Migration affected people's health and the epidemiological history of the Peninsula in two respects. The use of migrants as labour to open up new territory resulted in 'new' health problems among both the incoming and indigenous populations. Migrants introduced into local populations the infections of which they were host, and in turn were exposed to and infected by local endemic diseases. The extent to which Malay populations were subject to new pathogens and hence suffered changes in morbidity and mortality is unclear, and population movement prior to the large-scale migrations of the late nineteenth century must have already introduced various microbial and parasitic infections. Sections of the population, however, would not have had prior exposure because of their relative isolation in the hinterland, the geographic concentration of earlier settlers and visitors (i.e., at ports), and the fact that the smaller population of the Peninsula in previous centuries may not always have been sufficient to maintain a reservoir of infection. Population expansion and its penetration of the Peninsula introduced or at least sustained certain pathogens. As Denoon notes for Papua New Guinea, 'colonialism did not simply permit the introduction of entirely new diseases ... but also allowed the more even redistribution of endemic infections' through the introduction, dissemination, and redistribution of infection as labour was mobilised for mining, plantation work, and general employment by the colonists.[9] This mobilisation of the population was supplemented by voluntary circular migration and some early rural to urban migration, so that population movement as a 'mechanism was much more effective than the frantic attempts of the health authorities to stamp out epidemics once they occurred'.[10]

Immigrant workers to Malaya were not protected against diseases endemic in the region. The incidence of severe cases of fever and the high death rates from fever among railway workers and plantation labourers, for example, suggests that they had not been exposed and hence lacked acquired immunity to the virulent *Plasmodium falciparum* malaria. Both southern Chinese and Indian labourers were recruited from malarial regions, but the malaria to which they had prior exposure was often *P. vivax*; this difference in parasite would have accounted for the high mortality rate among plantation labourers and railway workers. In addition, of course, a proportion of labourers would not ever have been infected before, and so were vulnerable. Medical officers knew enough about malaria to recognise that semi-immunity developed among adults and to differentiate types of malaria clinically, but they did not make the parasitological distinctions and consequently did not understand why labourers from endemic areas would suffer so seriously from falciparum malaria.

The health of migrants and transients who called at the ports, including sailors, traders, fisherfolk and pirates, was ill policed, despite efforts to systematise notification and quarantine procedures from the mid-1860s (see further on this, below). However, quarantine provisions ensured that common highly infectious diseases were identified and interventions taken to reduce the risk of transmission, and although the potential introduction of infectious diseases such as smallpox, cholera, and the plague remained, the absolute number of cases was small. The most significant *epidemic* disease in Malaya, as elsewhere, was influenza in 1918–1919 (see below), but the geographic distribution of other endemic diseases such as syphilis and tuberculosis were also affected by population density, location and movement, and affected a much larger number of people. Further, malaria was by the far the most important disease, contributing to around 25 percent of morbidity at any time.

Above a distinction is drawn between Indian and Chinese labour immigrants and Indonesian circular migrants, but most immigrants, including those recruited from southern China and India, were temporarily resident only. Pryor estimates that while four million Indians entered Malaya between 1860 and 1957, nearly three million left the country in the same period, and that of one-and-a-half million Chinese entering between 1911 and 1921, almost two-thirds returned to China.[11] Over the 150 or so years of British colonialism, Ooi estimates that 14.5 of around 17 million Chinese were repatriated.[12] As already noted, most immigrants were men, who left their wives and children at home and travelled to Malaya as fortune seekers or to escape poverty, bondage or indebtedness. Women migrated primarily from the second quarter of the twentieth century in response to targeted government recruitment, and from then on, as the sex ratio improved and more marriages were contracted, immigrant communities began to reproduce, and the age dependency as well as sex ratio began to normalise.

Given the disproportionate sex ratio and high mortality rates of the nineteenth and early twentieth century, and the degree of outmigration or home returns, one might anticipate demographic stability in Malaya to around the 1920s, but this was not the case. There are a number of possible reasons for this, in addition to the scale of immigration: a higher population at the beginning of the nineteenth century than indicated by official statistics; the prevention of deaths from infectious diseases, especially malaria, from the early 1900s; and a higher birth rate than the statistics suggest. Closer examination of the demographic and epidemiological data for the period provides us with some clues to population changes during the colonial period, the impact of particular diseases on morbidity and mortality, and the efficacy of disease control measures and the delivery of medical services.

The nineteenth century

Population enumeration was an administrative imperative as the colonial regime extended control over the Malay States, and was systematised during the nineteenth century in tandem with the development of population science. In Britain, the collection of population statistics was promoted by William Farr, and under his direction, the General Register Office (GRO) from 1837 collected demographic and epidemiological data. The 'consistent, central aim' of the GRO from 1837 to 1914 was, Szreter claims, the identification of preventable diseases and the development of appropriate public health interventions to reduce these. GRO reports highlighted the variation in health outcome and life expectancy within the United Kingdom, and the correlation of higher life expectancy with improved sanitation and related social variables.[13] The establishment of the GRO therefore marked the beginnings of a public health sensibility, by demonstrating relationships between morbidity and social and economic circumstance which provided the impetus for policy changes and reforms.[14]

In Malaya, the social basis of ill health was rarely made explicit until the end of the nineteenth century, when the first commission of inquiry into conditions of labour was conducted. However, the commission of inquiry into prostitution and venereal disease in the 1860s and a number of other smaller enquiries – in 1872, following riots by Chinese coolies in Singapore, and in 1876 into the conditions of employment and service of Chinese labourers, for example – anticipated these links.[15] In the meantime, procedural demands and bureaucratic goals sustained the collection of population statistics. The earliest figures for Penang, Malacca and Singapore are derived from police head-counts and educated guesses. No census was conducted until the 1830s, although local administrators regularly requested resources from the India Office for this purpose, as well as for maintaining registers of marriages, births, deaths, slaves, and the sale of land and houses.[16] Early population reports tended to underestimate, since not all births and deaths were registered and both Malays and Chinese resisted colonial 'interference' in such affairs.

According to police estimates, the population in Penang by 1813 was 32,333 and in 1825 it was 53,334, representing a population increase of

5.4 percent per annum over these twelve years.[17] Official statistics provide a breakdown neither by ethnicity nor sex, but the population increase was largely due to Malay immigration to Province Wellesley and Penang following Thai incursions into and control of Kedah and attacks on Perak, primarily between 1821 and 1825. The populations of Malacca and Singapore, as a result of more precise census reporting, are better documented.

The Singapore figures are revealing in terms of the categorisation of individuals and the social construction of race. 'Armenians' and 'Europeans' are differentiated, for example; Chinese are categorised as a single ethnic group despite their regional, linguistic, clan and cultural differences; the status of 'troops and followers' and 'convicts' renders ethnic affiliation irrelevant or perhaps strips individuals of their rights to it. The figures highlight the gross disparity between men and women, even among indigenous and local immigrant populations (that is, among Malays, Buginese and Javanese), and draw attention to the fact that the indigenous population was already a numerical minority in this settlement. According to these early records, at the beginning of 1826 Singapore had a population of 13,762 which was steadily increasing; this excluded an itinerant native population (on vessels) of around 2500 throughout the year.[18] Chinese already predominated (see Table 2.1). In 1829, the population had risen to 18,819 with a 'surplus of Chinese' over

Table 2.1   Population of Singapore, 1 January 1827

Ethnicity	Men	Women	Total
European	69	18	87
Armenian	16	3	19
Native Christian	128	60	188
Arab	18	—	12
Chinese	5,747	341	6,088
Malay	2,501	2,289	4,790
Bugi	666	576	1,242
Javanese	172	93	265
Natives of Bengal	209	53	262
Natives of the Coromandel Coast	772	5	777
Coffrees	2	3	5
Siamese	5	2	7
Sub-total	10,305	3,443	13,742
Troops and followers	492	122	614
Convicts	248	4	252
Total	11,045	3,569	14,608

Source: SSR N1, 1826, p.75.

the previous year, largely accounted for, according to police, by migration from Riau.[19] Malacca's population in contrast was two-thirds Malay
and half female, but was also expanding steadily. [20]

In less than two decades, the total population of the settlements had
almost doubled and was 209,091 by the end of 1846.[21] No mortality or
fertility rates are available for this period, and hospital admissions and
case fatalities usually lack information of cause of death. Detailed
statistics were only collected for native troops, women and children after
1862,[22] and registration of births, deaths and marriages was provided for
legally only following the transfer of power from the India Office to the
Colonial Office in 1866.[23] Since birth and death rates were not included
in early population reports, the extent to which changes to migration,
mortality and fertility contributed variably to population expansion
during this period remains a matter of conjecture.

The census of 1871 provided the first comprehensive information
describing the population with respect to age, sex and ethnicity. According to data collected (see Table 2.2), nearly 50 percent of the total Straits
Settlements population were peninsular Malay, although in Singapore
Chinese dominated and Malays constituted only 20 percent of its
population. Among Chinese and Indians, the sex ratio showed marked
distortion. The returns identified as 'nationalities' some 28 different
groups of people,[24] counting separately 'British and Indian military' and
'local and transmarine prisoners' whose language, ethnicity or nationality was not specified. Later census reports gave greater detail of
nationality, distinguishing ethnic Chinese by language group, identifying
further 'nationalities' from the Indian subcontinent, and distinguishing
further also among various European sojourners. However, despite the
apparently polymerous nature of the settlements, they were in fact
largely Chinese and Malay communities, characteristically populated by
adult men. This had significance in terms of incidence of disease as well
as public health policy from the turn of the century.

The figures are highly suggestive of the numbers of people whose
needs were not met by contemporary health and medical services.
As described in the previous chapter, medical services in colonial Malaya
were established and operated primarily for European officials and
troops (about two percent of the population), then extended to those in
direct association with the colonial state, people such as Indian
labourers working on the railways and plantations, and Chinese working
in mines or in trade or service industries in the port towns. A few had
access to medical services as a result of individual initiative of which
there were presumably examples both in the settlements and the states:
for example Legge, an apothecary based in Sungei Ujong in the 1870s,
provided 'very useful' basic clinical care to Chinese miners as well as

Table 2.2 Population of the Straits Settlements by nationality and sex, 2 April 1871

Nationality	Singapore		Penang and Province Wellesley		Malacca		Totals		
	M	F	M	F	M	F	M	F	Total
Europeans and Eurasians[1]	2,155	1,459	891	878	1,084	1,188	4,130	3,525	7,655
'Kling' (South Indians)	7,664	1,633	5,136	1,687	1,556	1,318	14,356	4,638	18,994
Other Indian[2]	666	316	8,224	2,755	56	20	8,946	3,091	12,037
Chinese	46,631	7,467	30,168	6,214	9,850	3,606	86,649	17,287	103,936
Malays	10,041	9,209	35,501	34,963	28,102	29,372	73,644	73,544	147,188
Other Indonesian[3]	4,546	2,320	2,536	2,064	411	143	7,493	4,532	12,025
Other	345	230	697	471	173	168	1,215	869	2,084
Military									
British	481	115	58	18	3	—	542	133	675
Indian	412	3	191	—	186	—	789	3	792
Prisoners	529	3	290	—	99	—	918	3	921
Transmarine	878	8	457	31	416		1,751	39	1,790
Totals	74,348	22,763	84,149	49,081	41,936	35,815	200,433	107,664	308,097

1 Europeans, Jews, Armenians and Eurasians.

2 Andamanese, Bengalees and other natives of India not particularised, Hindoos, Parsees, and Singhalese.

3 Boyanese, Buginese, Dyaks, Javanese, Jaweepakans (i.e. Jawi Peranakan). The allocation of 'Straits Chinese' to this latter category is largely based on their established presence in the Malay Peninsula, use of Malay language and adoption of Malay dress.

Source: GB, *Colonial Reports 1871*, Return of the Population of the Straits Settlements, 1871 (London: HMSO, 1872).

meeting the needs of European residents,[25] and both Pauper and General Hospitals provided acute care to 'natives'. However, only around 30 percent of the population enjoyed physical access to hospitals and clinics which were concentrated in the towns, and most people, including the majority of Malays, lived in rural areas. In practice far fewer were served directly, and medical care was provided for and availed by only a tiny elite of settlers, colonial officers, and others in contact with them. This inequitable distribution of services and technical resources is characteristic of colonies, of course.[26]

Given that not all people had access to or used hospital services, the information derived from hospital inpatient returns and case fatality rates needs to be interpreted with extreme caution. Even so, it provides some indication of prevalent diseases and changing fortunes. The hospital in Butterworth, Province Wellesley, for example, in 1874 treated 454 patients of whom 22 percent died. Admissions included a number who had been victims of homicidal attacks or had been injured (16 percent of all admissions, including a case of intestinal goring by a buffalo), 'common diseases' – such as ulcers, diarrhoea, dysentry – 'debility' and venereal infections, 'fever' (often malaria) and rheumatism, with the high mortality rate attributed to 'a low form of diarrhoea, the result of a debilitated and broken-down state of the constitution of patients'.[27]

Hospital returns for Penang and Province Wellesley, published in the Colonial Report for 1878, indicate that only 3.2 percent of the total population of the settlement, or 4298 patients, were admitted during the year, including a number of sick coolies who had drifted to Penang from Dutch plantations in Acheh, Sumatra.[28] The figures are not an accurate picture of community health, case mortality or morbidity patterns, but even so, the data summarised for Penang Island, the adjacent area of Province Wellesley and Malacca (see Table 2.3), are instructive, because of the disparity of admissions between the two settlements not accounted for by the larger population of Penang/Province Wellesley alone, and because of the absence of women from the record. Figures by sex are given only for Sungei Bakup Hospital, where 5 percent of admissions were female of a total of 569 patients, of whom most (93 percent) were estate coolies.[29] Since even the unreliable statistics of the 1871 census tell us that 35 percent of the total settlement population and 24 percent of 'Kling' (South Indian) estate workers were female, then the gender differences are extraordinary, credible not as variations in morbidity or biology, or both, but as an indication of difference in access to and use of services.

Other issues arise from these returns. Firstly, whilst smallpox and cholera are given considerable attention for reasons that relate to the metaphoric weight of these diseases rather than their incidence (see below), the returns indicate that diarrhoeal disease and acute respiratory infections were the predominant causes of admission and death; sexually

Table 2.3 Hospital returns for Penang, Province Wellesley and Malacca, 1877

Hospital	Total admissions	Deaths	Notes
Penang	**2,483**	**347**	32% of 'native patients' police cases; 19.5% native deaths from beri-beri
General Hospital			
European patients	138	10	
Native	549	41	cholera outbreak
Lock Hospital	111	[not stated]	
Pauper Hospital	985	239	73% deaths from cholera . Poor condition of patients on arrival
Pulau Jerajak	64	16	
Dato Kramat			
Gaol Hospital	636	41	
Province Wellesley	**1,815**	**376**	21% admissions diarrhoeal diseases, 66% case fatality
Bukit Mertajam	406	83	Prevalance of pneumonia and syphilis
Birtam	258	54	
Bukit Minyak	517	110	
Sungei Bakup	569	129	43% admissions malaria
Malacca	**719**	**63**	
General Hospital	171	7	
Prison Hospital	106	0	
Lock Hospital	87	0	82.8% cases gonorrhea[1]
Pauper Hospital	355	56	22.4% admissions ulcers
Total	**5,017**	**786**	

1 This refers to cases of gonorrhea treated, not reason for admission.
Source: CO, Papers Relating to Her Majesty's Colonial Possessions (London: HMSO, 1879), pp. 326–329, 348–349.

transmitted diseases, malaria, beri-beri and ulcers were also prevalent. Secondly, according to the report, coolies were often admitted to hospital in a 'very debilitated and hopeless state', and although this was especially true of those who had travelled to Penang from estates in Sumatra, it was true also of local estate coolies received as prisoners and then transferred to hospital 'in a very wretched condition, and ... physically incapable of work, being debilitated and anaemic'.[30] The report refers also to the overcrowding and insanitary conditions of gaols and lock hospitals, resulting in the rapid spread of highly infectious diseases such as cholera; comments about the poor condition of gaols and other detention centres

Table 2.4 Population increases by decade, states and settlements, 1881–1921

State or settlement	Total population					Percentage of increase or decrease			
	1881	1891	1901	1911	1921	1881 to 1891	1891 to 1901	1901 to 1911	1911 to 1921
Singapore	139,208	178,253	220,344	311,985	425,912	+28.0	+23.6	+41.6	+36.5
Penang	190,597	231,224	247,808	278,003	304,335	+21.3	+7.2	+12.2	+9.4
Malacca	93,579	91,582	95,100	124,081	153,522	-2.2	+3.1	+30.5	+23.7
Straits Settlements	**423,384**	**501,059**	**563,252**	**714,069**	**883,769**	**+18.3**	**+12.4**	**+26.8**	**+23.7**
Perak	NO FIGURES AVAILABLE	214,254	329,665	494,047	599,055	NO FIGURES AVAILABLE	+53.8	+49.8	+21.2
Selangor		81,592	168,789	294,035	401,009		+106.8	+74.2	+36.3
Negri Sembilan		65,219	96,028	130,199	178,762		+47.2	+35.5	+37.2
Pahang		57,444	84,113	118,708	146,064		+46.4	+41.1	+23.0
Federated Malay States		**418,509**	**678,595**	**1,036,999**	**1,324,890**		**+62.1**	**+52.8**	**+27.7**
Johore	NO FIGURES AVAILABLE			180,412	282,234	NO FIGURES AVAILABLE			+56.4
Kedah				245,986	338,558				+37.7
Perlis				32,746	40,087				+22.6
Kelantan				286,751	309,300				+7.8
Trengganu				154,073	153,765				–.2
Brunei				21,718	25,451				+17.1
British Malaya	NO FIGURES AVAILABLE			**2,672,754**	**3,358,054**	NO FIGURES AVAILABLE			**+25.6**

Source: Nathan, *The Census of British Malaya*, p. 18.

in the colonies recur throughout the period. Finally, it accounts for at least some patient absconsions (20 percent of patients admitted to Bukit Minyak Hospital) as the result of touting, whereby 'crimps' in league with hospital servants induced patients to desert and take up service on newly opened Dutch plantations in Sumatra.[31]

Morbidity and mortality at the turn of the century

By the turn of the century, the population had expanded dramatically, almost doubling in Singapore from 1881 to 1901 with its development as the administrative, financial and commercial capital of the colonies. Penang's population had increased by around 25 percent, and while Malacca's population was comparatively stable at this time, it increased 30 percent during the years 1901–1911 with the growth of the rubber industry. Baseline data for the FMS is not available before 1891, but thereafter population expansion – if the numbers reflect true increases in the population rather than improved reporting – was extraordinary: Selangor's population more than doubled from 1891 to 1901; the combined population of the states doubled within fifteen years and had trebled by 1921 (see Table 2.4).

The age (a simple indication of dependents and workers), sex and 'nationality' of the populations of the settlements in 1901 (Table 2.5) provide a fuller picture of the way in which the demographic composition of the population was shaped by the colonial economy. Even in the FMS – and rather surprisingly, even among Malays – the sex and age structure of the population was distorted. This possibly reflected, and certainly would have reinforced, contemporary emphasis on men's rather than on women's or children's health, and documentation of and commentary on women's and children's health was notably absent.

A review of the processes of collection of population statistics from around 1866 to 1900 indicates that although sometimes information was collected relatively systematically and in great detail, the quality of vital statistical and epidemiological data was poor and incomplete even by contemporary standards, due to official incompetence, poor compliance from populations, reluctance of estates and mines to comply and report sickness and deaths, and understaffing. For example, infant and child deaths in Jeram District, Selangor, were not recorded in 1899 during an epidemic reported to have resulted in high child mortality, due to the absence of a police officer-in-charge to compile the statistics.[32] Information collected by native police and chiefs was often incomplete, and hospital-based data was itself suspect where the cause of death was reported by an unqualified dresser and was proximate.[33] Morbidity data are even more impressionistic. Malaria and intestinal parasites were said

Table 2.5 Population of Straits Settlements by age, sex and ethnicity, 1901 (continued on facing page)

Nationalities	Singapore							Penang, Province Wellesley and Dindings						
	Over 15		Under 15		Total			Over 15		Under 15		Total		
	M	F	M	F	M	F	Total	M	F	M	F	M	F	Total
Europeans and Americans	2,273	833	346	372	2,619	1,205	3,824	587	313	122	138	709	451	1,160
Eurasians	1,189	1,239	826	866	2,015	2,105	4,120	529	557	400	459	929	1,016	1,945
Chinese	118,196	23,956	12,171	9,718	130,367	33,674	164,041	65,295	16,275	8,481	8,373	73,776	24,648	98,424
Malays	15,128	10,373	5,132	5,447	20,260	15,820	36,080	31,581	32,390	21,446	20,583	53,027	52,973	106,000
Tamils	12,761	2,417	1,584	1,061	14,345	3,478	17,823	22,829	7,911	4,109	3,202	26,938	11,113	38,051
Other nationalities	953	1,075	316	323	1,269	1,398	2,667	1,113	897	315	302	1,428	1,199	2,627
Grand Total	150,500	39,893	20,375	17,787	170,875	57,680	228,555	121,934	58,343	34,873	33,057	156,807	91,400	248,207

Table 2.5 cont.

Nationalities	Malacca							Grand Total		
	Over 15		Under 15		Total					
	M	F	M	F	M	F	Total	M	F	Total
Europeans and Americans	48	19	6	1	54	20	74	3,382	1,676	5,058
Eurasians	423	503	331	341	754	844	1,598	3,698	3,965	7,663
Chinese	13,179	2,775	1,882	1,632	15,061	4,407	19,468	219,204	62,729	281,933
Malays	17,820	21,813	16,804	16,541	34,624	38,354	72,978	107,911	107,147	215,058
Tamils	785	227	140	124	925	351	1,276	42,208	14,942	57,150
Other nationalities	38	27	13	15	51	42	93	2,748	2,639	5,387
Grand total	32,293	25,364	19,176	18,654	51,469	44,018	95,487	379,151	193,098	572,249

to be universal,[34] but the absence of population-based data, the low use of medical services by Malays, and the reported tendency of all people, excluding Europeans, to delay presenting to hospital until they were critically ill, distorts our understanding of morbidity. Even in Singapore, where about one-quarter of all deaths occurred in hospitals or were certified by a qualified medical practitioner, the diagnosis and establishment of cause of death remained problematic.

Still, available data point to the vulnerability of particular communities and to the implications of this in terms of population structure. As one contemporary commentator on the 1891 census noted:

> Absolutely accurate returns of this nature are impossible, as no strict record of either births or deaths, of emigration or immigration, have been kept; and the census returns are not perhaps entirely reliable. But there can be little doubt that the mortality among the Malays is severe enough if not to threaten their distant extinction at least to greatly retard their growth and multiplication in a country which needs, above all things, a settled, vigorous and spreading population.[35]

State data give further indication of health trends. In Negri Sembilan in 1899, when the total population was estimated at 82,678, the Malay birth rate was around 36 per thousand (births among other groups were insignificant and their rates not computed). The total death rate was 26 per thousand, amongst Chinese 27 and Malays 24, 'nearly one third less than the birth rate' and regarded as 'very satisfactory given that they are using their own treatment'.[36] But among Tamils, the death rate was 68.[37] In 1900, the death rate had risen to an average of 38 per thousand: for Chinese from 28 in January to 52 in December, for Malays from 24 to 26, and for Indians from 68 to 144 largely as a result of the malaria-related deaths of Tamil labourers working on the railways.[38] Fever, dysentry and bowel complaints each accounted for 25 percent of deaths; beri-beri, 'infantile disorders', accidents and pulmonary infections stand out as the other significant causes of death. The infant mortality rate, conventionally regarded as a sensitive index of general health status, and here representing deaths for children from 0 to 5 years, was 101 for Malays and 193 for Tamils.[39]

Despite their inaccuracy, hospital records supplement this data. In Negri Sembilan in 1899, Chinese comprised 75 percent of hospital admissions, representing an admission rate to the total population of 116 per thousand. By contrast, the European/Eurasian rate was twelve; the Malay rate one – that is, virtually no Malays presented to hospital. The Tamil rate was a remarkable 513 per 1000 and Tamils accounted for 6 percent of all deaths while constituting only 2.3 percent of the total state population. The main causes of death in hospitals and within the community were recorded as fever, dysentery, diarrhoea, and beri-beri, the last accounting for 66 per thousand of Chinese admissions and nearly one-third of all hospital deaths. But this is a low figure, apparently, to be treated sceptically: less than one-tenth of all beri-beri deaths occurred in hospital, and possibly 20 percent of all deaths were caused by beri-beri.[40]

The 1900 report for Negri Sembilan indicates a decline in hospital treatments but an increase of inpatients (from 3,915 to 5,016), of whom 72, 24, 1.6 and 1.9 percent respectively were Chinese, Tamil, Malay and 'others'. Dysentery and diarrhoea accounted for 56 percent of hospital fatalities, 'debility' 12 percent, pneumonia 8 percent, and beri-beri 4 percent. But the medical officer writing the report warns:

> The diagnosis in many cases rests on the opinion of unqualified dressers, it cannot but be that here are many inaccuracies. In especial [sic] is this the case with regard to the very important section [of statistics] of malarial fevers. The return as it stands is, I am sorry to say, completely worthless, as regards the types of fever met with. I have been unable as yet to thoroughly instruct the dressers or to provide them with proper means for the differentiation of the various forms of malaria.[41]

Like Negri Sembilan, other larger populations had very high mortality rates: Pahang's infant mortality rate, for example, was estimated at 161.2 in 1899 and 334 in 1900, with an estimated maternal mortality rate (in 1899) of eleven.[42] In Selangor the picture was slightly different, possibly due to the larger number of immigrant labourers and hence the distinctive age and sex structure: a crude birth rate 10.48 and crude death rate 47.44 in 1902. In the UFMS, the data are less reliable due to poor statistics, the limited provision of medical services, and the very small proportion of sick people presenting for medical care. Kelantan in 1904, for example, had a hospital case mortality rate of 7.65, but derived from a total of 184 patients only;[43] in 1907 it was 19.1 percent of a total 475 admissions. To labour the point somewhat, at around this time the fatality rate of hospital admissions in private hospitals in Pahang varied, depending on disease, from 68.5 to 90 percent.[44] Morbidity and mortality rates also varied between districts and created the illusion of epidemics, even of non-infectious disease; the local constellation of specific diseases, infections and other health problems made extrapolation impossible and at best reflected the concentration of population by industry.[45]

Mortality rates remained high in the first decade of the twentieth century. In the FMS in 1908, the general Tamil death rate was 65 per thousand, while the total death rate on rubber estates was estimated to be 79.6, indicating high mortality rates on the estates; in 1910 the estimated death rate for all indentured labourers was 94.6, although less than 80 for unindentured labourers.[46] Both Sandhu and Jackson suggest that around 60–90 percent of estate labourers died within a year of arrival. Estate-specific mortality rates, despite marked seasonal and local geographic fluctuation, support this claim, which may indeed underestimate deaths since sick labourers often voluntarily left or were discharged from the estate, and repatriated, when ill.[47]

From around 1910, mortality rates fall fairly consistently primarily due to measures to reduce the transmission of infectious diseases and to increase health surveillance and early treatment of sickness. Beri-beri, as discussed in Chapter 3, ceased to be a significant health hazard by the 1920s; deaths from fever, ulcers and dysentery and diarrhoea all began to decline. The decline in adult mortality was gradual (see Table 2.6); among infants it was dramatic as a result of the supervision of deliveries and postnatal care, hence a reduction in stillbirths and deaths from neonatal tetanus (see Chapter 7).[48]

Table 2.6 Crude death, birth and infant mortality rates, Straits Settlements, 1901–1937

Year	Deaths per 1000	Births per 1000	Infant mortality rate	Year	Deaths per 1000	Births per 1000	Infant mortality rate
1901[1]	39.85	25.46	230.86	1919	33.04	30.29	212.42
1902	42.96	24.98	246.59	1920	33.20	29.63	194.86
1903	39.49	26.35	245.06	1921[1]	31.54	32.62	179.23
1904	39.00	25.59	250.05	1922	30.68	30.59	195.22
1905	40.51	28.57	256.29	1923	27.80	30.43	200.73
1906	37.82	25.23	255.02	1924	27.42	32.29	194.57
1907	39.07	26.11	250.91	1925	27.26	31.98	194.00
1908	43.06	28.75	265.63	1926	31.81	32.85	214.79
1909	37.58	26.69	263.67	1927	33.55	35.13	224.04
1910	41.88	27.55	268.93	1928	28.76	36.03	193.69
1911[1]	46.46	25.38	270.47	1929	26.10	37.20	188.61
1912	39.01	28.26	267.21	1930	27.32	38.25	200.19
1913	34.93	26.87	271.34	1931[1]	24.47	26.98	185.15
1914	34.13	29.09	250.23	1932	21.39	35.83	166.42
1915	29.15[2]	29.25	236.68	1933	24.26	40.95	172.72
1916	30.70[2]	28.15	216.72	1934	26.54	40.65	175.43
1917	36.98	30.65	266.92	1935	25.11	41.76	165.28
1918	43.85[3]	28.64	232.38	1936	24.91	44.33	170.85
				1937	22.45	42.13	155.80

1   Census years
2   Several thousands of Chinese were repatriated in 1915 and 1916 as a war measure
3   The influenza pandemic.
Source: SSAR 1937, p. 182 (Table IV).

Epidemics and control

I now turn to look at two epidemic diseases, smallpox and cholera, and the provisions that were instituted to control their transmission. Outbreaks of smallpox and cholera and control measures for them were well documented, for they were dramatic in onset and devastating in outcome. They were highly feared because of high case fatality, although their incidence was relatively low compared with other endemic diseases such as malaria, beri-beri, respiratory infections and diarrhoeal diseases other than typhoid. Other less prevalent diseases and chronic infections also took a heavy toll on the population. Yaws, leprosy and filariasis, for example, caused gross disfigurement, and even common ulcers from cuts and wounds could have final devastating results: 'In some instances so rapid is its progress that the patient sinks in 10 or 12 days, and sometimes in a shorter period, the limb below the knee becoming one slough and the muscular parts appearing like slimy rope yarn, and eventually a black mass of gangrene'.[49] Cholera and smallpox, however, captured popular and official imagination.

Quarantine provisions were important to prevent such epidemic diseases as smallpox, cholera and plague. Provisions were introduced in colonial Malaya in 1858 under the Native Passenger Act, but were regarded as inadequate by the Conférence Sanitaire Internationale, held in Constantinople in August 1866 to prevent the introduction of cholera to Europe.[50] A new Quarantine Ordinance, introduced in September 1868, applied to all vessels, including pilgrim ships, using Straits Settlements ports, and set out sanitary regulations for ships and mechanisms for the surveillance of infectious disease.[51] The ordinance was opposed by the Straits Settlements Association, representing merchants and developers, primarily due to its fear that the legislation would inhibit commerce. Lobbying of the governor to rescind the ordinance, however, was based on the argument that the 'Chinese, Hindoos and Mahomedans' of the colonies were 'tenacious as to the disposal of the bodies of their dead', that government intervention constituted an invasion of privacy, and that the control of ships would not prevent the spread of diseases such as cholera.[52] Arguments about the efficacy of quarantine continued locally and internationally, resulting in a tour in 1912 by the Chief Health Officer of the Straits Settlements to Java, Australia, South Africa, Siberia and Japan to study public health and quarantine conditions; his report advocated the establishment of a bureau in Singapore to collect and disseminate information regarding infectious disease in the ports and countries of the region.[53]

Smallpox

Documentation available for the nineteenth century provides limited information even about epidemics, but smallpox was most likely to result in commentary, given its dramatic spread and preventability.[54] For colonial Malaya, its relative impact on morbidity and mortality compared with other diseases is unclear. Both cholera and smallpox were significant in small settlement populations, and smallpox devastated closed communities: an epidemic on the island of Banka at the beginning of the nineteenth century, for example, was reported to have killed half of the population and led to the flight from the island of many able-bodied freemen and voluntary slaves.[55]

Vaccinations were provided from the early nineteenth century, with children being used for live (arm-to-arm) transmission. Problems with supply and quality of lymph led to a high proportion of vaccination failure, however, and outbreaks continued sporadically. The epidemic of 1824, according to the acting secretary to the Governor of Penang, 'extended its ravages among the population of this Island' leading to a 'considerable diminution' of the population.[56] Contemporary reports of smallpox suggest that infants and children were its major victims. Although numerically the number of direct deaths was small – 128 deaths, mostly of children, from smallpox in Province Wellesley in 1829, for instance, in a fixed population of 25,043[57] – there is some evidence that the prevention of smallpox had a far wider impact on infant and child mortality than the simple prevention of one disease; Aaby, extrapolating from measles vaccination data, argues that smallpox vaccination may have reduced all-cause mortality by some 10 to 15 percent.[58]

Vaccinations were not provided systematically until 1870, but thereafter coverage was increased with the employment of special purpose vaccinators. The first vaccinator in Singapore commenced work in the town area in May that year, a second worked in country areas of the island from July.[59] The first mass vaccinations included 2,876 children from all major ethnic groups, and successful vaccination was confirmed for 70 percent of inspected cases. Standard procedure in Singapore, and later elsewhere in the colonies, was for police to assemble children on a given day, and for vaccinations to continue until all children in the area had been covered. Parental objections to the procedure were ignored initially. However, with extension of vaccinations to the FMS, the issue was politicised, and the Residency Surgeon sought the public support of the Sultan and other members of the Malay royal houses. An example from Kuala Selangor illustrates some of the tensions as colonial officers tried to implement public health policy while avoiding offending local political authorities:

The Collector and Magistrate of Kuala Selangor was reprimanded by the Resident for summoning and punishing the men of Raja Mahmud of Kuala Selangor, taking an action that was regarded as 'somewhat injudicious and unnecessary'. In his defence, the Collector argued that the people of Pasangan were opposed to vaccination but had agreed to comply in the event of being so ordered by the Sultan. An order from the Sultan, and a notice by the Collector advising the time and place of the vaccination, was duly posted. However, Raja Mahmud counter-ordered that his children not be vaccinated, and they and the children of three of his men were taken to his house for protection. The men 'spoke rather impertinently', were fined, refused to pay, and so were gaoled for four days. On release they were told to bring the children forward for vaccination, again they refused on order from Raja Mahmud, again were fined, refused to pay, and so were gaoled for a further six days. No other children were brought forward for vaccination in consequence.[60]

In many areas people were reluctant to present their children, and occasional epidemics of smallpox continued well into the twentieth century in areas with low coverage.[61] Vaccination failures also occurred because parents covered rather than left exposed the innoculated wound, and applied local medicines resulting in 'large sloughing ulcers'.[62] Malay rulers also resisted hospital treatment of people with smallpox and in some cases infectious patients were taken home by relatives, although home care, while permitted in Malacca, was not regarded as generally viable. By around 1900 hospitals had largely overcome resistance to hospitalisation by allowing two or three relatives to stay with a patient and to provide food for them. This was not the only problem, however. Inadequate staff were available to vaccinate, and batches of lymph were often heat-affected after arrival when left on wharves or in godowns,[63] and insufficient supplies of lymph for vaccine inhibited state ability to control the spread of disease until relatively late. Consequently smallpox continued to be a problem; in 1927, for example, despite the increase in vaccinations that had occured during the preceding years, an epidemic in the FMS resulted in a total of 237 cases and 24 deaths, including 170 cases and 4 deaths in Selangor and 63 cases and 20 deaths in Negri Sembilan (Table 2.7).

Table 2.7   Smallpox vaccinations, Federated Malay States, 1924–1927.

State	1924	1925	1926	1927
Perak	54,278	86,125	88,539	106,865
Selangor	11,745	26,369	14,256	65,091
Negri Sembilan	6,563	8,268	5,392	64,639
Pahang	5,821	5,543	5,727	32,914
Total	78,407	126,305	113,914	269,509

Source: FMSAR, 1924–1927.

Cholera

An outbreak of cholera demanded immediate measures, which meant maximum control over the population. Because it was epidemic and the deaths spectacular and frightening, the disease had dramatic impact on both individuals and the landscape. An account of a cholera epidemic in Malacca in the late nineteenth century illustrates this. E. W. Birch, Magistrate and Collector of Land Revenue in Malacca from February 1888, recalls:

> We had a terrible cholera epidemic in Malacca. It was a worrying time in which Dr J. T. Leask worked indefatigably, often sleeping half-dressed ready to answer a night summons. Mr Copley of the Municipality and an Inspector of Police gave splendid assistance. Between the four of us, the entire Town was inspected every day – sulphur fires were kept burning at most street corners, all who were sick with the scourge were removed to a segregation hospital, three Police Constables who drove the hospital ghari died. Everyone begged for the corpses of their relatives to be handed to them for burial and the necessary refusal was very distasteful ... The leading towkays complained to the Resident Councillor ... that my fines for breaches of the regulations for the removal of cholera patients was too severe. They said, in my presence, that the hospital was not fit for a bullock ... [They were taken on an inspection of the hospital and] saw many patients, some in the last stage of collapse, some dead and not yet removed for burial.[64]

Outbreaks occurred sporadically, particularly at the end of dry seasons as the concentration of *Vibrio cholera* in local waterways increased in both urban and rural areas. A small outbreak among sampan men in Kuala Lumpur occurred in 1885, for example, due 'without doubt (to) the disturbing of the old drains of the town to make way for new brick ones. The mud from those drains emptied daily into the river, the water of which the sampan men use for drinking'.[65]

The case fatality rate of cholera was also high and hence the demand for medical assistance was heavy. The state hospital in Kelantan, for instance, was placed under considerable pressure in 1912 as a result of both smallpox and cholera epidemics, and despite claims of popular resistance to services, 8,194 of the 12,937 outpatients were said to be Malay.[66] In the sampan epidemic in Kuala Lumpur and in other outbreaks of cholera and unconfirmed 'pseudo-cholera' caused by polluted well or river water, public health and sanitation procedures were relatively straightforward: control at source by an application of quick lime and carbolic acid or permanganate of potassium, distributed free of charge to ensure wide coverage, health education notices in Malay and Chinese posted with instructions for treatment of severe diarrhoea and vomiting, and requests for all cases of diarrhoea to be reported. In Kuala

Lumpur, bottles of a 'Board of Health Cholera Mixture' and other remedies were provided to all police stations for free distribution. Use of disinfectants in wells and drains, and distribution of posters for health education, were standard, and from the early twentieth century, village headmen and Malay *bomoh* assisted authorities in disinfection and case notification.[67] Government officials could also quarantine individuals with dangerous infectious disease, and this measure was used at times to enforce segregation with outbreaks of cholera, smallpox, plague or occasionally dysentery.[68] Population movement was circumscribed particularly to prevent cholera from ships spreading to land, by preventing the disembarcation of cases or contacts from ships. However, this was often disregarded. The Singapore Colonial Secretary shared the view of ships' officers that quarantine was 'a fight in the dark',[69] and cancelled regulations that prevented boats with cholera cases on board from anchoring in local harbours, leading to outrage from some residents who claimed that this showed 'the most sublime and callous indifference to the well-being of (the) colony and an insulting contempt for (the) discretion of the local authorities'.[70]

Cholera was never as widespread here as it was elsewhere in the region, and the punitive actions (burning houses, segregating contacts in concentration camps, mass burials) that occurred in the Philippines, for example, in the 1880s or in 1902 in light of thousands of deaths, were not replicated in Malaya.[71] Still, outbreaks were common enough (in Singapore, eight severe outbreaks from 1895 to 1914), hence the concern with sanitation and prescriptions regarding the management of epidemics as reflected in Gimlette's memorandum, published in Kelantan in 1911.

Gimlette, at the time Resident Surgeon for Kelantan, provided advice specifically to Europeans on remote outstations.[72] He regarded as appropriate prophylaxis drinking highly acidic drinks such as 'sulphuric acid lemonade', avoiding eating river fish, not eating fruit and vegetables without other foods, drinking only a moderate amount of alcohol, and guarding against chills – a 'cholera belt', a cummerbund worn at night, was believed to prevent chilling and therefore to protect against cholera. In the event of severe diarrhoea or cholera, Gimlette recommended castor oil, laudanum or chlorodyne, brandy and bed rest, and upon recovery from persistent diarrhoea, the gradual introduction of invalid foods such as rice water, barley water, diluted condensed milk, and patent infant foods. Phenol, Jeyes' fluid or carbolic acid was used to disinfect areas possibly polluted by faeces or vomitus; excreta and dead bodies were buried in dry earth away from any water supply. A quarantine period of seven days was advocated.

Gimlette's provisions regarding disinfection, care of the sick and disposal of bodies applied to the Malay population and to wage labourers;

Table 2.8 Community-based cholera cases, Federated Malay States, 1902–1946[1]

Years	Cases	Deaths	Case fatality percentage	Cases/state
1902–7	133	97	73	Selangor 41 Pahang 39 Perak 53
1910–15	1,685	1,114	60	Selangor 237 Pahang 280 Perak 1,121 Negri Sembilan 1 Trengganu 46
1918–20	186	140	80	Selangor 1 Pahang 1 Perak 184
1924–27	132	85	64	Selangor 13 Perak 119
1945	287	216	75	Perlis 287 (June 1945)
1946	221	182	82	Kelantan and Trengganu 221
Total	**2,644**	**1,834**	**69 (mean)**	

1 Figures for Kedah and Johore not available.
Source: IMR, *Studies from the Institute of Medical Research*, p. 241.

instructions to *penghulu* and other Kelantan government officials were set out in a circular distributed to all headmen. Gimlette cautioned European officials against unnecessary burning of dwellings, argued that the population be discouraged from panicking and scattering with their sick, and suggested that, given Malay distrust of hospitals, a local isolated house be used for the segregation of infected persons. In general his recommendations emphasised the importance of maintaining local confidence and goodwill: allowing burials to proceed without interference, encouraging the local distribution of tea and the donation of *kualis* and other pots for water to be boiled in segregated houses, supporting local *bomoh* practices and massage, and so on.

Like smallpox, typhoid fever and plague, cholera tended to occur in small epidemics. These tended to leapfrog and were usually contained locally due to control of population movement: in 1926, for example, there was a small outbreak of 13 cases and six deaths in Selangor, but none elsewhere; in 1927 none in Selangor but three in Perak resulting in 114 cases and 74 deaths, the largest involving 57 cases and 40 deaths. The figures (Table 2.8) give some idea of the distribution of cholera by time and place of the disease; although they exclude some 1,175 cases held at Port Swettenham Quarantine Station, most occurring in the quinquennia 1916–1920 (530 cases, 340 'eaths) and 1923–1927 (619

Table 2.9   Typhoid fever, Federated Malay States, 1901–48

Year	Cases	Deaths	Years	Cases	Deaths
1901–03	39	23	1922–24	218	54
1904–06	196	59	1925–27	429	87
1907–09	174	62	1928–30	610	184
1910–12	108	35	1931–33	724	189
1913–15	201	72	1934–36	753	163
1916–18	168	58	1937–39	1,357	256
1919–21	103	35	1946–48[1]	2,379	513

1   Figures for 1946–8 are for the Federation of Malaya
Source: IMR, *Studies from the Institute of Medical Research*, p. 261.

cases, 238 deaths).[73] From the mid-1920s, largely as a consequence of water and sanitation control, there were few cases.

Other epidemic diseases were devastating although they affected a smaller population and were easier to contain. Plague was uncommon but feared because of its high case fatality, and cases were reported under provisions of the International Sanitary Convention.[74] For the entire period 1900–1950, there were only 765 cases of plague and 712 deaths in Singapore, 200 in the Malay States, and 7 in Penang, with the greatest number of cases occurring out of Singapore in Perak in 1915 (53 cases) and 1927 (33 cases, see Chapter 4).[75] Typhoid was also uncommon and geographically contained until the late 1930s; there were serious outbreaks in Penang, Perak, Negri Sembilan, Johore and Singapore in 1938, again during the Second World War in 1942, and in the immediate post-war years (see Table 2.9). Whilst the epidemics of the 1940s fit with a picture of the risks of typhoid coincident with a breakdown of services and surveillance during a period of great civil and political disruption, the 1930s epidemic, reputedly transmitted by an ice-cream seller,[76] occurred when hygiene and sanitation controls were well developed, when health inspections were routine, and civil circumstances good.

The influenza pandemic

As argued already, endemic diseases such as diarrhoeal diseases, respiratory infections and malaria were most important in terms of both morbidity and mortality through the nineteenth century, and continued to be so for the remainder of colonial rule. However, the influenza pandemic was a major one and worldwide, and it is useful to consider briefly its impact in British Malaya to continue the discussion of changes in morbidity and mortality in the twentieth century.

An account of the pandemic in the settlements and the FMS has yet to be provided that would allow good comparison with other countries where health status and infrastructure were comparable.[77] But in Malaya as elsewhere the pandemic was dramatic and its management therefore exacted a rather different response from the government than was provided for endemic diseases and, indeed, other epidemics. Influenza reached the Peninsula around September 1918; the toll was greatest the following month. Institutionalised populations were especially vulnerable: the Malay College of Kuala Kangsar was closed on 13 October after virtually all 135 boys were infected, and remained closed until 24 November; most vernacular schools also had closed by mid-October.[78] Under Section 3 of the Quarantine and Prevention of Diseases Enactments of 1903, restaurants, theatres, cinemas and public halls were closed for usual purposes, although entertainment centres were not closed since poor attendance at the height of the epidemic had already reduced the risk of transmission and infection. Toddy shops on some estates were closed also to prevent the congregation of people and reduce infection.[79] Special hospital wards were set aside and in some places temporary wards were built to accommodate increased admissions; closed cinemas were also used as hospitals.[80] Medicines were distributed to village headmen, school teachers and local police to provide palliation to those who were sick.[81] Public health leaflets were distributed from mid-1919 in Malay in both *rumi* (Roman) and *jawi* (Arabic) scripts, and in Chinese, Tamil and English, warning of the dangers of congregating in public places. Similar messages were printed in the local press.[82] People were advised to keep fit, avoid fatigue, chills and alcohol, to gargle and wash out the nostrils with a mix of warm water and salt, to go to bed at the first sign of infection, to minimise transmission by using paper rather than cloth handkerchiefs, and to avoid crowds for a week after recovery.[83]

Direct recorded deaths from influenza were relatively low, in the Straits Settlements accounting for 844 deaths in 1918 and 344 in 1919. But these figures, as government officers noted, bore little relation to the actual toll of the epidemic. The annual report of the Medical Department for the Straits Settlements claimed that in 1918, when excess deaths of pneumonia, bronchitis, phthisis and fever (not specified) were included, influenza had caused the death of some 3,500 people;[84] the registrar in Perak maintained that at least 10,000 deaths could be attributed to influenza, most occurring within a six-week period (October–November 1918), with the heaviest toll among 'natives of India'.[85] The pandemic resulted in some increase in mortality for the years 1918–1920, varying from state to state, although recovery to rates around the level of 1917 had occurred in all states except Johore by 1920 (see Tables 2.6 and 2.10).

Table 2.10   Death rates[1] 1911–1920, Federated Malay States, Kedah and Johore

Year	Federated Malay States Death rate	Kedah Death rate	Johore[2] Death rate
1911	39.11	17.50	—
1912	37.80	17.34	—
1913	34.00	19.45	—
1914	34.31	30.20	38.05
1915	28.92	19.50	35.24
1916	30.60	20.00	45.23
1917	34.17	23.32	63.39
1918	52.85	21.72	78.68
1919	29.37	38.49	54.36
1920	32.34	26.14	59.65

1 Deaths per 1,000 population.
2 The Johore death rates are calculated on the 1911 population and are
    therefore of no utility for comparison with the rates in the Straits
    Settlements, Federated Malay States and Kedah.
Source: Nathan, *The Census of British Malaya*, p. 18.

Births and infant deaths

Statisticians such as Vlieland gave far greater attention to the broad trends
in births, deaths and migration than to case-specific mortality, and
Vlieland in fact argued that the 1921 census had created a 'false picture of
British Malaya as a country in which the birth rate is so curiously low and
mortality so disgracefully high that the population is only saved from
gradual extinction by continual replenishment from outside'.[86] He
maintained that all statistics were unreliable, but also that no account had
been taken of male migration in an attempt to determine the population
growth rate, nor of the current population structure consequent upon
migration policy: 'the population is debited with the deaths of a large
excess of males who have no influence whatever on the number of
births ... It would in fact have been surprising if there had been an
appreciable excess of births over deaths between 1911 and 1921'.[87]

   Whilst the collection of vital statistics had become considerably more
sophisticated by the time of the 1921 census, even these figures and others
used to identify and monitor demographic trends were treated – at the
time of their production and later – with some scepticism. Nathan,
Vlieland and Del Tufo, respectively the authors of the 1921, 1931 and 1947
censuses, were all cautious of the preceding returns and their own,
inconclusive in relation to their ability to explain or interpret demographic changes, and often in conflict with each other in terms of their
interpretation. Nathan concluded that between 1911 and 1921, deaths
were largely in excess of births in all areas; that this was due to the high

mortality rate from all causes as well as to specific epidemics such as influenza in 1918; and that, 'were it not for the stream of immigrants from China and India and the Islands of the Malay Archipelago, there would have been a decrease in the population'.[88] Vlieland had, as noted, argued that this interpretation failed to take account of the artificial excess proportion of males. Assuming a colony-wide death rate of around 30.8, equal numbers of men and women (that is, for 1911 figures, debiting the number of excess males for computational purposes), and assuming a rather low infant mortality rate of 200,[89] Vlieland argued that the population of British Malaya would in fact have increased at around 2 percent per annum during the decade 1911–1921.[90] Hence, rather than immigration replacing a dwindling population, Vlieland suggests that the male bias of migration provided a check against rapid population growth.

Vlieland then turned to the birth rate, flawed by under-reporting both in Singapore and in outer areas. The Kelantan and Trengganu figures for the years 1927 to 1930 illustrated his point. Officially Kelantan had some 3500 births annually during the period 1927–9, but in 1930 over 6,000; in Trengganu, with half the population of Kelantan, there were some 4,500 births per annum in 1927–8, over 6,000 births in 1929, and slightly under 6,000 in 1930. Over the decade, Kelantan's population appeared to have increased by 53,000, without the substantial bolstering from migration enjoyed by the FMS, but Vlieland argued that this simply highlighted the unreliability of the baseline data: if one were to accept the population increase, 'we would be forced to conclude that the population was practically immune from death'.[91] His own estimate was that around 1911 in states and settlements such as Singapore, where government authority was tightest and population registration most accurate, births were under-registered by around 35 percent, in 1920 by 20 percent, and in 1931 still by 10 percent. Given this, he suggested that the birth rate for Singapore in 1930 was at least 39 per thousand but perhaps as high as 58.[92] Birth rates remained unreliable, and as late as 1936 government officials complained of parents' reluctance to register their newborns and of bureaucratic confusion over the identity of children:

> The birth notifications are obtained from the various police stations, but to find the child is another matter. As enquiries for the baby usually elicit the reply 'which one' or 'there are many over there a little distance'; further endeavours may result in walking 2 miles or more through mud, climbing over tree trunks, crossing rivers either by raft or by bamboo bridges and heading through padi fields, and at the end to find no new-born baby because the names of the parents mean so little – there are many Ahmeds and Fatimahs.[93]

Infant mortality rates were, according to Vlieland, less suspect, although he was critical of their use as an index of 'deadliness',[94] since

Table 2.11   Infant mortality rates,[1] Straits Settlements, by ethnicity and
settlement, select years, 1904–1934

	1904	1909	1914	1919	1924	1929	1934
Settlement							
Singapore	316	309	256	236	203	188	165
Penang	282	231	228	177	158	150	165
Province Wellesly	144	181	170	137	143	112	147
Dindings	165	178	221	168	139	174	244
Malacca	256	230	364	260	252	247	203
Labuan	—	—	270	128	218	223	311
Ethnicity							
Europeans	—	58	57	43	15	29	25
Eurasians	—	309	164	167	170	134	123
Chinese	—	291	237	246	184	166	154
Malay	—	248	271	204	217	228	235
Indian	—	273	256	241	—	154	145
Japanese	—	—	—	—	47	99	—
Other/not known	—	134	225	21	119	482	66
Mortality rate (mean)	**252**	**264**	**250**	**212**	**195**	**182**	**172**
Stillbirths, percentage of births	4.82	4.35	4.30	4.76	4.82	4.35	3.81
Crude birth rate	25.50	26.70	29.09	30.29	32.29	37.20	40.65
Crude death rate (adult and infant)	39.00	37.60	34.13	33.04	27.42	26.10	26.54
Total no. of deaths	10,937	23,925	25,906	27,957	26,358	29,544	28,051
Percentage deaths in hospital	24.6	15.7	18.2	20.6	19.5	17.0	23.2
Percentage certified by medical practitioner	—	9.1	9.8	12.7	14.0	20.2	11.8

1   Deaths per 1,000 live births.
Source: SSAR, select years.

under-registration of births, although probably offset by the under-
registration of neonatal deaths, may have inflated the rate. The major
contributing cause of infant death was neonatal tetanus, although most
infant deaths not seen by a medical practitioner were reported to police
as due to *sawan* (convulsions).[95] The data indicate extraordinary
variation by ethnicity and colony, and the decline was neither regular
nor rapid (see Table 2.6 above). In 1914, for example, the rate in the
Straits Settlements ranged from 56.7 for Europeans to 270 for Malays,
and varied by state: 364.32 in Malacca and 169.98 in Province Wellesley.
By 1922, the range was 25 (European) to 202.75 (Malay), but while
Province Wellesley again had one of the lowest rates (154.64),
Singapore's was one of the highest (233.98).[96] For the quinquennium
1921–5, the rate had dropped 226.[97] But over ten years later, after two

decades of energetic and extensive infant welfare work, in the FMS, the IMR was 139 for 1931, and had dropped by one-third for the period 1927-1931 due to the extension of maternal and child health programs.[98] There were again discrepancies by ethnicity and by place, the latter a reasonable indication both of the availability of services and of the predominant ethnicity.[99]

The infant mortality rate remained high among most groups in the UFMS, suggesting that access to care was an important factor, although the reasons for variations among groups were complex. In Kedah in 1928, for example, the rate was 111.95 for Malays, 136.72 for Chinese and 262.96 for Tamils; in Perlis in 1930, it was 110.66 for Malays, 153.33 for Chinese, and an extraordinary 381 for Indians.[100] In Trengganu in 1934, it was 221.33 for all groups, an increase of around 30 percent over the previous year.[101] In the UFMS the proportion of supervised pregnancies and births was low – 5 percent of all births were in hospitals in Perlis in 1928–9, for instance – although even in 1937 in Singapore, only around 30 percent of women were delivering in hospitals and government officials were fairly cynical of the efficacy of the training of local midwives to supplement hospital services.[102] Ethnic variation in the rates, moreover, could not be well explained by reference to service provision. In any case, the lack of consistency of the downward trend led to the postulation of a variety of possible factors which contributed to the IMR other than the presence or absence of midwifery services, including 'native disposition', prevalence of malaria, housing, nutrition and the employment of women:

> Racial differences seem to be of little importance in determining the infant mortality rate. Different races in the same place have fairly similar infant mortality rates, and the problem here is to explain the variations in different places, for the same race ... The places where the population is spread out in kampungs in the rice fields have the lowest rate. Infantile beri-beri is certainly a factor, and it may be more important than crowded housing. In most of the places where the rate is high, the two exist together ... [but also] there is some relation between the need for labour and the rate, so that it is possible that the rate of employment of women to a more than usual extent leads to a higher rate, and conversely where the women are not employed but are not destitute the mortality is less.[103]

Despite its understatement of ethnic variability, the above quote suggests that access to care of any kind may have been more important than its quality (that is, village *bidan* versus hospital services), and the association between low infant death rates and place of dwelling (*kampung* versus 'crowded housing', that is to say, urban cubicles or plantation labour lines) suggest in the end a distinction that reverts back to race/ethnicity, with ethnicity also standing for a mix of social, economic and other circumstances.

Table 2.12   Stillbirths and maternal mortality rates,[1]
Straits Settlements, 1928–1937

Year	Stillbirths	Maternal mortality
1928	45.5	10.7
1929	43.5	10.2
1930	39.4	10.1
1931	37.2	9.9
1932	35.5	9.8
1933	33.1	8.6
1934	38.1	8.3
1935	35.5	6.7
1936	35.5	8.0
1937	32.6	6.7

1 Stillbirths and maternal deaths per 1,000 live births.
Sources: SSAR, 1928–1937, pp. 1080–1081.

Data on maternal mortality rates and stillbirths create a confusing impression too, for if we accept the role of maternal and child health programs in reducing the infant mortality rate, the same general trend might be expected to be reflected in the maternal mortality rate and stillbirths. This was the case in the Straits Settlements where some series data are available (Table 2.12). However, whilst Province Wellesley and the Dindings in 1931 had the lowest infant mortality rates in the Straits Settlements,[104] the proportion of stillbirths to live births in these two settlements was by far the highest – 6.55 and 10.33 respectively, compared with a mean of 3.72.[105] These rates compare with that for 1905 of 4.57,[106] but antenatal care and the reduction of infectious diseases that might have contributed to poor foetal outcome, both of which occurred during the intervening period, should have reduced this rate further. The pre-existing health of mothers was also a determinant, and malaria, nutritional and other anaemias, and syphilis were all implicated. The maternal mortality rate was also high and discrepant, although sufficiently small to have little impact on the general demographic trend. Mortality rates were particularly high among very young Malay and Indian women. Among Indians in the FMS in 1936, for example, whilst the sex ratio of the population was two men to one woman, this was reversed in the mortality rate – that is, two women died to every one man: 'The only explanation of this would appear to be a low standard of nutrition, early marriage, and lack of proper attention during pregnancy and childbirth'.[107] This high maternal death rate contributed to women's higher general mortality rate, and there is some evidence to suggest that throughout the period and in all states women's health and nutritional status was poor and their access to health care limited. Only five percent of all hospital admissions in Kelantan in 1916 were women, for example,[108] although this is not reflected in any significant skewing by sex of uncertified deaths. District level data from Perlis provide corroborating evidence of women's disadvantage, and it was claimed that mortality from fever was higher for women than men because of poor access to medical services and greater reluctance on their part to present for treatment.[109]

Adult deaths and diagnostic puzzles

The decline in the crude (adult) death rate was also uneven, despite clear improvements over time due to the relative efficiency of public health measures.[110] The immigration of young adult labourers, presumed healthy at the time of their recruitment, would have depressed the death rate, although the extent to which this occurred is difficult to establish.

Deaths were often registered by unqualified persons and proximate cause was often merely an educated guess. Even in the settlements where medical services, infrastructure and communications were best developed, still in 1929 less than 37 percent of deaths occurred under the care of a registered doctor and so were certified, and a further 23 percent only were examined postmortem by a doctor or coroner for certification. The remainder were registered by local police officers and accordingly were even more inaccurate;[111] in Trengganu in 1935, for example, only around one percent of death certificates were signed by a qualified medical practitioner and most deaths were certified by deputy registrars with little or no medical knowledge.[112]

In addition, nosology was not consistent. Consider, for example, deaths in Singapore in 1907 (Table 2.13); although this is an early year, the categories used were largely maintained thereafter.

Each of these categories ('Infective Diseases', 'Diseases of the Nervous System') includes various symptom complexes and discrete pathologies that derived from the then contemporary understandings of the etiology and pathology of various illnesses. The infective diseases, for example, included beri-beri, cholera, diphtheria, dysentery, enteric fever, erysipelas (acute streptococcal infection with rash), leprosy, malaria, measles, phagadaena (an ulcer spreading from a necrotic or gangrenous area), plague, pneumonia, pyraemia (blood poisoning with fever), pyrexia (fever), rheumatic fever, septicaemia, smallpox, syphilis, tetanus, and tuberculosis; general diseases not included in other classifications included anaemia, diabetes, unclassified fevers, other general diseases including 'age' and debility, and certain morbid conditions 'incident to various parts' (that is, non-malignant and malignant growths and cysts). Diseases of the nervous system covered both physical and mental ill-

Table 2.13 Deaths in Singapore, 1907

Disease classification	Number
Infective diseases	7,386
Diseases of the nervous system	719
Diseases of the circulatory system	293
Diseases of the respiratory system	2,434
Diseases of the digestive system	759
Diseases of the lymphatic system	66
Diseases of the urinary system	136
Diseases of the generative system	61
Diseases of the organs of locomotion	25
Diseases of the connective tissue	53
Diseases of the skin	88
Injuries	154
Poisons	8
Parasites	19
Natural causes	74
Unknown	66
Total	**12,341**

Source: SSAR 1907, p. 401, Table L.

nesses of various etiologies and included infantile convulsions, meningitis, myelitis, abscesses of the brain, haemorrhage of the brain, sclerosis of the brain, puerperal convulsions, mania, dementia, and so on. Diseases of the generative system included extravasation of urine, gangrene of the penis, sloughing of the scrotum, inflammation of the uterus, post-partum haemorrhage, shock after delivery, and 'other'. There were clearly problems with these classifications: non-infectious diseases, and changes in health status unrelated to disease such as 'aging', were included under 'infective diseases'; distinctions were made without clear indication of the clinical (or pathological) basis for doing so (for example, the distinction betwen pyraemia and septicaemia); diseases might be classified in more than one category (pneumonia, for example, was included as an infective disease, but bronchitis and broncho-pneumonia were listed separately as diseases of the respiratory system; tuberculosis was an infective disease, but phthisis – pulmonary tuberculosis – was included as a disease of the respiratory system); and so on. An alternative tabulation of these statistics, which links together many of these diseases, gives a rather different picture of probable causes of death in Singapore in 1907, suggesting that around 23 percent of deaths were from malaria and other fevers, 12 percent from respiratory infections including pneumonia, and 17 percent from tuberculosis.

Morbidity statistics were even less reliable since only a small proportion of sick people sought care from colonial medical services. Clinical diagnosis was often inaccurate and laboratory confirmation not always possible or reliable; illnesses were frequently treated by dressers with basic skills only who were not able to differentiate between symptoms or to recognise specific symptom complexes. Returns from rubber estates were especially suspect,[113] and contemporary evidence, such as that given by G. W. Scott to the Commission of Inquiry into the Health on Estates (1924), suggests that there was some pressure on dressers to suppress information as well as making inaccurate diagnostic guesses:

> I never trust the dressers entirely. What I mean is this. A dresser, once he finds out what type of infection pleases his doctor, will provide that type, and he must be continually watched on that account. For instance, if I tell him in a rather sharp manner that there has been a great deal of malaria the previous week, the likelihood is that the next time I go he will tell me there has been no malaria. The dresser is liable to conceal sickness for the sake of pleasing the master. It does not constitute altogether a scandal; it is due to the subordinate's desire to please.[114]

Lack of a clear picture of the prevalence of particular diseases made the development of intervention strategies difficult. Lack of data on malaria, for example, resulted in a proposal to the Malaria Advisory Board in 1921 that medical practitioners be paid one dollar for each case of clinical malaria notified and referred for serological confirmation.[115] In 1936, the board again drew attention to the problems associated with epidemiological surveillance – 'No statistics are available of patients treated in their homes nor of the many thousands of *kampung* sufferers for whom little treatment is available'[116] – and figures of community morbidity gave poor indication of the true prevalence of parasitic infection.[117] Further, as discussed earlier, hospital returns are imperfect indicators of health status. Hospitals were unevenly distributed in the Federation, serving especially urban populations, and admission policies differed from hospital to hospital according to availability of bed space and staff. In addition, leading and selected causes of death masked other diseases, and the criteria for the selection of a particular disease is not always clear.

Causes of death, 1900–1938

The task now is to describe briefly, notwithstanding gaps in the data, what we know of cause of death for the period. Table 2.14 sets out cause of death in the Straits Settlements for select years 1904 to 1934; Table 2.15 provides details for the years 1928 to 1937 for the most important of these. Malaria was always the premier disease, although it reduced in importance over the decades as a result of environmental management,

Table 2.14   Cause of death, Straits Settlements, select years, 1904 to 1934
(percentage distribution)

Cause	1904	1909	1914	1919	1924	1929	1934
Convulsions	10.3	12.9	14.8	15.3	14.5	15.9	14.7
Bronchitis	2.6	3.2	2.5	2.3	1.6	1.7	2.9
Malaria	30.4	10.8	13.6	17.3	13.3	15.7	2.8
Other fever*		20.0	16.5	8.0	10.5	6.4	16.4
Dysentery	2.3	5.2	4.2	4.3	3.2	2.3	1.6
Diarrhoea/	4.4	2.2	2.2	1.3	2.1	4.7	5.2
enteritis		+1.4	.5	2.8			
Plague	.1	.0	1.0	.1	.1	.0	—
Cholera	.0	.3	.1	1.1	.0	—	—
Smallpox	.1	.1	5.7	.6	.0	.0	—
Beri-beri	9.8	6.3	1.3	5.1	3.5	3.2	3.3
Heart	.8	.9	10.7	1.0	1.4	1.7	2.5
Tuberculosis	10.9	11.1	.5	11.1	9.1	9.2	8.2
Head	.2	.2	.7	.6	1.2	—	—
Injury	1.1	.6	5.6	.6	—	1.1	—
Debility and							
old age	10.0	5.0	—	6.3	8.0	7.6	10.4
Syphilis	—	—	—	—	.2	.7	1.0
Childbirth	—	.9	.9	.9	2.7	1.4	—
Pneumonia	—	3.8	—	5.1	—	8.5	7.8
Other/not known	16.6	15.2	20.5	16.2	31.5	19.9	12.8
Total deaths	**23,233**	**23,925**	**25,906**	**27,953**	**26,358**	**29,544**	**28,051**

* Includes typhus, blackwater fever, remitted fever, and fever not specifically
classified

Source: SSAR, select years.

chemoprophylaxis and chemotherapy (see Chapters 3 and 5). Tuberculosis was also a major cause of death, particularly in urban Singapore
and Penang, and it barely decreased during the colonial period, reflecting difficulties in improving urban conditions (see Chapter 4). Convulsions were also a major cause, but this was not a disease-specific category,
and among adults may have been due either to cerebral malaria or
cerebral tuberculosis. Other acute respiratory infections (pneumonia,
broncho-pneumonia, and bronchitis) were not registered as major
causes of death in the early 1900s. By 1928 the number of deaths from
tuberculosis and pneumonia were more or less comparable, and from
1934 the acute respiratory infections predominated (see Table 2.15).
Scharff, in 1937 Registrar of Births and Deaths of the Straits Settlements,
regarded this as an indication both of increased incidence and more
accurate diagnosis; he noted also that neither tuberculosis nor
pneumonia had appeared to 'yield' to methods of control and that there

Table 2.15 Deaths and death rates for malaria, beri-beri, tuberculosis and pneumonia, Straits Settlements, 1928–1937

Year	Malaria (Fever unspecified)	Rate per 1,000 Mal. (F. unspec.)	Beri-beri	Rate per 1,000	Pulmonary tuberculosis	Rate per 1,000	Pneumonia	Rate per 1,000
1928	5,798 (1,636)	5.29 (1.49)	1,146	1.05	2,727	2.49	2,679	2.45
1929	4,648 (1,768)	4.11 (1.56)	944	0.83	2,710	2.39	2,502	2.21
1930	5,018 (2,013)	4.29 (1.72)	1,047	0.90	2,795	2.39	2,343	2.00
1931	3,506 (1,513)	3.15 (1.36)	911	0.82	2,461	2.21	2,373	2.13
1932	2,601 (2,051)	2.27 (1.79)	725	0.63	2,081	1.81	1,860	1.62
1933	1,747 (2,821)	1.68 (2.72)	723	0.70	2,027	1.95	1,976	1.90
1934	814 (4,506)	0.77 (4.26)	912	0.86	2,120	2.01	2,181	2.06
1935	1,698 (3,787)	1.52 (3.39)	916	0.82	2,077	1.86	2,541	2.27
1936	1,315 (3,562)	1.13 (3.05)	1,080	0.92	2,181	1.87	2,624	2.25
1937	1,185 (3,319)	0.95 (2.66)	853	0.69	2,268	1.82	2,712	2.18

Source: SSAR 1937, p. 1084.

was likely to be little change 'under existing social and economic circumstances'.[118] Beri-beri was high in the first decade, and thereafter declined in response to state interventions to control the availability of polished rice. Gastrointestinal diseases remained relatively constant. It should be restated, too, that major epidemics were rare, and that deaths were due increasingly to 'other' non-communicable diseases. Data for the FMS are poor by comparison, and even more fragmentary for the UFMS. In general, however, the trends follow those of the Straits Settlements, but with the incidence of tuberculosis lower due to lower urbanisation and crowding.

The expansion of medical services

The mortality rate declined in Malaya during the interwar period (1919–1939) with the rapid expansion of clinical and preventive health services. Official accounts for this period provide extraordinary detail of public health activities: quinine tablets distributed, vaccinations against smallpox given, campaigns for the administration of salvarsan injections for yaws, and stools collected, worms counted, populations dosed, shoes distributed and toilets built to reduce ankylostomiasis (hookworm). People from all communities were encouraged to use outpatient departments, travelling dispensaries (by road and river) were increased in number to improve the provision of acute care in remote areas, and so on. The bureaucratic accounting that flowed from these campaigns was an end in itself, the increased delivery of services a measurable outcome of government efforts to improve people's health.[119]

The government was lucky, perhaps, that there were a number of highly prevalent diseases that responded well to contemporary treatments and for which the strategies for prevention and cure were simple to administer and relatively acceptable to the population: hence the efficacy of innoculation against smallpox and the successful mass treatment for yaws, in contrast to the frustration and equivocal success of malaria control strategies. Even here, however, efforts were increased; travelling dispensaries went to schools and supplied teachers with quinine tablets to treat children presumptively, estates were visited by health officers and estate hospitals inspected. There was some resistance to these invasions. Joe Allgrove, a planter in Malaya from 1920 to 1953, recalls that liquid quinine was often administered: 'It is horrible and the horror lasts some time. Many labourers would try to miss their dose by hiding in the "rubber", it being still dark at 5.30. Many having had their dose, would squat in the roadside drain and retch violently.'[120]

In all areas, the quantitative measures of public health interventions and the provision of health services were impressive. In the FMS in 1929,

Table 2.16 Health and medical services, Straits Settlement and Federated Malay States, 1936

	Population	Beds	Dispensaries Outdoor	Dispensaries Travelling	Dispensaries River	Infant Welfare Centres Centres	Infant Welfare Centres Sub-centres	Infant Mortality Rate (per 1000 births)
Straits Settlements								
Singapore	603,163	1,753	5	1	—	5	6	169
Penang	205,994	680	3	1	—	6	2	152
Province Wellesley	148,406	400	3	1	—	6	1	150
Malacca	202,828	500	2	2	—	10	—	189
Total	**1,160,391**	**3,333**	**13**	**5**	**—**	**27**	**9**	**mean 168***
Federated Malay States								
Perak	830,093	2,312	12	8	2	3	—	142
Selangor	575,775	1,475	12	4	—	9	—	137
Negri Sembilan	249,853	966	4	5	—	1	—	144
Pahang	192,230	1,980	8	4	1	3	—	153
Total	**1,847,951**	**6,733**	**36**	**21**	**3**	**16**	**—**	**142**
Grand Total	**3,008,342**	**10,066**	**49**	**26**	**3**	**43**	**9**	**mean 162**

* Includes Dindings and Labuan

Source: SSAR 1936, p. 909; FMSAR 1936.

for example, 150,239 women and children attended the five infant welfare clinics then operating, and 116,019 home visits were made, 31,468 by trained European nurses. This focused work was supplemented by that undertaken by four European hospitals, 34 district hospitals with outdoor dispensaries, three women's hospitals, two leper asylums, five gaol hospitals, one mental hospital, one Pasteur Institute which primarily functioned to provide rabies vaccine, four vagrant wards, 30 dispensaries not attached to hospitals and five VD Clinics. In total 117,639 inpatients were treated, of whom 9,764 died; a further 878,158 people received outpatient care from hospitals, clinics, travelling dispensaries or the dispensary boats that operated on the Perak and Pahang Rivers.[121] For any year and for any of the states or settlements, this kind of list could be made, with steady progression over time (see Table 2.16). This is not related to overall improvement in living conditions, health or the subjective experience of illness, however, as the following chapters illustrate.

CHAPTER 3

Biology, medical ideas and the social context of illness

Doctors and other colonial administrators perceived their best efforts to reduce mortality in controlling infectious disease, but at the same time they saw the role of the state in extending clinical services throughout the colony. A growing number of practitioners were attracted to Malaya, and these included medical practitioners, dentists, vaccinators, midwives, dispensers, nurses and dressers: a total in 1911 of 2,312 people, 52 percent of whom were doctors and the vast majority male.[1] Most worked out of government hospitals and outpatient clinics, primarily in large towns; the extension of medical services to smaller populations through clinics and home visiting occurred particularly in the 1920s and 1930s. Small hospitals were also built for special purposes. In Perak, a number of district hospitals were built in the early 1880s in response to mounting death rates from beri-beri. Government hospitals provided the institutional focus of clinical medicine, but these were supplemented by private hospitals established in towns and on mines and estates. The Yeng Wah hospital, for example, supported by a tax on adult Chinese men of one dollar per annum, was established in Taiping around 1882 for sick miners who previously had been 'turned into the jungle or filthy outhouses to die without any care, shelter or attendance'; it was hoped that hospitalisation might have a 'civilising effect' on coolies through contact with Europeans.[2]

Medical services were also provided privately by European, Indian and Japanese doctors with partial or complete medical training,[3] and by government outdoor dispensaries, that is clinics staffed by either dressers or medical doctors. These latter included the travelling dispensaries which operated both on roads and waterways, introduced first in Perak in 1896 to address the distance between worksites and hospital facilities that occurred as development activities expanded, and to save labourers 'the trouble' of going to hospital. Travelling dispensaries were relatively cost-efficient compared with hospitals,[4] although services were often 'rough and ready',[5] discouraging attendance by those they were meant to serve. Minimal medical services were also provided by apothecaries to those too remote to present at a hospital when sick. From the 1870s too a number of police stations held supplies of medicines; their role in providing basic medical advice and free medicines was regarded as an important means 'to increase the power and influence' of the state.[6] Medicines held by police stations included Epsom salts, calomel, powder of rhubarb, tincture of rhubarb, cream of tartar, sulphate of quinine, laudanum, bicarbonate of soda, chalk powder, lotions for the head and eyes, cholera mixture, ammonia, Friars' balsam, dilute sulphuric acid, liver pills, opium pills, chlorodyne, dysentery pills, cough mixtures and a variety of other embrocations, creams, ointments, pills, powders, syrups, inhalants, antipyretics, antiseptics, sedatives and tonics known by such simple descriptors as blue powder, blue pills, grey powder, stomach mixture, and so on.[7] The drugs were popular, according to police and district officer reports; posts usually received supplies in bulk and ran out, due to local demand, well before new stock had been delivered.[8]

Use of services rarely matched the expectations of providers, however, and commentators sought to explain continuing high death rates in terms of native reluctance to take advantage of biomedical services. High hospital case fatality rates in both the settlements and FMS were accordingly attributed to delays in presentation, refusal to be admitted, absconsions, or a combination, though there is little consistency in official accounts of the use or non-use of Western medical services. Many medical officers insisted that Malays, Chinese and Indians were equally reluctant to take advantage of clinical services whether provided in major urban centres such as Penang, Kuala Lumpur and Ipoh, or in small towns and on estates. People were frightened of hospitals, which were often crudely constructed and were smelly, isolating, unfriendly and sickly places; given the high case fatality rates it was not surprising that the hospitals were perceived as places in which to die rather than recover; crowding allowed rapid spread of infectious disease within the hospitals, despite isolation procedures; nosocomial infections were not uncommon;[9] and hospital dressers and medical officers could be rude and racist. Figures from Pahang make this point neatly. There were 1,153 admissions to private hospitals in 1900, 70.6 percent of whom had beri-beri, with a reported case fatality rate of 79.9 percent. Case fatality for diarrhoea was 84.6 percent, for dysentery 90 percent, for malaria 68.5 percent. In the Chinese hospital at Bentong, overall mortality of hospital admissions was 74.7 percent, and the estimated population mortality rate of adult males was 222 per thousand.[10] Given this, it was hardly

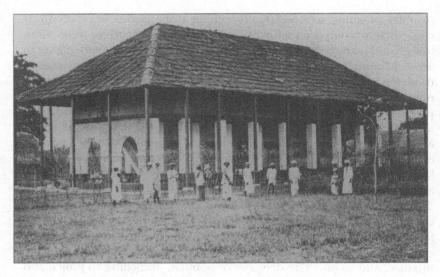

Figure 3.1 General Hospital, Butterworth, Province Wellesley. Printed with permission of Arkib Negara Malaysia, Kuala Lumpur. N 114/78, Album 1, p. 249.

surprising that hospitals were regarded as 'death houses', to be avoided if at all possible.

. Contemporary reports, whilst relatively agnostic about or disinterested in the provision of care, were occasionally revealing about the basic facilities, including of those provided for Europeans which were supposedly far better than those for 'native' patients.[11] The first hospitals were often converted from buildings of other purposes. The hospital in Larut in 1875, for instance, was housed in an old residence and part of the court house, and lacked light, ventilation and adequate drainage.[12] Even European wards in the nineteenth century were often poorly maintained; Frederic Brine, for instance, reported that at the General Hospital 'the Chinese servants throw all the slops and clean all the utensils in the lavatories' and bathtubs were used for a variety of purposes of which bathing the sick was but one.[13] From the turn of the century, government hospitals were arguably better built and maintained, although for decades it was claimed that many were 'ill-equipped and grossly inadequate' and that conditions for 'natives' were 'austere and primitive'.[14] On estates and at mines, hospitals were often simply sheds with stretchers for sick coolies, without trained dressers or doctors in attendance (see Chapter 5 below).

Issues of quality of care rarely emerged in relation to poor use of medical services, however, and reports focused instead on the apparent intransigence of Malays and immigrants in seeking early treatment. Chinese patients, it was claimed, were brought to hospitals in a 'moribund' state so that they 'may not die at home and bring bad luck upon the home',[15] hence hospital case fatality rates were unduly inflated: 'Many of these patients are picked up at the roadside in a dying state by the [ambulance] cartmen and though it is doubtless better that they should die in the Hospital rather than in the public roads, the Hospital death rate must suffer unfairly thereby'.[16] It was also argued that Chinese 'of the poorer classes ... still look askance at Government Hospitals and western methods and medicine', and preferred to patronise Chinese medical hospitals,[17] although there was also some suggestion that parsimony guided their actions: 'The Chinaman, as a rule comes into hospital as a last resource, after he has been ill for a long time and probably spent all his money. He eventually finds his way to the pauper hospital unless he has friends who will pay his hospital fees'.[18] Malays were also said to be reluctant to present for care:

> It is very difficult to get them to come into hospital. This is not on account of any difficulty with regard to their food or religious custom. The Pathan, who is a much stricter Mohamedan [than Malays], readily comes into hospital when he is sick. People of other nationalities in the FMS are immigrants and have left their families at home. The Malay is eminently a family man and objects to come into hospital unless he can bring his wife and children with him.[19]

Resistance to hospital and other medical services was considered especially characteristic of Malays in the UFMS where health services were few and rudimentary. The high infant mortality rate in particular was blamed on women who retained their faith in 'native treatment' and refused to seek medical attention for sick infants.[20] Official commentary on such resistance tended to be rather truculent, as the following comment on the response of the population to the yaws campaign in Kelantan suggests:

> It has been usual, during the last few years, to comment on the popularity of treatment for this disease but it is strange that it is not even greater. The fact that young children are allowed to remain untreated in villages near dispensaries, even now that the success of the treatment is universally known, can only be ascribed to laziness on the part of the parents or total disregard to the disfigurement which will be brought about by letting the disease run its course. It is disappointing that in spite of all the trouble taken by the Government to carry treatment to these people, young children are still seen with large patches of ulceration on their mouths and noses which will lead to disfiguring scars which could have been prevented by the injection of Salvarsan, and it is irritating to be met with an entirely disinterested attitude in the parents when their attention is drawn to this fact.[21]

However, these views were by no means consistent, internally or between commentators. Evans, author of the above quote, also wrote contrarily of the number of Malays seeking surgical treatment for severe yaws and willing to submit to amputations if necessary;[22] and others referred to the extent to which 'kampung Malays' were attracted to biomedical services, primarily as a consequence of the successful campaign against smallpox and the later one against yaws.[23]

In general, reports from the settlements and the FMS drew on stereotyped notions of native belief and practice to explain suspicion of Western medical services, and people's use of, resistance to and non-compliance with medical services. This worked either way. That is, people either failed to use medical services for essentialist, racially characteristic reasons, or they took full advantage of the services for more or less the same reasons. The *1937 Report of the Medical Departments*, for instance, represents Tamils as compliant subjects of the planters, without agency or self-interest, whilst

> [m]ost Malays are still rather sceptical about the benefits of Western medicine, but they are not opposed to it. They have been convinced by the experience of vaccination, and the dramatic effect of arsenical preparations on yaws has made them keen to have injections. They come willingly to the travelling dispensaries for the treatment of malaria, worms and skin diseases, but they still have a distrust of surgery, and they do not like hospitals ... The Chinese gladly accept Western medicine, without giving up their belief in their own medicaments, which are often taken at the same time. They come to hospitals willingly, but usually they wait until their illness is far advanced. As long as they are able to work they carry on, they do not object to surgical interference, and usually they are ideal patients, too fatalistic perhaps, but long enduring, cheerful, and grateful in an undemonstrative way.[24]

But demand for treatments and increasing patronage of Western hospitals and outpatient clinics suggests that this was an exaggeration. As noted already, from the 1870s and thereafter, there is contradictory evidence of the demand by *kampung* Malays for medicines supplied to outstation officers, customs officers and police, and of 'advice and medicine frequently sought in the case of illness by the different Penghulus of districts'.[25] In general, it would appear that people took advantage of treatment provided by outdoor dispensaries, outstation officers and at police stations,[26] and some had sufficient faith in the skills of Western doctors that they went to considerable length to receive medical attention:

> One old Malay man from Sungei Bulu walked from there a distance upwards of 30 miles to the dispensary at Kwala Lumpur seeking advice for an overgrowth of conjunctiva [which] interfered with his vision. This man

informed me that he had seen ninety six bulan puasa or rhamadan that is to say that he was in his ninety seven year (sic). I mention this incidence as it shows the longevity of some Malays.[27]

Other reports also challenged the assumption that Malays were reluctant to use medical services. The Perak Medical Report of 1899, for instance, maintained that poor use of hospital facilities by Malays was primarily a consequence of distance, together with preference to be nursed by kin.[28] In 1912 in Kelantan, 63 percent of the 12,932 outpatients were Malay and 'on many occasions it was necessary to refuse admissions to Malays for want of room in the wards'.[29] This was also the case among the Chinese. J. L. Welch, the District Surgeon in Kuala Lumpur in 1889, maintained that '[s]o far from finding that the Coolies were adverse to availing themselves of the advantages afforded them by the State Hospitals, I found them as a rule most anxious to do so'.[30]

Miasma, race and disposition

In the colonies, the structure, management and delivery of medical services and disease control were motivated by imperial goals. In turn, however, the content of these programs was informed by contemporary and changing understandings of various diseases, and of the susceptibility of different populations to infections. Notions of race and gender filtered colonial understandings of the etiology and epidemiology of disease and risk factors of infection. European commentators – administrators of the colonies and scientists – distinguished between expatriate and 'native' (indigenous and immigrant Asian) communities, and between men and women, adults and children, and explained differences in morbidity and mortality in this light.

Prior to major breakthroughs in microbiology in the last quarter of the nineteenth century, understandings of the cause and distribution of disease derived from belief in the relationship between climate, geography and health, specifically, that air and soil could be contaminated by miasmas, poisonous vapours from putrefying organic matter and stagnant water. Such beliefs were reinforced by the experiences of everyday life, as Carlo Cipolla describes; the offensive smells of the pre-industrial age – excrement and decomposing corpses, domesticated animals and rotting slaughtered carcases – provided people with plenty of reason to believe in the correlation between foul smells, disease and death.[31] The towns of nineteenth-century Europe as well as Asia were foetid. In Britain, until the widespread use of water closets, people either defecated in lanes or fields, or used chamber pots and threw urine and faeces out of the window or front door of their dwellings. Water supplies were badly contaminated by seeping sewage, and food was frequently highly contaminated or rotten at time of eating. Industrialisation and urbanisation, occurring rapidly and resulting in chronic overcrowding, compounded health problems.[32]

Original understandings of health and illness in the colony were influenced by ideas of 'miasma', that is, that disease was transmitted through telluric and atmospheric vapours (hence the term malaria – bad air). The dominant view from the sixteenth century was that the tropical climate was restorative and sustained good health, but by the early nineteenth century this had yielded to the obverse view.[33] Little, writing in 1848, held that 'wherever there is much moisture there is a corresponding increase of diseases' and that the combination of heat and moisture led to 'a universal relaxation of body and mind, especially of body, which creates a preternatural susceptibility of external impressions' causing catarrh, diarrhoeal diseases, gonorrhoea and leukorrhea, among other things.[34] Mid to late nineteenth-century accounts gave credibility to the immunity and resistance of 'native races' and 'native troops', although Colonel Woolley, in 1870, argued that native (Indian) troops 'deteriorated' in the second year of service and that colonial interests would be best served if all troops were European.[35] Others conceded too that 'though hot and damp, the climate of the Straits has not the bad effect upon the European constitution that might be anticipated', that a consumptive patient might, unless severely ill, benefit from residence in the colony, and that in general a year in a cold climate after a period of service was sufficient to restore health and fit a person for a further period of service.[36] Climate, however, was seen to have major effect in facilitating the spread of disease: the increased incidence of beri-beri in Negri Sembilan in 1899 was attributed to the 'excessive wet', although also to the fact that new Chinese coolies had arrived, who, 'being non-acclimatized', would have contracted beri-beri in an endemic area.[37]

By the end of the century, miasmic theory had largely been displaced by biomedical understandings of disease causation and therapy, and practising doctors and epidemiologists argued that most infectious diseases were 'dependent on removable conditions and habits', that fevers were 'not *essentially* dependent on any of the factors that go to make up climate', and that the only real climatic were sunstroke and frostbite.[38] Developments in microbiology and parasitology gave Western medicine the edge over other medical systems and therapies both as a result of direct interventions (that is, vaccination and chemotherapy) and public health interventions (quarantine/isolation hospitals, clean water, pure food, slum clearance).[39]

Even so, contemporary medical scientists maintained that temperature and humidity played a preconditional role in disease transmission by providing an environment to sustain particular vectors and microbes. The publication of Manson's *Tropical Diseases* in 1898 provided the first coherent and extensive presentation of 'tropical medicine', whereby pathogenesis and climate were represented as dependent, or, at least, that heat and moisture provided an optimal environment for certain diseases to survive, even if – as was the case for both malaria and leprosy – they had a prior history in a colder climate and could alternatively be explained as diseases of poverty rather than place.[40] Late-nineteenth-century doctors and research scientists maintained too that climate affected metabolic rate and therefore health, and did not therefore dismiss entirely the links between climate and disease.[41] Many continued to argue not only that the tropical climate was debilitating, but also that different races adapted with greater or lesser alacrity to the constancy of heat and humidity; as late as 1929, staff at the King Edward VI College of Medicine in Singapore were conducting research on the effects of muscular work in the tropics, in order to acquire information 'for the maintenance of efficiency in the tropics'.[42] Woolcock suggests that climate remained an organising feature of germ theory as it had previously been for miasmatic beliefs, both because of the effect of environment on pathology – the conditions under which microbes and parasites might survive and reproduce, for example – and also in terms of medical practice and the role of climate in cures.[43] From this, the Malayan colonies, like India, gained their hill stations. Such faith in the value of altitude as well as cool weather was in certain instances reinforced by the absence of lowland endemic diseases, as tended to be true for malaria.[44]

Those who were believed to be most vulnerable, however, varied over time. In 1870, as noted above, Colonel Woolley argued for the replacement of 'native' with European troops, since European troops were better able to withstand the pressure of the environment on their health.[45] A number of articles appeared in the *British Medical Journal* and *The Lancet*, and in the local press, from 1860 to around 1900 on climate and its importance for imperial expansion, social progress and medicine, which sought to establish the correlation between climate, cause and treatment of various diseases. In this context, Australia for a while was heralded as offering the ideal climate for the prevention and cure of tuberculosis.[46] Yet others held that a tropical climate was detrimental to health and the depleted energy of Europeans, though not of those born in the area. Thus Dr M. F. Simon claimed of the Malayan colonies in 1890 that 'Europeans cannot do so much physical work out here as they do at home and yet keep in the same health. Europeans get run down and they cannot get better food here unless stimulants are used; the bread and meat procured here are not so good, whereas the coolie can get better'.[47]

White men in the tropics

Arguments that a tropical climate was physically, mentally and morally debilitating, particularly for women and children but also for European men who stayed 'too long', gained momentum and elaboration over time, providing the rationalisation for the establishment of the hill stations that characterised British colonial settlements.[48] Participants of a Medical Congress held in Malaya in 1898, for example, argued that no officer over the age of 50 'could be reported as entirely fit and well', and it was recommended that the retirement age be lowered, that the period of employment before long service leave be reduced, and that short vacations be allowed on an annual basis.[49] The author of the 1899 Negri Sembilan Medical Report similarly argued that deterioration of health in the colonies was the result of climate, high temperature, and lack of seasonal variation: 'Under the physical strain which this involves, the most vigorous system soon grows languid, and "run down"; and morale and mental efficiency pursue no less rapid a descent towards decay'.[50] Accordingly, he argued that '[n]o officer of European constitution [could] stand the brunt of 30 years' service in the tropics', that recruitment and conditions of employment needed to be adapted to ensure 'yearly draughts' of cadets from England 'caught young and early', and that 'access to the hills' be provided to enable locally the 'marvellous, almost magical, change which we perceive in decayed and dilapidated colleagues after a spell of long leave in England'.[51] Pamphleteers and government officials argued for a maximum posting of four to five years, emphasising both decreased resistance to disease and poor mental health, insomnia, depression, irritability, alcohol abuse, loss of memory and energy, and increased infections: 'a few years residence makes him (the European) realize that continual summer is enervating and bad for the nervous system and that to remain in good tone it is necessary for the body to be stimulated by cold. The tissues become lethargic and muscles and brain refuse to act with the vigour natural in a temperate climate'.[52] An article in the *Malayan Medical Journal* in 1926, picked up by the local press, made similar recommendations,[53] and the articles published in 1933 by Kenneth Black, Professor of Surgery at the King Edward VII College of Medicine in Singapore, maintained that 'the white man, when transplanted to the tropics is all day long receiving noxious stimuli', resulting in irritability, memory loss, loss of concentration, loss of self-control, alcohol abuse, mental breakdown, insanity and suicide.[54]

Hygienic rules of tropical life, 'individual and moral as much as medical',[55] paralleled the developments of a scientific medicine which emphasised biology and pathogen rather than personal behaviour as the major risk of infection. But preventive measures reflected a combination of folk and medical approaches to disease. Pamphlets directed to potential immigrants emphasised self-restraint: they were to live moderately, take plenty of rest, dress sensibly, and bathe cautiously. Europeans posted abroad and others planning to migrate were advised against going to the colonies until they were adults (20 years of age), and then to adhere to certain behavioural rules in order to survive. Advice in the mid-1930s to Europeans intending to go to the tropics was for people to be vaccinated for smallpox, typhoid and paratyphoid, to wear (pith) helmets and dark glasses, cotton clothing, and mosquito boots to avoid ankle bites; to eat cooked vegetables and keep alcohol consumption to a minimum; to sleep under nets, to take moderate exercise to keep fit, and to wear a 'cholera belt' or dry towel outside the pyjamas at night to avoid catching cold.[56]

Until well into the twentieth century, therefore, physical, mental and moral degeneration was regarded as an inevitable consequence of prolonged residence in tropical colonies. Only a few (missionaries, for example) were exempt[57] and women and children were especially vulnerable. Women, because of 'their more highly strung nervous systems', needed to return to a cold climate after three rather than four or five years; children, whilst not at all affected in infancy and early childhood, from around six would become 'thin and anaemic' and so should be returned to a cold climate to avoid physical and mental arrest. Conveniently, the impairment of child development by exposure to a tropical environment coincided with the usual age at commencement of schooling, and so the child might be sent from the care of an *amah* in Singapore to boarding school in England.

These ideas on the effect of climate were used by colonial administrators and others to explain differences in the health of Asians and Europeans, and it is important to understand that notions of race, vulnerability, immunity, infection and culture powerfully influenced ideas about health risks, appropriate medical care, social and cultural factors associated with poor health status and illness, and the provision of health and medical services. Others have documented a shift in ideas through the nineteenth and twentieth century, from ideas of the immutability of genotype, whereby inherited immunity gave 'natives' the advantage in the tropics, to ideas of acquired immunity and the role of the native as 'carrier', the latter view positioning colonial subjects as a far greater threat to the colonists, since now the health and well-being of the latter was directly threatened by invisible pathogens. These shifts in ideas can be traced in public health thinking in colonial Malaya as in the Philippines,[58] but they were neither universal nor immediate. Other older ideas of immunity and climatic preadaptation existed concurrently with notions of germ theory, and with public health practice that constructed non-European cultures as a risk and that was designed to clean up people's habits and their surrounds.

Native resiliences and weakness

Notions of the colonial subject as the carrier of disease were compounded by evolutionary ideas that ranked peoples and societies in terms of technological development, material culture and intellect. These were premissed on a belief that European civilisation (and in this case, nineteenth-century England) was superior to others. Representations of race varied depending on individual experience and prejudice, but were invoked to explain health status, risk of infection, progression of illness, health-seeking behaviour, and response to medical services. Tamils, Malays and Chinese, then, were represented as stupid, lazy, dirty, ignorant and obdurate against the advantages of biomedical clinical services, public health interventions and public health education messages. According to variants of this argument, either because of the enervating effects of heat and humidity at any time, or because genetic adaptation had resulted in people being 'by nature' lazy, climate contributed to indolence.[59] Further, belief in native vulnerability to infection, as evidenced by higher morbidity and mortality levels, was consistent with the contemporary ideas of social evolution influenced by the writings of Spencer and Darwin,[60] or rather the popularisation of their ideas in terms of 'fitness' and 'natural selection'.

These ideas in turn were influenced by other essentialist representations of race, fed by imperial reports, travellers' tales, early anthropology and other stories of a mythic, fantastic, fetishised 'orient'.[61] Edward Said has argued that creation of the Orient in discourse and scholarly endeavour was produced and sustained by imperialism; and that the 'idea of the Orient' shaped concrete political, economic and social relations between colonising states and their territories. Certainly it influenced everyday relations between colonists and colonial subjects, and colonist interpretations of corporeal experience. The writings that emerged at the time conventionally portrayed the people of colonised territories as morally as well as physically degenerate:[62] this, recall, was the risk that white men faced too if they stayed in the tropics too long.

The high morbidity and mortality rates suffered by indigenous and immigrant labouring communities, in contrast, were rarely simply attributed to climate.[63] Rather, as already suggested, Europeans understood the incidence and spread of disease amongst the peasantry and labourers as the consequence of various co-factors, including genetic predisposition, 'cultural' factors (the particular personal – hygienic and food – habits and customs of various groups), and socio-economic and political circumstance.

Genetic difference was only one of these factors, and notions of genetics, inheritance and race were broad and unsubtle. Sinclair,

Residency Surgeon and Medical Officer in 1890, for instance, claimed that 'dark-skinned coolies [were] as a lot very much stronger and healthier, and not so liable to get fever as the light-skinned ones'.[64] Mr J. E. Romenij, who was in charge of the recruitment and placing of coolies for Mansfield and Company, maintained that, in contrast with other Chinese such as 'Hai-lok-hons and Te-chius ... [g]enerally speaking the Khehs are miserable specimens' and 'a miserable tribe', and that their quality had 'fallen off' in recent times;[65] Chin Fui Lan, a depot keeper and broker of Chinese coolies, maintained too that Kheh coolies were especially 'weak and bad ... the dregs of the market', and that if miners did not buy them, no-one else would.[66] Cretch, some 40 years later, contrasted the Chinese, who he said 'have an extraordinary resistance to disease and their life history bears evidence of racial robustness, a healthy active life and a normal life span', with Tamils, guilty of 'wholesale in-breeding' due to village endogamy, 'physically degenerate', with poor resistance to disease, limited intelligence and powers of endurance, and a low expectation of life compared with other groups. However, he also referred to the 'inherent laziness and filthy habits' of Chinese miners whose dwellings, if not supervised, would soon become 'most insanitary and repulsive'.[67]

A number of early reports argued that the poor health of immigrant labourers, both Indian and Chinese, derived from poor selection procedures, hence any 'racial difference' might be associated with pre-existing poor health, although such a view still begged the question of genetic predisposition or circumstantial cause of poor health. An 1855 article claimed that 'diseased paupers and criminals' were intentionally recruited by 'Mandarins' to get rid of them.[68] Turn-of-the-century reports also indicated that the poor and sick were most likely to be recruited, and a report on Indian immigration to the Colonial Office in 1900 led to the conclusion that many men brought to the Malay States to work on the railways had been inappropriately recruited:

> In many instances large batches arrived from India who ought never to have been sent, their emaciated condition was highly suggestive of their being famine stricken before they emigrated; others were old decrepit men who should never have been allowed through the depot in India. Can it therefore be a matter of surprise that numbers of these coolies succumbed to bowel complaints, when they were put to work in somewhat unhygienic surroundings, such as rail head, irrigation works and new estates must be?[69]

The more common view held by colonial medical officials in the late nineteenth century was that Indians from non-agricultural castes were recruited, people who were unused to manual labour, whose poor physique at point of recruitment was compounded with lack of familiarity with the work required, who accordingly 'lose heart and strength, deteriorate into "hospital birds", and swell the death rate' after migration.[70] Others, including both planters and non-medical colonial officers, interpreted labourers' ill-health as a combination of 'fretting' because of unfamiliarity with the work and discontent at the level of pay.[71] Along these lines, William Duncan of the Caledonia Estate, in giving evidence to the 1910 inquiry into conditions of indentured labourers, argued that Javanese indentured labourers were 'the best' in the FMS because 'their health is very much better. The Javanese comes from a climate similar to that of the FMS, is more able bodied, and has worked under conditions more alike'.[72]

These views yielded to those more likely to associate illness with 'intelligence' and cultural factors. A *Straits Times* editorial in 1920, for example, held that Tamil labourers should be treated 'very firmly' for 'many of the coolies are little more than children', and that 'health preservation is of the utmost importance. Not much fuss is made when a coolie dies of fever, but the news of his death goes all over the district he came from ...'.[73] Tamil dietary inadequacies associated with food preferences, and their reported reluctance to spend money on food, was mentioned often. Cretch, for instance, claimed that Tamils spent only 50 percent of what Chinese spent on food, and were consequently poorly nourished; Orde-Browne, on the basis of his inquiry in the colonies in 1939, also maintained that the nutritional deficiences of Tamil labourers were due to their inclination to 'economise at the expense of [their] stomach[s]', while the Chinese were better fed, healthier, and capable of sustained hard work (see also Chapter 5).[74]

Other factors compounded the effect of limited expenditure on foodstuffs. It was consistently maintained that dietary changes concomitant with urbanisation and the import of manufactured and refined foods had led to a decline in the nutritional status of all non-European groups.[75] Alcohol consumption was also reputedly a problem among Tamil labourers and other Indians which influenced resources (for food purchases) and health status in general, but it was also regarded as a growing problem among Chinese workers: an increase in alcoholism was used as an argument against restrictions on opium use by Chinese labourers and artisans.[76] There was also concern, by some, that rates of pay, conditions of housing and sanitation correlated with poor health.

The relative ranking of factors associated with high mortality varied according to the context of the commentary. The association of both the inferior physique of Tamil labourers, and their reluctance to spend money on mosquito nets and food,[77] suggested the predetermination of illness whilst locating the blame on the workers themselves. The low rate of malaria in Malacca was attributed to the fact that labour was chiefly

Chinese and supplemented by Malay workers.[78] In this case there may have been an empirical basis to the observations, since Malay workers may have had acquired immunity to malaria and Chinese were reportedly more willing than others to use bed nets to avoid bites. However, this was an area also where environmental control measures were extensive. The use of broad racial categories rather than a more subtle exploration of possible causal factors of low morbidity perpetuated stereotypes that many others held about different peoples in the region. I return to these points in subsequent chapters, particularly when I focus on estate labourers (Chapter 5). In the section which follows, I address in general terms conditions of employment and living, social change and declining health status.

Conditions of employment

Conditions of employment in the settlements and states were variable. People worked in the burgeoning towns as day labourers, pedlars, and gardeners; in the country as tin, iron and gold miners, as labourers on sugar plantations and as rubber tappers, and as railway labourers under government employ. All were vulnerable to malaria, dysentery and diarrhoea. The incidence of dysentery tended to be especially high among railway workers, although estate labourers and miners were also vulnerable as a result of poor water supply, provision of ground-level huts for housing, and bad drainage. Around the turn of the century dysentery and diarrhoea combined were the major cause of death in the Malay States.[79] The worst mortality was among indentured labourers, although this varied between estates as it did between administrative areas (87.60 per thousand in 1902 in FMS, 84.64 in 1903, for example)[80] and prognosis following an episode depended both on the availability of medical care and employer practice with respect to the sick. Labourers working on the railways were sent to hospital or put to work in a town area until they were better enough to go back to the railway head; others were able to spend the period of acute illness resting in a sick shed or in the lines. Cretch reported that whilst estates provided a 'medical man' and a hospital for coolies, labourers on mines were 'left more or less to their own resources and for the most part the conditions under which they live are deplorable'.[81] Other plantation and railway workers were turned out or drifted from employment when sick. Late nineteenth-century practice had been to arrest beggars and others apparently homeless and unemployed, and to place them in the vagrant wards of district hospitals, but demands on hospital services led to the closure of these wards, resulting in turn to increased vagrancy and homelessness.[82] By the turn of the century there were numbers of Tamil vagrants staying in tenement houses or sheltering in temples in Kuala Lumpur, often sick with

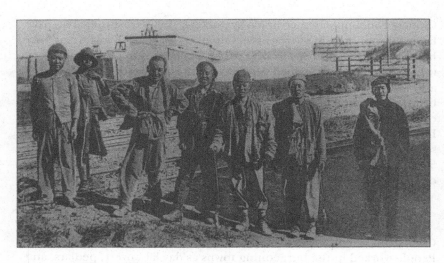

Figure 3.2 Chinese railway coolies. Printed with permission of National Archives, Singapore. Photograph No. 29448.

malaria.[83] Indigence was increasingly frequent with the end of indenture – the system was abolished for Indians in 1910 and for Chinese in 1914 – and as a result of depressions in the early 1920s and 1930s (see later).

Conditions of employment and living were poor for all workers, although here I discuss briefly the conditions of Chinese miners. In the late nineteenth century coolies working on contracts in mines were supplied with opium as well as food and other supplies, were expected to work eight hours per day and were punished for breaches in work; *towkays* who did not enforce this were also subject to fines or imprisonment.[84] Contract conditions varied. In Pahang, miners received $30 in the 1880s, of which $14 was withheld to cover food and clothing; if indebted at the end of the contract period the coolie was retained for $5 per month plus food until the debt was repaid. In Perak and Selangor mining coolies were paid $22 biannually, with free food and clothing; if indebted at the end of the period of indenture they were retained at the wage rates of free labourers. Indebtedness was common. The 1890 inquiry recommended the establishment of a procedure for routine government inspection of Chinese coolies employed in the settlements and states; the abolition of licensed depots and brokers and the substitution of this with a government depot and government recruitment; and granting full sanction for immigration from the Chinese government to avoid forced migration and kidnapping.

Miners were recruited – and many allegedly kidnapped – in Swatow or Hong Kong, brought to Singapore and examined by a government medical officer there, then placed in a coolie depot until taken by a mining company. In 1900 there were 7,462 indentured Chinese labourers working in mines; by 1909 this had dropped to around 864 and the method of recruitment was unpopular; European employers preferred free labourers because they said they were physically healthier. The total number of indentured labourers in 1910 in the FMS was 3,700, compared with 17,687 free labourers, of whom fifteen percent were women. Wages were around 5 cents per day. Since the system pertained whereby provisions were purchased for the labourers and deducted from their pay at the end of the period of indenture, indebtedness was common. In most cases surveillance of residential areas was sufficiently lax to enable mistreated miners to abscond from mines, but this often put them at subsequent risk (in face of capture and return). Information put forward at a trial in 1909, and evidence to a second commission of inquiry conducted in 1910, suggested that at least in some areas miners continued to live in 'mere hovels' and to work under conditions of 'disguised slavery' where they were ill-treated and ill-fed:[85] 'A Chinese miner is permitted to treat his coolies just as he likes, he puts him into a kongsi built on the edge of a swamp, with no provision for water, the jungle growing almost up to the hut; the kongsi is usually overcrowded and a quantity of rice and salt fish is supplied'.[86] Although the 1907 Report of the Chinese Secretariat maintained the contradictory view that mining kongsis were 'very satisfactory from a sanitary point of view'[87] and Cretch agreed that they were 'airy, cool and comfortable but often overcrowded with poor drainage and sanitation,'[88] more commonly housing was described as situated at the edge of or close to the excavation, dirty and crowded, with defective ventilation and damp floors. Spitting resulted in high prevalence of tuberculosis within the mines. Latrines were described as primitive and unsatisfactory, surrounding grounds grubby and flies pervasive, due, Sinclair claimed, to prejudice, superstition, and 'an inherent spirit to evade the laws especially of sanitation'.[89] Malay mines, in contrast, were reported to be cleaner and smaller.

Occupational health was also an issue. Workplace injuries were not always reported, and unless they resulted in death, rarely appeared in health statistics. The evidence points to regular accidents, however. The death of Chin Kee, a 'weakly man who smoked opium', is a case in point. On 24 November 1899 Chin Kee, with four other men, was bailing water out of a mining shaft around 12–13 fathoms deep, and fell in after he lost his balance when he found a bucket of water too heavy. He was recovered from the shaft, but had a head wound and was taken to Sungei Besi Hospital, where he died soon after admission.[90] Earth falls were also common and led to a number of deaths. An extract from one of the monthly reports of the Mines Department in 1915, for example, noted:

On the 21st March a fall of earth occurred in the open mine on Mining Lease 2600 Ampang which killed three coolies. On the 28th March a fall of earth in the Sungei Besi Company's mine caused slight injuries to a coolie. On the 29th March a fall of earth in the Sungei Besi Company's mine caused injuries to two coolies. On the 29th March a shafting coolie was killed by a basket of earth which fell off the hook and hit him on Mining Lease 2613 Kuala Lumpur.[91]

In Selangor, some provisions were provided for miners permanently disabled, many blinded, others with paralysis or amputations due to workplace accidents and injuries. Hospital care of acute cases, most frequently diarrhoeal disease, was provided by the Tah Wah Fund, set up under legislation in 1902, supported by contributions from miners and government, and administered by a committee that included the State Surgeon, the Protector of Chinese, district surgeons and members of the Chinese community – over 100 at any time.[92] In general, however, provisions were poor and their availability uneven.

The high mortality rates among indentured labourers led in 1910 to an inquiry into conditions in the FMS which, unlike earlier enquiries, was limited to Chinese and Javanese labourers working on estates and in mines.[93] Despite these inquiries and the apparent improved surveillance by the Chinese Secretariat, deaths from accident and violence were common, and both injuries and disease frequent. Malaria contributed to continued high morbidity and mortality at mines especially in relatively isolated areas. As an example, Table 3.1 on morbidity and mortality at mines in Trengganu in 1934 indicates nearly 55 percent morbidity from malaria at the Freda and Bundi Mines, Kemaman; at Kajang mine the percentage rate was even higher, suggesting prevalence rates similar to those on rubber estates around 1910. Estates were obliged, under the Estate Labourers' (Protection of Health) Enactment, and subsequently the Labour Code, to provide for employees' health, but provisions for mines were more general: accommodation was supposed to fulfil 'reasonable sanitary requirements', and management was required to send sick labourers to the nearest government hospital.[94] On-site hospital facilities at the mines were not required, however, regardless of distance from a government hospital. In the UFMS there were even fewer requirements: the Trengganu Labour Enactment 8, for instance, was only introduced in 1934 (AH 1353) and stipulated simply that employers provide medical attendance for employees and cover any costs of hospitalisation or treatment.[95] As late as 1937, the Kajang Tin Mine in Trengganu, which employed around 120 to 150 miners, had only one dresser who closed the dispensary whilst on a month's leave in Singapore; there were no other keys for anyone else to inspect or use the medical supplies, and no provisions for alternative attendance.[96]

Table 3.1 Morbidity and mortality on mines in Trengganu, 1934

Mine	Average total monthly pop.	Deaths	Injuries	Malaria cases
Nippon Mining Co, Dungun	1,504	12	3	31
Ishihara Sangyokoshi, Kemaman	306	5	—	134
Freda and Bundi Mines, Kemaman	693	11	—	375
Sungei Ayam Mine, Kemaman	157	—	—	88
Kajang Mine, Kemaman	117	1	—	157

Source: BATr 481/1935, *Annual Medical and Sanitary Report for the Year 1934*, p. 11.

In other respects too the health on mines was poor. The *Straits Times* in one article assessed conditions as being 'hideously dangerous, [the] miners were like dumb-driven slaves'.[97] Physical isolation affected not only access to medical care and general health, and nutrition, but also had a wider social and health impact: the British Adviser of Trengganu estimated that 20 percent of all opium in Trengganu was consumed at one tin mine upriver from Dungun, and saw no way of reducing this dependency until communications systems were improved and miners had activities other than opium smoking for relaxation and amusement.[98]

Housing and sanitation

Housing and sanitation were common themes in government discussions of the health of Malay, Chinese and Indian communities. As described above, government commentaries maintained that particular races were 'by nature' insanitary and unhygienic, or that Asian standards of health and hygiene were different from (and inferior to) those of Europeans, or that Asians were ignorant of hygiene and sanitation measures. Less frequently it was argued that the material circumstances of the labourers were such that little better was possible.

Housing and sanitation on rubber estates was under the surveillance of the Labour and Medical Departments. In general conditions were poor.[99] Dr Fox, Acting State Surgeon of Perak, commenting in 1906 on the death rate among the Tamil population, the high prevalence of malaria, dysentery, alcoholism among men, and puerperal fever (sepsis) among women, suggested that money spent on a good water supply and proper medical provisions would be money well spent, and noted that:

> The primitive points of hygiene have not been observed [sic]. Lines have been built on or near swamps, wells have been dug in places where the refuse from the cooly lines and washings from storm water have been able to pollute

the supply, no latrine accommodation has been provided, everything has
been left to happy chance, with disastrous results always to the coolies and
frequently to the European in charge.[100]

Both estates and mines should have been supervised on a regular basis
by medical officers, but there were inadequate staff for this to occur with
sufficient frequency 'to be of any practical value', and medical officers
were said to have their time 'fully occupied'.[101] In rural areas, extreme
overcrowding was absent, but reports even so were critical of conditions
in tin mines, rubber estates, and from the late 1800s, rural Malay
kampungs as well as in towns. As noted above, Chinese *kongsi* houses were
rudimentary and sanitary conditions were poor, and *kampung* houses
were also described as inadequate in terms of ventilation, sanitation and
crowding.[102] Houses in Langat district, for instance, were reported as
'dilapidated', and many were untenanted and required demolition
rather than renovation.[103] The poor condition of *kampung* houses, as well
as the inadequate provision of potable water, sanitation and refuse
disposal, remained a constant theme,[104] as reflected by the District
Officer's description of a house in Jeram, occupied by three families and
fifteen people: 'The filth of the place was indescribable and the children
were suffering from sores the result of the unsanitary surroundings. In
another house close by there were also three families ... The surroundings of Datoh Sluman's house were most disgusting and the stench
absolutely overpowering'.[105] However, Cretch's description suggests that
the objections were aesthetic as much as hygienic:

> [Malay housing] is cool, comparatively clean but dark, badly ventilated and
> often overcrowded ... The floor of the house is raised some five or six feet
> above the ground and the space below is usually devoted to all sorts of
> accumulated rubbish. The small livestock inhabit this shady retreat and the
> poultry are confined there at night. To add variety to the nastiness, kitchen
> refuse is thrown from above and there is a hole cut in the floor of the dark
> verandah to serve as a latrine for children and sick elders. The Malay
> homestead certainly does not conform to English ideas of sanitation but
> tropical rains and a powerful sun seem to exercise a disinfection.[106]

Access to health services in rural areas varied too. Where economic
development activities (plantations and mines) were concentrated, basic
clinical services were provided with reasonable regularity by road- and
river-travelling dispensaries, and these were supplemented by district
hospitals in larger towns and, on the larger estates, by estate-run
hospitals. But the least developed states, predominantly the UFMS, had
few trained medical staff and few health posts, and the populations not
in regular contact with colonial enterprises were largely bypassed except
during epidemics. Travelling dispensaries provided some firstline

treatment, but were infrequent – in Kelantan until around 1930 most *kampungs* would have been fortunate to have had one visit per month from a travelling dresser.[107] Conditions in villages in all states resulted in sporadic outbreaks of infectious disease – an outbreak of suspected cholera in Pasir Tumboh and Limbat Districts of Kelantan in 1918 was one case that led the state's Senior Dresser, L. I. Devosa, to remark that 'an infective agent which sets up a simple diarrhoea in a healthy person may induce a much graver disturbance in one whose nutrition is faulty or who is living under imperfect sanitary conditions', where housing, surrounds, and water are all dirty.[108]

Public health work was introduced in a cavalier fashion. Where the Sanitary Board was able to operate effectively, village sanitation and 'conservancy' was conducted. This included house-to-house inspections; arrangements for 'village scavenging' (rubbish removal and general environmental management), removal and disposal of night soil, control of piggeries in Chinese villages and cattlesheds and dairies in Indian villages, in towns surveys of hygiene and sanitation provisions of markets, surveys of building plans and sites, and the control of water supplies; and sanitary inspection of police stations, schools, rubber estates and factories. Such measures worked best where the population was dense and the sanitation staff and infrastructure well in place (hence Singapore especially), and despite the terminology 'village conservancy', sanitary inspections rarely extended beyond small towns. In the UFMS, sanitary measures were only enforced when diseases such as dysentery occurred, when they became both necessary and expected, and major developments were largely delayed until the 1950s.[109]

Malaria

Malaria affected all populations and typically accounted for around 30 percent of hospital cases in any year from 1900 to 1940. I discuss the incidence of and state responses to malaria here, although a more detailed discussion in relation to the health of plantation labourers is provided in Chapter 5.[110]

Malaria has been characterised very much as a rural disease, in colonial contexts occurring in association with rural development. To an extent this was true for Malaya. However, *Anopheles* mosquitoes, vectors of malaria, bred in the urban and peri-urban environments also, as environmental changes due to the rapid growth of towns created ideal conditions for breeding, and the population density of town areas ensured that a human reservoir of infection was maintained, facilitating transmission. The first efforts to control malaria took place in towns; the first comprehensive strategies to control mosquitoes were also urban-based. From there the state extended its work to the countryside.

Ronald Ross's study in 1896–7, incriminating the mosquito as the vector, led to his early calls for environmental measures to reduce the risk of transmission, and he was extremely bitter at the reluctance shown by government to take up his recommendations.[111] Malcolm Watson, however, introduced environmental controls in 1901 in Klang and Port Swettenham, the old capital and port towns servicing Kuala Lumpur, and the success of these measures is hailed as the first successful anti-malarial work in the British empire, providing corroboration of Ross' claim of the effectiveness of vector control to reduce disease.[112]

In 1901, of a total population of 3,500 in Klang and Port Swettenham, 582 died; of these 368 were regarded as dying from malaria, the remainder dying from a range of other proximate ailments – diarrhoea, abscesses, and convulsions – but all were parasitaemic and had had a prior attack of malaria. In the first twenty days of November alone, the *Straits Times* reported, 52 coolies had died, and while the State Surgeon claimed this was a gross exaggeration, it was clear that there was a serious problem of transmission and that this had political import.[113] The General Manager of the FMS Railways complained that 'no sooner has a man learnt the duties of his special post than he falls sick and another (if available) has to take his place and start afresh'.[114] Chinese business houses closed their shops for three days for religious ceremonies and processions through the streets; the High Commissioner reprimanded the government of Selangor as irresponsible in allowing development of the port area to proceed before measures had been taken to drain the area, and ordered the closure of the port.[115] Drainage and filling of swampy ground commenced in February 1901, with some 37 miles of drainage put down; in a year cases and deaths from malaria and all causes had dropped dramatically (Table 3.2). Diarrhoeal diseases, for example, declined too, since to an extent anti-malarial measures addressed also issues of hygiene and sanitation.[116]

Measures used in Klang and Port Swettenham were extended elsewhere in the colonies, with the emphasis placed on environmental

Table 3.2   Fever and other deaths in Klang and
Port Swettenham, 1900–1905

Year	Fever	Other	Total
1900	259	215	474
1901	368	214	582
1902	59	85	144
1903	46	69	115
1904	48	74	122
1905	45	68	113

Source: Watson, *Some Pages from the History of the
Prevention of Malaria,* p. 4.

management and involving the Medical and Public Works Departments, the Engineering Branch of the Railways, the Sanitary Boards, from 1911 the Malaria Advisory Boards, from 1921 the Mosquito Destruction Boards, and the Public Health Education Committee of the FMS. Preventive strategies varied according to the habitat and breeding behaviour of the *Anophelene*. In Port Dickson, where the first extensive control measures were instituted, waterways with evidence of *Anophelene* breeding were oiled once every eight days, with oil spread over exposed water surfaces to inhibit breeding after the *mandor* (foreman) of an oiling team collected a sample of larvae for identification. Benzine was sprayed on the surface – work that was 'arduous and unpleasant'.[117] On days when no oiling took place, ditches were cleared and new ditches, drains and sub-drains were dug sufficiently deeply to accommodate heavy rain without causing overspill or erosion, or both, with the intention of draining swamp land and preventing subsequent surface water problems. In addition, community work was undertaken among villagers to encourage the maintenance of ditches and to fill or oil old wells harbouring *A. maculatus*. Selective use of larvivorous fish was appreciated as early as 1899,[118] and in the 1920s, a larvivorous fish (*Haplochilus panchax*, known in Malay as *ikan mata timah*) was used for areas of water (for example, a mosque pool) where oiling would have been unacceptable.[119] These measures were effective for the control of mosquitoes in conventional waterways and swamps, but were unable to take account of the creation of breeding sites as a result of the penetration of the hinterland, the construction of roads and railways, and the establishment and continued work on plantations, farms and at mines. Hence while some *Anophelene* bred in streams, either in semi-shade or in full sun, larvae might develop 'in the smallest holes, such as those formed by the hoof of a bullock, ruts cut in a road by wheels, and upwards through all sizes of puddles, swamps, ponds, mine holes, old surface wells, and even in an artificial lake'.[120]

Beyond the environmental measures of oiling, draining, ditching, and filling, preventive measures included routine and special surveys for adult mosquitoes and larvae; the distribution of quinine tablets to dispensaries, schools, police stations and *penghulus*; and direct notification of fever cases to the Mosquito Destruction Committees of the Sanitary Boards, excepting on large estates where notification was made on a monthly basis by the estate managers. Depending on the state and resources, estate labourers and school children were also periodically examined by medical officers for signs of anaemia and enlarged spleen.[121]

Malaria control was complicated because of the number of vectors and differences in vectorial habitat and behaviour. This affected urban as well as rural transmission and morbidity. Malaria was not as extensive in towns, and the epidemic peaks were not as dramatic, but even so the toll was heavy: the high crude death rate of 85.8 per thousand in June 1911 in Singapore, for example, compared with the annual rate for the year of 50.91, was solely the result of seasonal epidemic malaria.[122] In Batu Gajah, Perak, morbidity among shop-house dwellers in the town following the apparently successful control of *A. maculatus* led to the possibility that people living near low 'ing swampy areas, near breeding places of *A. barbirostrus*, were acting as a reser ···.   f infection; a control strategy followed aimed primarily at improved drainage but included dredging and deepening the Kuta River, filling the swamps, and introducing flood control measures.[123]

In Kuala Lumpur, anti-malarial work undertaken by the Sanitary Board included clearing, digging ditches, maintaining existing drainage, oiling, inspecting for larvae and gradually providing concrete drains and subsoil drainage. The chairman of the board could authorise control measures, but this was not systematic. Occupants of land were required to keep down 'useless vegetation', prevent the collection of stagnant water and sullage, and dispose of unnecessary water containers (tin shells, coconut husks etc.).[124] Quinine hydrochloride was supplied to schools, post offices, and police stations to enable treatment of presumptive malaria. In 1923, some 32 towns and villages of the FMS, and all major towns of the settlements, had subsoil or open drains for antimalarial purposes;[125] by 1932 in Singapore alone there were 41.25 miles of concrete channels, 72.63 miles of subsoil pipes, and over 300 miles of earth ditches, supplemented by the application of nearly 19,000 gallons of larvicide; this was regarded as the primary reason for the declining death rate from 51.23 per thousand in 1902 to 19.66 by 1933. Antimalarial work was intensive and expensive.[126]

Malaria was endemic peninsula-wide and led to various inquiries. Dr C. Stiskland, an entomologist, toured Kelantan in early 1917 and was 'impressed' by the extent of malaria infection and by increases of blackwater fever.[127] Like others before him, his diagnosis of health problems extended well beyond malaria – in particular he was to identify on estates gastrointestinal ailments due to contaminated tinned milk and inadequate provisions for the disposal of refuse.[128] Malaria, however, was the major problem and concerned state authorities because of its presumed effect on people's general health status:

> Malaria, by lowering the resistance of the population, *raises the death rate from all causes* ... Without wishing to be considered alarmist, the present Medical Officers are of opinion [sic] that unless malaria is controlled in Kelantan. the health outlook is going to be serious ... I personally consider that there is far too much apathy in this matter, the prevailing idea being that malaria and other mosquito-borne diseases have always existed in this part of the world, and that we have got on fairly well in spite of them.[129]

Stiskland argued that the root cause of malaria was economic, and that the problem might be addressed in part through education: 'The mortality rate of malaria among native infants must be very high. The main difficulty in the eradication of malaria is the economic side. Something may, however, be accomplished by instructing school children in such matters of elementary tropical hygiene as a causal connection between the life of the certain kind of mosquito and malaria.'[130] This, however, was an unusual position to take. In response to the report, it was proposed instead to introduce rules for estate sanitation to ensure the provision of clean water, dwellings and surroundings to prevent cholera, typhoid, and plague as well as malaria.[131] In the FMS, meanwhile, the establishment of the Malaria Advisory Board served to concentrate government interest on environmental control, and much of the work of the board was to monitor the maintenance of these measures and to remind estates, periodically, to undertake them. In conducting this task, there was a certain amount of jurisdictional tension between the board and other government instrumentalities – the town sanitary boards, the Mosquito Destruction Board, individual estates, and health officers.[132] Tension became more marked in the early 1930s as budgets were cut to save costs. The Chief Health Officer (FMS) wrote to the Chief of the Malaria Advisory Board in April 1930 stating that sanitary boards (that is, at local government level) were not willing to be responsible for anti-malarial measures on government reserves and state land, and had no funds to do so, as a consequence of which board advice to continue selective clearance of jungle was being 'universally disregarded'.[133] A notice in the press, subsequently placed by the board, stressed the importance of maintaining these measures, as 'loss of labour from sickness and death will inevitably result in estates where anti-malarial works are neglected'.[134] This was considered to be especially important during the Depression, when other public work projects involving environmental management were frozen.[135] For economic reasons, however, the measures themselves were modified: for instance, oiling was reduced from once every seven days to every ten days. The Chief Health Officer was to regard a subsequent decline in cases in malaria 'as a tribute to the co-operation of estate managers, visiting medical practitioners and the Health Branch during the difficult period of economic depression', although as he also observed, at least part of the decline was related to the repatriation of Indian estate labourers (in 1932, numbers were reduced from 216,303 to 170,285).[136]

Beri-beri

Chamberlain, Medical Adviser to the Colonial Office in the late 1890s, noted that 'malaria, black-water fever, yellow fever, and other afflictions brought death, sickness and debility, at an appalling rate, to the Empire's officials and traders, as to the hapless natives' and that 'sudden burials, repeated invalidings, and chronic enfeeblement made regular administration difficult and continuous policy impossible'.[137] However beri-beri, according to Chai, was one of the most serious of ailments at this time, 'decimating one of the most valuable sections of Malaya's population, the Chinese miner'.[138] It remained a major cause of death in the early twentieth century.

Its etiology – lack of anti-neuritic micronutrients (vitamins B_1 and B_2) – was not established until 1926.[139] Original speculation linked the incidence of beri-beri to environmental and climatic conditions (heavy rainfall and flooding, for example), miasma (as a 'place disease'),[140] or in association with the consumption of rice, a germ, mould or poison, the toxicity of which may be influenced by the 'quality' rather than quantity of poison consumed.[141] Favoured thinking by the 1900s was that beri-beri was an infectious disease spread among consumers of polished rice. Braddon in 1901 suggested that this was due to a toxin, probably fungal, which would explain the absence of the disease among Europeans and Tamils who ate 'Bengali rice'.[142] The Institute of Medical Research in 1906 had planned to undertake a case-control study, importing 200 coolies from China to work on Sungei Lembing mines, of whom 100 were to be fed on a diet of parboiled rice and 100 on polished rice; the experiment did not proceed when the mining company decided not to employ more indentured coolies.[143]

The highly focused distribution of the disease attracted early attention: it affected predominantly poor Chinese and Javanese, especially miners, but not Indians or Malays; it was also 'almost entirely confined to the new-comers who have been employed under European supervision'.[144] Incidence was often high: in one gold mine in Kelantan in 1905, for example, in one 'epidemic', 105 of a total 400 Chinese miners had beri-beri and 17 died. Its absence among Indians was associated with their preferred consumption of parboiled rice, among Malays to the use of home-milled rice. However reports from Trengganu in the 1930s indicated that towards the end of the northeast monsoon when there were food shortages and an increased dependency on purchased foods, beri-beri also occurred among Malays and particularly among women observing post-partum food proscriptions.[145] Beri-beri was also more common in coastal areas where less home-milled rice was eaten.[146] Further, available cash was sometimes used to purchase refined and imported foods for adult and infant consumption. Part of the attraction of polished rice, it should be noted, was its longer shelf life, which influenced stock policies of provision shops.[147] In a memorandum on the Report on Nutrition in the Colonial Empire, Haynes noted the 'large and growing consumption of sophisticated and purified foodstuffs' and cautioned that

[W]e must guard against this being extended ... The countryman who goes to work in the town is tempted in this direction. I have myself seen the tendency amongst the Malays, not only town-workers, to change over to white polished rice, white bread, and tinned salmon for their home-pounded rice, home-grown vegetables and fresh fruit. It is more convenient; and Europeans eat such food. In that event the reproach against us would be not merely that trustees had allowed their wards to suffer malnutrition, but that the trustees had actually caused it.[148]

In consequence, therefore, beri-beri probably occurred wherever diet was limited and highly milled rice was used as the staple; to some extent, given the availability of the rice, the geography of beri-beri mapped onto that of colonial penetration and development. This was a point not lost on colonial administrators, who recognised the general poor health status of those who became sick with beri-beri; the Medical Department Report for the FMS for 1927, in commenting on an outbreak of beri-beri during the year, while deploring increased consumption of white rice, observed too that 'the outbreak ... proves how narrow the margin is amongst Asiatics between health and disease, and also how they immediately react to any interference with the vitamin contents of the food supplies'.[149]

Interventions proceeded prior to a clear answer as to etiology. In 1911 a tax or restrictions on the import of polished rice was proposed, through a system of licensing dealers in rice, although this was opposed by the British Resident in Selangor because of the risk of corruption, its impact on small dealers, the shortage of rice, and the need firstly to establish an adequate supply of undermilled rice.[150] The Food Production Enactment in Selangor in 1918 specified areas of state land to be used for the cultivation of vegetables, and 500 acres in Batang Berjuntai Mukim and 7,800 acres in Tanjong Karang were gazetted.[151] Haynes also claims that at around the same time he had proposed that contracts for the supply of rice in the FMS contain a clause binding contractors to undermill some rice, and proposed the opening up of a small shop for the sale of this rice in the Malay settlement in Kuala Lumpur, where only white polished rice was readily available.[152]

The concern with beri-beri predates a wider interest in health and nutrition, and the relationship between the two. Publications appeared from the late nineteenth century on beri-beri, and on infant feeding a decade later. Although nutritional science gained momentum in the inter-war years, underpinning colonial office concern regarding subjects' health and nutritional status,[153] concern with diet and nutrition in Malaya related not only to beri-beri, but to a wider concern with immigrant labour health and efficiency and the cost-benefits of improved nutrition. In the words of the Principal Medical Officer of the FMS in 1911:

> It is important that the advantage of a generous diet should be carefully considered by all employers of labour ... It is most essential to build up and strengthen new arrivals who have very little reserve force to call upon either for work or to resist illness ... not only from the human point of view but also from the business aspect it is necessary that this supply [of food] is adequate. Expenditure on prevention of illness is soon repaid with large interest; stupid ignorance or wilful neglect of this important duty means unnecessary wasteful extravagance as well as loss of life.[154]

Depressions and food shortages

Workers were laid off following the 1921 recession and were vulnerable to fluctuations in the tin and rubber markets. Although it would be inaccurate to characterise Malayan economic history as one that simply faithfully tracked that of the industrialised West, the crash of 1929 was simply a moment in a far longer period of economic peaks and troughs driven by industrial demands.

During periods of low employment, vagrancy was reported to increase, but wages were always low and people were often forced to supplement cash with other economic activities such as horticulture and fishing. Streams in Krian, Perak, were used extensively in the mid-1920s by Chinese and Tamils for fishing, and everywhere wage labourers as well as peasant farmers used forest and water resources to supplement subsistence agriculture.[155] From around the mid-1920s, too, there was growing interest by government departments in labourers' supplementing food bought from wages by agricultural production, and in addition there was some discussion of recruiting women immigrants to boost food supplies and to meet several other purposes, including reproduction of the labour force and reduction of venereal disease through their presumed monogamous and permanent partnership with single men (with an expected decline in the use of prostitutes as a result). In this context, the relationship of family formation to diet was set out by the Secretary of Chinese Affairs:

> All that we can do is to render this country as attractive as possible to female immigrants. A great many of them came down here to find work and are attracted by vegetable gardening, poultry and pig-rearing, etc. If a man can get a home down here for his family he will bring them. Here I am in favour of the allotment of definite areas for squatters for vegetable growing, pig and poultry farming on temporary licenses.[156]

The concern with diet, fired by economic changes, encouraged growing scientific interest in nutrition, and the Institute of Medical Research
established a strong research program concerned with malnutrition
and micronutrient deficiencies that built upon and extended the original research concerned with beri-beri (for example, on 'burning feet'
syndrome from vitamin B_2 deficiency, vitamin A deficiency among
Indian estate labourers, and so on).[157] A comprehensive assessment of
nutritional status in colonial Malaya, and a very clear statement of the
relationship between nutrition, health status and colonialism, occurred
in the context of the work of the Colonial Nutrition Committee and the
interest of the League of Nations Health Committee also in nutrition
(see Chapter 8); the Malayan Government Report to Colonial Nutrition
Committee in 1936 drew on the research of the IMR, and the early
nutrition surveys that were conducted.[158]

The 1930s' Depression led to continually worsening conditions, and
as their places of employment wound down or ceased operation, many
Tamil labourers and Chinese miners were repatriated. Others remained
in Malaya, squatting on land and subsisting from gardening and fishing,
or drifting to towns in search of casual employment. All states were
affected, and the coroner Bourne argued in 1933 that the number of
vagrants dying in the streets was limited only because police regularly
rounded up the ill and took them to hospital.[159] Whilst unemployed and
destitute workers were portrayed as the most 'severely and adversely
affected',[160] Malays as well as immigrant wage labourers were affected.
This was so particularly where they had shifted from padi production to
cash cropping, although in most cases, as crop prices fell, farmers
diverted back to producing rice and vegetables for domestic use, resulting in an apparent rise in nutritional status. Annual Reports of the Straits
Settlements and the FMS hence noted the improved health and nutritional status of both adults and children during the worst years of the
Depression, and a decline in health and nutrition as cash crop activities
resumed and men and women moved back into wage labour. The
possibility for Malays to move between cash cropping and domestic food
production appears to be an important factor in explaining their
differential experience of the Depression, and their ability to return to
subsistence was regarded by colonial economists as 'a great safeguard
against some of the worst social and economic fluctuations in the
income from money crops'.[161] But the maintenance of subsistence production also held down wages, and government and estate initiatives to
encourage gardening, although located within a rhetoric of welfare,
need to be considered in this light. Peel, Controller of Labour in Kuala
Lumpur from 1920, sought – against considerable resistance – to
encourage both planters and government departments employing

labourers (such as the Public Works Department) to allocate land to labourers to allow them to grow food: 'I used to stress the material value of a contented labour force and the desirability of getting them to settle on the land'.[162]

As suggested, the Depression was only one of a number of crises that affected food supply. Malaya depended upon imported rice to meet country needs, as a result of rapid population growth through immigration and the expansion of the non-food agricultural sector without a concomitant program to increase food production for an expanding local market. By the second decade of the twentieth century, the FMS was producing only one-fifth of the rice requirements of those states alone and depended on rice imported primarily from Burma. Fluctuations in food supplies at source had serious implications for Malaya. The First World War especially placed pressure on food-producing areas, and created a shortage of ships, resulting in the irregular importation of rice to Malaya. Government exhorted estates to supplement food supplies through their own exertions, and specified the kinds of vegetables they should grow.[163] Local rice shortages also were felt acutely. Reports in 1912 from Kelantan claimed that people were eating rice only once every three days, procured through the general store of the Duff Development Corporation, because of temporary disruption to the supplies to estates.[164] Local conditions – a rat plague in 1917, for example and foot and mouth disease in Kelantan around the same time – also affected food supply.[165]

In March 1919, as importing was regularised, crop failure and famine in India again reduced supply and the FMS government was advised that monthly rice supplies from Burma would be reduced by nearly half, from 13,000 to 7,000 tons. Rice from Thailand was costly due to an increased demand for Thai rice from Java, Japan and Europe, as well as currency fluctuations which affected local capacity to pay; and rice rationing was introduced from April 1919 to 1921.[166] Inflation in the cost of rice – top quality rice jumped from $6.50 per *gantang* (just over a litre) to $21.40 between 1914 and 1920 – resulted in price jumps in other foodstuffs also, leading to the subsidisation of rice and price fixing. According to Sir William Peel, the Food Controller, this was an instance of the beneficence of imperialism: 'this assistance, which inevitably saved many from starvation, may afford evidence that the British are not so callous as is sometimes alleged'.[167]

Rice shortages and inflated prices for all foodstuffs was a hardship felt by all groups and classes, as discussed later with reference to estate workers (Chapter 5). Those with money were able to supplement ration supplies with purchases from the black market. Peasants and labourers, however, reportedly had difficulty in buying adequate food to meet their needs, particularly as wages were static; in many cases total spending exceeded earnings, and those who could lived on credit. However, sources make no reference to the production and consumption of non-rice staples by Malays or others, and it would be surprising if corn, tapioca, yam and sweet potato had not been important foodstuffs in the 1920s and 30s, as they were to be during the Second World War. To say that lack of rice would result in starvation was, therefore, a statement of the cultural significance of rice and of ethnic identity, rather than one of genuine famine.[168]

Repatriation programs in the early 1930s arguably minimised the impact of the Depression locally, although policy varied. Indian workers who had migrated to Malaya with assistance from the Indian Immigrant Fund could be repatriated, but free migrants – clerks and artisans – could not, and sought assistance from the community; the Selangor Punjabi Unemployment Committee, for example, was established with this in mind, and there were a number of meetings between various delegations and the British Resident to seek government assistance for repatriation.[169] However, there was fluctuation rather than a general decline and then recovery: hence the pattern through 1932–34 tended to be one where small mines and estates would close then reopen, and while the workforce required might shrink in some areas, jobs would become increasingly available in others. In January 1931, for example, there were 23,917 mining coolies in Selangor and 4,673 in Pahang. The Selangor mines were hard hit initially and some 9,000 men had been deployed within six months, but by December there had been a slight recovery, a decline in labour needs again in early 1934, but a rise again at the end of the year. In Pahang, the number of mining coolies dropped to a low of 3,104 in October 1934, then recovered. Meanwhile employment on rubber estates rose: from 4,108 in Pahang in November 1931, for example, to 7,978 three years later.[170] The point is this: the labour market was unpredictable and in this context, sick and decrepit workers were laid off and rendered homeless; the fittest workers were kept on as skeleton staff, especially on the larger estates and mines, and were best able to survive the vicissitudes of the time.

Unemployment was a continuing problem through the 1930s, particularly in the rubber industry, although also in mining and agriculture as a consequence of incomplete recovery from the early 1930s' Depression. Changes in technology led to further displacement of certain workers, and the introduction of workers' compensation provisions led to a reduction in the employment of the elderly and physically handicapped. The government of Selangor also blamed women for unemployment – that is, wives of working men were taking the jobs of other men – and it claimed too that education and technical and training deficiencies made some workers unsuitable.[171]

CHAPTER 4

Public health and the pathogenic city

The colonisation of the late nineteenth century was distinguished from earlier imperial presence by the annexation of land. Previously Europeans worked in an environment which they shared with others, and while they sought to establish through technology and self-ascribed moral authority certain jurisdictive power over other subjects, they were themselves subject to pre-determined and pre-established authority, activities and the delineated spaces within which these might occur. Noyes argues that colonisation is not only the annexation of geographical territory, but that it is the 'totalizing control of representational and subjective space'.[1] Colonisation, in other words, defines the areas to be annexed, establishes control over those spaces, and declares their purpose; hence 'empty space' (not owned by Europeans, rather than uninhabited) is claimed for colonial capitalist purpose, named – that is, it becomes plantations, mines, jungles, farms, and 'vacant' or 'Crown' land – and given meaning as 'functional networks of discreet (sic) places'.[2] The process of naming, incorporating the allocation of functions, rights to and ownership of place, are important, since prior territories are in the process negated; they are, in Harvey's terms, 'reterritorialised' according to the convenience of colonial and imperialist administration.[3]

At the centre of the colonies were the towns, established nodes from which control was established and within which it was maintained materially, institutionally and ideologically. The town was a nodal point of colonial capitalism, in the terms used by Noyes to capture (and insist upon) the fact that place is imbued with geographic, spatial *and* subjective social meaning.[4] In Malaya, the ports and plantations as well as the towns were 'nodal points' of colonialism. The town also had a particular role in representing and maintaining the colonial presence because of the concentration of mercantile, financial, legislative, and administrative authority, and the activities of both capital and the state emanated from it. It is perhaps not surprising that the British chose the lightly populated areas of Singapore and Kuala Lumpur as the sites of the capitals for the Straits Settlements and the FMS, rather than impose the colonial state over both a pre-existing polity and its physical and social site.

The town was the most domesticated space, contrasting with the untamed, unpenetrated hinterland and the diseases that it harboured. The town reflected the colonists' best efforts to create colonial space out of, and in face of resistance from, place, and issues of the use and misuse of urban space were examples of their imperfect control over both place and people. The prevalence of diseases, particularly those of 'place', such as malaria (as understood in terms of early theories of the environment and later, vector density and habitat), highlighted and constituted part of the difficulty of establishing territorial control. But at the same time, use of space and human interactions with and use of both the natural and built landscape reflected the cultural tensions of colonialism. Obsession with hygiene and sanitation in the cities was part of this. There were good public health reasons to reduce risks of transmission of disease by ensuring potable water, clean food, and sanitation. But there were other cultural reasons for colonial insistence on sanitation, and for frustration at the inability of the state to maintain hygienic standards and to inculcate into the minds of others (immigrants and 'natives') British notions of cleanliness and order. The sewer and the well were sites of cultural conflict. Human waste in the towns of the colonies produced malodorous and visual assaults, sanitary transgressions that challenged European authority of human behaviour and urban space. Here was matter out of place.[5]

The ports and inland towns of British Malaya were centres of commerce, administration, and hospital and medical services. Whilst colonial entrepots are often written about as if Europeans, on arrival, simply declared the purpose of the place and transformed their use, in fact of course Europeans and others (Indian and Chinese merchants, for instance) superimposed their settlements and economic systems. Interaction between indigenous and other systems were often arbitrary and superficial, although the colonial capitalist project was to change this, and during the early years the systems were discrete rather than interdigitating.[6]

The old towns of the Peninsula were distinctive. As noted in Chapter 2, many had a history which long pre-dated the establishment of the colony, but they grew in response to the needs of this new polity and were subject to considerable change in terms of the use and political geography of space, and demography, as a result of rapid population growth and urbanisation. Kota Bharu for some centuries had been a centre of Islamic learning and publishing as well as administration; at times it included within its sphere of influence a substantial area of Siamese as well as Malay territory; its mosques and *madrasah* brought to it scholars from throughout the Indonesian archipelago, Egypt and Arabia. Johore Bahru was a powerful court city that through marriage and trade linked the Arab and Malay worlds. Malacca was a cosmopolitan city of Chinese and Indian merchants, ruled over by Malays, Portuguese and Dutch before its subjugation first to the East India Company then to British Straits Settlements administration. Despite the growing ascendancy of Penang and Singapore, in the nineteenth century Malacca continued to be an important link with China and India, and was culturally and politically dominated by *baba* (Straits-born) Chinese. By contrast, Singapore – by 1900 the premier city of the settlements in size, commercially, and politically – was at the time of British occupation a village of fisherfolk and peasant farmers; it and Kuala Lumpur, the administrative capital of the FMS, were essentially creations of colonialism. Other state capitals flourished with colonialism, and small towns grew in response to the rapid influx of people and money.

Penang, Singapore and Malacca were the first to expand. British and 'native' (Indian) troops were stationed in the settlements to establish a military presence in support of the interests of the East India Company. With the creation of the FMS, colonial presence was established in Kuala Lumpur in Selangor, Ipoh in Perak, Seremban in Negri Sembilan and Kuantan in Pahang, as well as in other strategically important towns – Klang, Port Swettenham, Kuala Lipis, Raub, Tampin, Kuala Kangsar, Taiping, for example. Growing numbers of immigrant labourers, petty merchants and shopkeepers settled in these towns to support hinterland development. Banks and business houses grew up amidst restaurants, coffee houses, brothels, provision shops, pharmacists and medical institutions, hotels, and the crowded boarding houses of the urban labourers. Inland, the railway and the railway hotel provided a focus of the business of colonial capitalism and settlement; on the coast, in the towns of the settlements, and in Klang and Port Swettenham, godowns stored tea, rubber and tin ready for the industries of Europe, and imported goods from Europe, India, China, and Arabia designed to meet the varied tastes of those settled in Malaya and wealthy enough to buy. The towns were to become the centres of European medicine as well as of commerce and colonial jurisdiction, as already noted, in response to one of the perceived duties of colonial government: the promotion of public health.[7] If they were centres of medicine, though, they were also centres of disease.

In this chapter, I describe the material conditions of the cities. The circumstances of everyday life – where people lived, worked, ate, bathed, slept and socialised – provided the physical context in which they contracted infections, sought cures, were nursed, and recovered or died. While the physical environment, like the biology of infection and disease, was (and is) mediated by culture, the built landscape and people's use of it was what attracted state interest. This was public health as interpreted during the period of high colonialism,[8] and while new discoveries in science were changing medical knowledge and treatment of disease, emerging knowledge of and belief and confidence in sanitation and hygiene were neatly calqued on older beliefs in the relationship between sickness and environment. In practical public health terms, the interest was in housing, water supply, and sanitation, reflecting public health developments in the United Kingdom. The model that was current from the 1840s explained epidemic disease as 'the product of dirt and decomposing matter', concentrated in towns and remedied by public health and sanitary engineering.[9] From the perspective of the colonial administrators, the extent to which the state might modify or manipulate the landscape or its man-made uses[10] directed ideas about disease and its prevention, and conversely, government response to death and disease was to look to matters of residence, water and sewerage. Medical and public health officers in late nineteenth-century Malaya developed policies in response to the risks that were presented by town life. Disease control and public health measures, as well as medical and hospital services, extended from the towns to the countryside, and so in a general sense public health in the city defined its rural practice also.

The social topography of the city

I describe the towns of the colonies in general terms first, and focus later on Singapore because of the extensive documentation and the acute conditions that pertained there. Extreme overcrowding and high morbidity and mortality rates, especially from tuberculosis, pneumonia and diarrhoeal diseases, resulted in two major housing enquiries, conducted in 1906 and 1917 respectively, and in continued debates about the most appropriate way to resolve housing shortages, crowding and poor sanitation. But Singapore in many ways is exemplary, and the ideas of transmission and control of disease through public health measures existed throughout the colony.

Although the use of the term 'town' is rather problematic, since the distinction between urban and rural can be slippery and the peninsular towns often were not dense settlements, populations in the major centres were sufficiently concentrated to result in the rapid spread of infectious disease; the most virulent spread from town to country. Government records document the most dramatic of these – smallpox, cholera, and plague – although in terms of absolute numbers infected or diseased they had little impact on the population. The management of these epidemics however gives us some insight into European approaches to the control of disease, as explored in Chapter 2 with respect to smallpox, cholera and influenza; in this chapter I consider plague as another disease that highlighted the approach taken. Other infectious diseases, such as measles, although probably important in terms of child mortality, received no attention by the administrations of the colonies; acute respiratory infections too received little attention until relatively late when pneumonia began to outstrip tuberculosis as the main cause of mortality in Singapore. Other communicable diseases in both towns and rural areas, such as diarrhoeal disease, malaria and tuberculosis – considered as 'social diseases' – were subject to various health interventions; tuberculosis is also discussed below.

As McGee, Butcher and others have described for colonial Malaya, and as argued in theory by Noyes and others, space is socially produced and culturally constructed.[11] That is, the meanings given to topography and ecology vary across cultures and according to social and economic formation. The colonial city operationalised European notions of the desirable aesthetic and climatic coalescence of altitude and ecology, in keeping with ideas of the correlation of altitude and disease. Urban space was stratified through the alignment of locality, function, class and ethnicity. In Malaya, in the absence of old established cities along European lines which incorporated an elite cordon in an inner residential area, the stratification operated in such a way that Europeans built their homes on hillsides overlooking the towns; at their feet, Chinese built, worked and lived in shop-houses in the heart of the town, Malays remained in rural-style villages on their periphery, and Indians were sequestered in areas where their own shops and stalls were concentrated, and in 'lines' provided by employers (the brick works, the railways, and so on). The towns evolved then to include 'Chinatowns', 'little Indias', and Malay kampungs in their midst.[12]

Nineteenth-century Malayan towns were, according to contemporary records, crowded, grubby and exciting places. They grew haphazardly and quickly; Singapore, for example, expanded from a population of a few hundred in 1820, to 97,111 in 1871 and 228,555 in 1901; Penang and Province Wellesley increased from 133,230 to 247,808 between 1871 and 1901; Malacca from 77,756 to 95,487 in the same period.[13] Both Chinese shop-houses and adjacent Malay kampungs became increasingly dense with new immigrants and others drifting to the cities, sick or displaced or in search of work and excitement. Accommodation was cramped and people therefore lived on the streets where possible. Food stalls cluttered walkways; provision shops spilled out onto the streets; people ate and drank at walkway stalls, then disappeared into the gaming and opium houses and brothels that gave individual streets and areas their unique character. Street life was noisy and at times violent, marked by petty theft, burglaries, fights, and occasional homicides, assaults and injuries, involving 'all classes of natives, who now perambulate the street at all hours of the night, brawling and shouting and generally disturbing the public peace'.[14] The occasional violence of the streets – brawls, assaults, robberies, homicides – were reminders of the desperation of many who lived in and on the towns. Occasionally but not entirely uncommonly, the corpse of a baby girl, or a still-living infant of five or six months, was a pitiful reminder of the fragile edge on which many women lived; men's lives were perhaps no easier.[15] By day, roads were congested by cart traffic, hack-gharries (i.e. hackney carriages) and rickshaws, with transport slowed by occasional accidents;[16] they were narrow and flanked by open drains that were, except during heavy rain, reported to be offensively smelly.[17]

Public space within the colonial towns acted as a constant reinforcement of the idea of the pathogenic city which characterised much of the medical thinking at the time.[18] Here, illness was produced in certain enclaves – prisons, ships, the harbour, asylums and hospitals, the urban space at large – the congregation of people maximised chances of infection, hence, while wary too of natural spaces and hidden risk, the value of 'ventilation' and 'air'. Crowding and the odours that emanated from refuse, decomposing rubbish, stagnant water and faecal matter led to complaints about these from (European) colonial subjects (though rarely others), and the invasiveness of (mal)odour and effluent challenged British aesthetics as much as colonial public health.

Public health and the nineteenth-century town

Few contemporary commentators spoke well of the colonial towns and cities, or of the health of the people who lived there. The Medical Officer of Kuala Lumpur in 1882 described people's health as being in 'a very unsatisfactory state' due to the 'notoriously dirty and filthy state of the town and the habits of the people', impure water, and drought leading to an outbreak of 'choleric diarrhoea' which stretched the facilities of both the General and Pauper Hospitals.[19] In all cities, inadequate and blocked stormwater drains, and canals overgrown with weeds and blocked with refuse, resulted in their flooding in heavy rain, sending dirty water through street-level shop-houses and obstructing

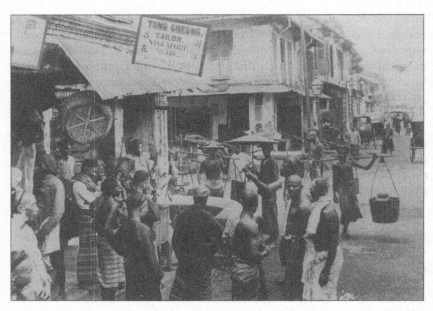

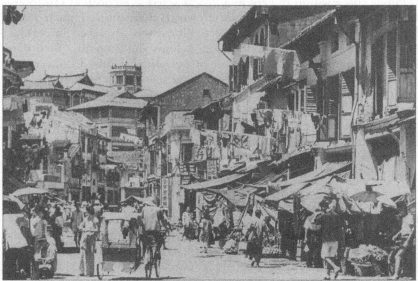

Figure 4.1 Singapore street scene. Printed with permission from the Royal Commonwealth Society, London. Files of the British Association of Malaya, BAM/1 – Singapore.

Figure 4.2 Crowding in Chinatown, Singapore. Printed with permission of National Archives, Singapore. Photograph No. 339, 11994/16.

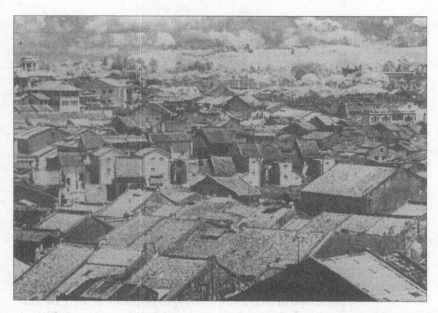

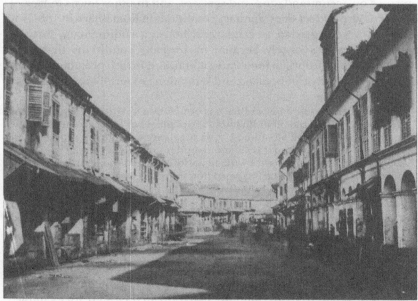

Figure 4.3 Singapore skyline, highlighting the construction of back-to-back houses. Printed with permission of National Archives, Singapore. Photograph No. 417, 14211/19.

Figure 4.4 Two-storey shop-houses in Singapore. Printed with permission of Arkib Negara Malaysia, Kuala Lumpur, N 141/78, Album 2, p. 315.

traffic.[20] There were complaints too about the standard of 'native' housing: dung spread on the floors of Indian dwellings, regarded as 'unsavoury and a nuisance to the neighbourhood',[21] and Malay houses built over mudflats so that the tide might carry away household rubbish and excreta washed through gaps in the floorboards.

Another description of Kuala Lumpur from the newly arrived President of the Sanitary Board, in 1902, gives a further idea of insanitary conditions. Town drains were in a 'deplorable condition' through poor construction and lack of maintenance: '[t]he cement rendering had been completely worn away and large holes formed by defective brick work causing stagnant pools of sewage at frequent intervals'.[22] In some areas conditions were especially bad. The Java Street house and road drains, for example, were considered 'in a disgraceful condition' and in need of repair. In addition, the steady increase of population and haphazard building of new housing placed pressure on the sewerage system, and there was no plan of town drainage on which basis to make improvements.[23] The problem in this case was a combined one of town planning, engineering, and the allocation of public monies. In other towns conditions were also poor, due in larger towns to rapid population increase and pressure on accommodation and services, and in other towns to lack of infrastructure and services. Sanitary conditions in Kota Bharu in 1881, for instance, were regarded as crude and housing rudimentary, but the problem here was largely because of *kampung* conditions that were regarded as inappropriate for a state capital, and British prejudices about appearance and style of housing and sanitation coloured their accounts:

> The only brick house in Kota Bharu is owned by a well-to-do Chinese called the Interpreter, all the other buildings are of planks or bamboo partition, the Sultan's palace is built all of wood … its streets are very narrow with heaps of litter here and there, and it is almost a wonder how human beings can live in such a state. The water used by the majority of them is taken from the river near the bank and it can be imagined how impure it is when thousands of the people make their latrines in the river.[24]

Wooden housing was not of itself a problem, and houses built for Europeans as well as Malays were also wooden and on stilts, providing ventilation and light which, it was argued, were essential to maintain good health in a tropical environment. Fire was a hazard, however, which spread quickly in areas where walls and roofing were of poor quality and where houses were set in close proximity. In Singapore in the 1880s, for example, fires broke out regularly in both Malay villages and in Chinese shophouses. In 1883, a fire in a dhoby's shop destroyed twenty houses in February; in May a woman was badly burned in a fire in a brothel in Hokkien Street, and a fire in Kling Street damaged the site and adjacent shops due to the delay between the outbreak of fire and the connection of water. In early July three fires occurred in one day – in an opium shop, a godown, and in Kampung Krabu near Bencoolen Street, where seven houses were completely destroyed; five days later there were further fires in this *kampung*, where 'a casual walk through the place – the houses, cooking-places, verandahs and all about them, being built of light poles and attaps, supplemented at times by the lightest and thinnest of plants' – provided the evidence of the risk of spilt cooking oil or a tipped paraffin lamp.[25] The major fire during this period occurred in Campong (Kampung) Kapor, near Rochore Canal Road, on 3 April as a result of a cooking oil accident; within two hours about 100 houses had been destroyed, as 'several small-pox patients were carried out on litters, and shelter sought for them among friends or relatives elsewhere; invalids and old people were supported by friends and forced to hobble away out of danger'.[26] Final assessment of the damage, following a Report to the Municipal Commission, was 116 houses burnt or demolished subsequently, some 1,020 people rendered homeless, and estimated damage of $846,843. The fire led to recommendations by the commission that houses be built of raised wood, with tiled roofs, lanes 30 feet wide to be positioned every 200 feet, and roads 50 feet wide.[27] Such recommendations were difficult to carry out, however, and *kampung* housing changed little.[28]

Much of the discussion about sanitation focused on domestic space and products, encapsulating European affront at the corporeality of the colonial subject spilling into colonial streets and streams. But public space was also poorly maintained. The central market in Kuala Lumpur, for instance, provoked continuous complaints, and in 1885 proposals to improve its cleanliness and 'general comfort and convenience' were prepared for the Public Works Department. They were not implemented since the Resident did 'not wish to spend more money on this market than is absolutely necessary',[29] leading to further complaints of 'intoler-able stench'.[30] Street stalls were also regarded as unhygienic and continu-ally offended European aesthetics and notions of order and hygiene:

> Street stalls caused the usual trouble in control, and whilst action was taken to remove the most unsatisfactory, it can never be accepted that any of them will at any time be satisfactory. They compete unfavourably with eating shops; their very nature makes it impossible for them to comply with the hygienic conditions called for in the production and handling of food; their structures on roadside and vacant land are a hindrance to improvement in the appear-ance of the towns, and they are frequently a source of obstruction to both pedestrian and vehicular traffic.
>
> Their entire elimination should be the ultimate object. No hardship need be involved … a number of holders of such skills could quite easily open suitable eating shops. Hawkers offer an even greater problem, and a gradual elimination of them is desired.[31]

Sanitary control and sewage disposal

Sanitary policy centred around the management of water supply, waste disposal, and housing. Whilst these appear innocent and innocuous objectives, they disguise a tension over prevailing 'Asiatic' practices related to domestic space, excretion and disposal of refuse. In colonists' eyes, residential patterns were insanitary, as discussed in detail below, in both physical and moral terms. People were at risk of air-borne infection because of the lack of space per individual in tenements, but were also 'morally' at risk (that is, close proximity to other bodies would lead to licentiousness, hence also to venereal disease). The disposal of faeces and urine were regarded as unaesthetic, visually and olfactorily offensive, and a danger to public health; in-leakage from drains to wells providing water for household use created constant concern for the risk of faecally transmitted infections.

Late nineteenth-century municipal sanitation regulations and practices reflected earlier government reluctance to intervene in the domestic environment, or to spend much in terms of public health. However growing concern with and embarassment regarding the high adult and infant death rates in the colonies propelled change. This was encouraged by pressure within Britain, notably following a deputation from the Chambers of Commerce, with Ronald Ross of the Liverpool School of Tropical Medicine and Hygiene, urging the appointment of commissioners to inspect and report on the 'sanitary performance' (provision of water, sewers, drains, and so on) of colonial governments.[32]

Sanitary Boards had been established in individual settlements and states by the end of the century, which were responsible for nightsoil and refuse removal, inspecting and issuing notices to abate nuisances, the repair of drains and public latrines, limewashing houses, and closing unused and dangerous wells. Dairies, markets, food stalls, bakeries and slaughter houses, hotels, lodging houses, eating houses and other places of public resort were all under their control. The boards were also empowered to inspect and where appropriate prosecute people for breaches in public health and hygiene: for keeping unregistered dairies, tampering with weights, failing to demolish cubicles in town houses, keeping laundries without licence, having filthy premises, and selling unwholesome meat. The boards and the Health Officer were also responsible for road surfaces, issuing various business and factory licences, the siting of public buildings, registering transport such as the hack-gharries and *jinrikisha*, disinfecting buildings during epidemics, controlling rats, and maintaining the supply of water for trade and domestic use.[33] Buildings which were considered to be dangerous to public health could be ordered to be demolished under the rules of the

Quarantine and Prevention of Disease Enactment.[34] The Health Officer was also empowered to inspect common lodging houses and to prosecute for overcrowding.[35] The boards were kept busy: in 1929, for example, the Kuala Lumpur Sanitary Board issued 15,134 notices to owners or occupiers of houses for failure to comply with Sanitary Board regulations.[36] The boards had jurisdiction also over various peri-urban villages, where problems were often exacerbated because of the difficulties of surveillance and control and allocation of resources: the location of wells and seepage from cess-pits into surface wells, the lack of systems of disposal for garbage and nightsoil, insanitary dairies, unventilated premises were all common problems.[37]

As indicated, European sensibility was particularly affronted by nightsoil arrangements, which, as Brenda Yeoh argues, were regarded as symptomatic of Asiatic domestic practices and hence symbolic of race.[38] Cholera, diarrhoea, dysentery, and other so-called 'filth' diseases were understood to be transmitted faecally, and waste disposal was regarded as not particularly salutary.

Sanitary arrangements in the Federated Malay States

Nightsoil disposal was a concern to town authorities because of infection both through direct contact with faecal matter and indirectly from flies. According to the graphic descriptions in official documents, nightsoil 'sometimes teems with pathogenic germs such as typhoid, dysentery, or Cholera, and where the excrement of thousands of people are concerned it can be taken as a certainty that some of it is infective ... flies feed on the material and deposit their eggs in it ... One moment they are feeding on faeces and getting themselves contaminated, at another they are crawling over the food on the table'.[39] Disease prevention was regarded as relatively straightforward however, through improved nightsoil collection and its proper disposal.

Arrangements for excretion and waste disposal in the town houses of late nineteenth-century Malaya were crude. Usually an open drain ran through the centre of the dwelling for household refuse and urine. Municipal council regulations specified that a latrine be provided in every house, with a bucket, usually wooden, to be put out each morning and emptied by the town scavengers. The bucket was kept in the kitchen area, often located near the household well where surface water, polluted by the effluent from the drains and buckets, was collected for cooking, drinking and washing. Few houses abided by the rules:

In some houses if there is insufficient latrine accommodation one small closet in a corner of the kitchen being considered enough for 50 or 60 people. In some instances the tubs are too small and quite inefficient. In others the tubs had not been emptied at all for days and had even fallen to pieces where they stood; while in others again no tubs had ever been introduced at all but the bricked space in which it ought to stand was the only receptacle, this having … perfectly free communication with the well.[40]

Even where basic procedures (the use of the tubs) were followed, faeces and urine might remain exposed to air and flies for up to 24 hours; contents were spilt as the tub was removed. Householders would also often drain off urine into the central kitchen drain to minimise slopping as the bucket was carried through the house and out the door for collection.[41] In most cases all waste from the kitchen, bathing area and latrine ran to the front rather than the back of the house, then into the street.

A description of one block of ten houses in Kuala Lumpur in 1899 provides an elaboration of this. One drain ran from house to house, its condition in reasonably good order despite some odour, 'the sewage coming as it does from the kitchen and bathing place to it'. The drain traversed the length of the houses through narrow brick drains, liable at any time to become choked up, then into the open street. Channels at the back of houses were provided for run-off water, but were often clogged, creating stagnant pools 'offensive in the extreme form'.[42]

Latrines in private houses were supplemented by a limited number of public latrines and bath houses. In Kuala Lumpur in 1908, there were only ten public latrines supposedly emptied three times daily, two public bath houses in Klyne and Sultan Streets, and 264 dustbins located around the central city area for other refuse.[43] The latrines were modified with the use of a slow filter, through which effluent was discharged into the river; septic tanks were introduced later and were rare.[44] Elsewhere, bucket latrines were used: in Penang in 1938, only 49 of 189 public lavatories had flush toilets and the rest were bucket latrines emptied by municipal workers; the town also provided 86 bath houses. Bucket latrines remained the predominant domestic system also, although over the period there were some improvements. In Pahang by 1931, for example, some towns used single but others double buckets, and septic tanks were provided in European quarters in larger towns like Raub and Bentong.

Nightsoil was collected by contract scavengers. Cattle were used to draw the carts, and they added to street pollution; carts were often spattered and wet faeces and urine spilt on the road.[45] Arrangements for the disposal of nightsoil after its collection from households and public latrines varied, but frequently, as noted already, it was discharged into rivers or the sea; some was used in horticulture. The Medical Department in Kuala Lumpur did not approve of this latter practice and claimed that it attracted flies and caused cholera, typhoid, fever, bacillary and amoebic dysentery and ankylostomiasis; and prosecutions could be brought against people illegally removing nightsoil. In 1913, despite objections from the Sanitary Board, the collection and disposal of nightsoil in Kuala Lumpur was brought under the direct control of the Health Officer in order to improve the delivery of the sanitary services and improve efficiency.[46] A memorandum in 1914 from the Principal Medical Officer of the FMS, Charles Sansom, claimed that as a result conditions were in Kuala Lumpur 'relatively good' compared with other towns, and did not contribute to the high infant mortality rate, which he associated with maternal ignorance and malaria. After 1915, the system of disposal was changed and nightsoil was buried in shallow trenches; gangs of up to fifty were alleged to raid the trenches at night to steal the nightsoil for agricultural use.[47] Prosecutions occurred sporadically; the Resident of the FMS felt that the public health risk of nightsoil in agriculture was overstated and he was disinclined to prosecute, arguing instead for its value in improving agricultural productivity, people's employment and the food supply.[48]

Other large towns in the FMS had concrete or earth drains carrying wet waste into streams; in some, from the turn of the century, brick drains were provided.[49] In many towns particularly in the UFMS, however, facilities were quite inadequate. In Kota Bharu for example, the Sanitary Board had claimed improved services in 1931 when it could provide 454 nightsoil buckets to an estimated population of around 15,000 occupying 2,412 dwellings – hence one bucket to every 33 people.[50] Conditions, at least until the 1920s, were no better in Singapore (see below). Elsewhere too conditions remained poor, and Dr J. T. Clarke, Health Officer in Kinta, maintained that in many towns 'the main streets ... are so filthy that I do not think there is any need to look into nightsoil disposal methods nor to go inside or to the back of the houses to find out the reason for the high Infant Mortality Rate'.[51]

Refuse, rats and plague

Town administrations provided for 'scavenging', the collection of household refuse, on a regular basis, using brick incinerators for the disposal of solid waste. All houses in Kuala Lumpur were reportedly provided with rubbish bins by 1915, and rubbish was supposed to be collected every morning. But people threw out rubbish at all times, leaving it uncovered through the day or simply throwing it into the drains.[52] Vacant land in Petaling Street (near Pudu Road), near the central markets and in one of the densest areas of settlement in the city, was used as a garbage dump and the exposed decomposing refuse smelt.[53] In addition, the Inspector of Nuisances maintained that there were not enough coolies to help him with the work to ensure regular collection.

The real problem was rats, which bred in these garbage dumps, in the market places, and in crowded tenement houses. Outbreaks of plague, transmitted from rat fleas infected with the plague bacillus, *Yersinia pestis*, occurred sporadically throughout the Peninsula, and while only a few people were infected in any year some rats were infested with infected fleas, and the risk of an epidemic was real. Rat-catching was introduced as a control measure in 1903, surprisingly early given that the first paper suggesting the association between rats, fleas and disease, by Paul-Louis Simond, had only been published in 1898, its findings rejected by the Indian Plague Commission in its 1902 Report. While the Director-General of the Indian Medical Service still regarded the work as 'promising' in 1905, public health campaigns in Malaya had already been instituted on the assumption that the theory was correct.[54]

Local rat populations were supplemented by vermin jumping ship in the ports of Singapore, Penang and Port Swettenham, and their prolific breeding meant that aggressive control measures were required. This was primarily achieved by offering a bounty on rats caught and brought to the Sanitary Board. A bounty – of four cents per head – was first introduced in Kuala Lumpur in 1904. By the end of the year a total of 34,673 rats had been brought to the destructor employed by the Sanitary Board, 4,476 of them in December alone. The large numbers of dead rats brought in led to a change of system: dead rats' tails only were inspected, tallied, chopped up to prevent fraud, and burnt, the disposal of the remainder of the corpse now being the responsibility of the rat-catcher. The bounty, a generous amount against contemporary wage rates (about 25 cents per day), fluctuated – two cents in 1908, three in 1911 – but remained a relatively effective control.[55] A bounty was also used for a while in Singapore to control the rat population, although the Municipal Council was suspicious that some people were breeding rats for the purpose,[56] and by the mid-1920s, it had replaced the policy of mass extermination of rats with one of monitoring flea infestation and flea infection rates, supplementing this by routine rat-trapping. The Municipal Health Officer argued that the only efficient and permanent method of control was through food hygiene, however, but that this was not feasible given current housing conditions:

(W)here food is allowed to be prepared in any insanitary coolie house and hawked about the streets without let or hindrance, where the conditions of overcrowding are so terrible ... the wonder is not that we have so few cases of plague, but rather that so many escape it, where most efforts directed to improving conditions generally are met with apathy if not opposition ... there is plenty of evidence that rat plague has a fairly firm hold in different parts of the town.[57]

Elsewhere 'abourers were employed by the municipality or town board to control the rats: in Penang as late as 1938 still one assistant supervisor and six coolies were engaged full-time on rat eradication, killing 6,512 that year.[58] But epidemics were rare and there were mostly isolated cases not leading to further infection. Between 1900 and 1933 there were 765 cases in Singapore, of whom 712 died; in the same period there were 200 cases in the FMS, over half in Perak.[59] In many years, there were few or no cases, but even small epidemics caused considerable concern. In 1924, for example, in Singapore, there were 20 cases of plague, four contracted from rats in residential huts in the Serangoon Road area. Hence it was the metaphoric rather than epidemiological weight of the disease that propelled public health action. Where plague occurred, action was severe: although the rats caught in Serangoon Road were not infected, the huts – 'mere hovels with mud floors' which could not be disinfected – were burnt down, with compensation paid to the residents.

Housing in the Federated Malay States

Housing provoked almost as much criticism and concern as did nightsoil disposal, primarily because of the association of crowded living and sleeping conditions with pulmonary tuberculosis (phthisis). The condition of houses in Singapore was reputedly the worst (see below). But town lay-out, building styles and standards were replicated throughout the colony, and general concerns regarding poor quality housing, lack of light and ventilation, overcrowding, and urban mortality and morbidity, were constantly voiced.

In Kuala Lumpur housing issues became important as the town grew. The Conference of Residents of 30 January 1902 called on the British Resident of Selangor to draw to the attention of the Sanitary Board the need to encourage suitable houses for poor classes in towns and villages. Building regulations, it was claimed, had resulted in high rents that were the cause of overcrowding: 'There appears to have been a tendency hitherto for Sanitary Boards, taking a pride in the appearance of their Towns, to insist on all houses being built in accordance with plans the cost of carrying out of which necessitates a charge for rent which the poorer classes of the community cannot afford to pay'.[60] Rent was reputedly also high because of the high cost of land,[61] and because demand exceeded supply. The towns were the first points of call for in-migrants, and houses served social functions as centres of employment and points of return for sick or unemployed labourers. While the late nineteenth and early twentieth century were relatively prosperous times for Malayan investors, both the tin and rubber markets were vulnerable to market fluctuation, and workers carried the burden of these shifts;

there were continual waves of unemployed workers who would drift to towns in search of work and housing. In addition, lack of hospital bed space limited the number of inpatients. In Ipoh in 1908, for example, sick workers were continually being transferred from one hospital to another, then to available cubicles in workers' houses: 'The general depression in the State that followed on the fall in the price of tin threw many coolies out of employment. This consequently meant want and disease. In the larger towns vagrants with impaired health were prominent. The admissions to the hospitals rose, especially in the mining centres, and taxed the available accommodation.'[62]

In Kuala Lumpur, conditions were especially bad. In 1907, the population was estimated at 39,998, occupying 2,791 houses and additional huts and attap dwellings – an average of 14.3 people per dwelling.[63] Among these dwellings were some 51 common lodging houses, mostly badly overcrowded, where indigent workers sought shelter.

In 1910 the crude death rate in Kuala Lumpur was 32.2, and concern with this 'appalling' statistic in comparison with other towns in the FMS (for example, around 11 in Ipoh) led to growing pressure on the government to improve ventilation, lighting and drainage, and to employ more sanitary inspectors to do this.[64] Inspectors were empowered to visit houses to ensure adherence to basic hygiene standards. According to the Federal Secretary, the sanitation by-laws governing lighting and ventilation were 'strictly enforced' in Kuala Lumpur although not in other towns, and the fine for breaches – one dollar in 1910 – was considered 'a very small one for a man who allows his house to get into an absolutely filthy state'.[65] Prosecutions had little effect, however, and authorities recognised that the real problem was one of insufficient housing;[66] and over the next decade health indices worsened, leading the board to claim in 1920 that overcrowding was the major contributing factor to the high incidence of tuberculosis, other infectious diseases, and the high infant mortality rate.[67]

Overcrowding was most acute in the areas where rickshaw depots were situated, and in Kuala Lumpur and other towns there were no rules to enforce the provision of suitable accommodation for the drivers by rickshaw owners:

> At present a rikisha depot is usually run by some men (sic) who rents the house and makes as much profit as he can out of the pullers. He is usually a man of straw and it is to his interest to allow overcrowding as much as possible ... The existing state of affairs here is appalling. There are 3243 coolies licensed as pullers and the houses which were licensed in 1911 only provide accommodation for 1532 men.[68]

In 1911 in Kuala Lumpur, around 53 places designated as rickshaw depots were estimated to be overcrowded – from between 1 and 40 people too many. By 1929 conditions had deteriorated despite fines to limit occupancy, and it was estimated that rickshaw depots were by this time overcrowded by as much as 272 percent.[69] This reckoning alludes to extraordinary crowding – men sleeping in the same beds or sleeping platforms in three or four shifts, ten or twelve men sharing a room of around eight feet square.

This was as true in the UFMS as in the FMS and settlements. In Kota Bharu lines 'of a very poor type (were) springing up all round the town'; cubicles in townhouses were overcrowded and insanitary; open areas were roofed in for additional shelter and unauthorised extensions were added to existing houses. Drains were full of refuse. The town had no building inspector, and urgently needed it.[70] Strang, Chief Medical Officer in Kota Bharu in 1936, recommended that the old 'slum type of houses' be demolished since both structural and sanitary improvements were impractical:

> In the old town area, which unfortunately was not completely burnt out during the fire of 1929, main streets are narrow and the centre of the blocks or squares formed by shop houses are occupied by groups of Malay houses, the majority of which abut against the back walls of the shop houses themselves; and render the construction of back lanes impossible.[71]

Official reckoning of overcrowding (like 'hygiene' and 'filth') is confusing. It varied from town to town and was based on estimated space, allocated per person but with the measurement not made explicit in reports. Data are available for licensed boarding houses and depots, registered with (and hence the responsibility of) the Sanitary Board, but are not available for private housing in the FMS or elsewhere. However, reports from about 1900 suggest that overcrowding was probably under-estimated, since with forewarning occupants would move out: Sanitary Board inspectors tried to circumvent this by making night inspections.[72]

A report of housing in Sultan Street, Kuala Lumpur, based on inspections in 1927, illustrates the problem further. Clerks, hawkers, fitters, shopkeepers and assistants, miners, stallholders, 14 Chinese physicians, 3 teachers, 3 fortune tellers, 2 dentists and 2 priests lived there; many others worked in the street.[73] One hundred shop-houses accommodated 410 families or household units – 2,975 people, of whom 2,309 were adults. The number of persons per house ranged from one to 71 people, but in only 19 were there less than ten; in 56 there were 40 or more people. Ninety-five of these shop houses were divided into 915 cubicles. The cubicles were temporary structures, subdividing interior space while allowing limited light and air through the gaps between the floor and foot of the screen, and the ceiling and top of the screen: usually the partitioning for the cubicles commenced about six inches from the floor and left around the same space at the top. Cubicles might house seven or more people and many were only around 7 to 8 feet square – enough for bed space only. The openings between the cubicles allowed air-borne infections to spread easily, and overcrowding increased exposure and the severity of infections.[74] The ratio of latrines to people on Sultan Street was 1:24. Authorities were faced with the difficulty that rental on any new housing would exceed people's capacity to pay, and the Sanitary Board in Kuala Lumpur felt that the only way around this was to build coolie lines with minor improvements which would cost little more than the 'more primitive types of lines' – semi-permanent or temporary buildings to alleviate the housing demand.[75]

Accommodation and crowding in Singapore

In Singapore, housing was especially tight, overcrowding intense, and morbidity and mortality from infectious disease high from the late nineteenth century to well after the Second World War. The first major inquiry into housing and urban health occurred in 1906, although it followed the work of an earlier committee, appointed by the Governor and was comprised of the Principal Civil Medical Officer, the Municipal Health Officer and the Municipal Engineer, which had recommended changes in building regulations to ensure back lanes to houses. In June 1905, the Colonial Secretary, E. L. Brockman, wrote to the President of the Municipal Commission, E. G. Broadrick, regarding death and disease rates, and the need for action regarding housing. Broadrick in reply referred to 'the ignorance and apathy of a great part of the Asiatic population', the prohibitive cost of rebuilding where housing was structured back-to-back, and the lack of power given to the municipality to control building standards.[76] The Governor, Sir John Anderson, subsequently called for an inquiry into the increased number of deaths from tuberculosis, resulting in the appointment of Dr William J. Simpson to conduct the inquiry. Simpson, who in the 1890s had been Health Officer in Calcutta and had been a member of the Indian Plague Commission,[77] visited Singapore July–August 1906; the report was released in mid-1907.[78]

The report was extensive, and highlighted the abnormally high adult as well as infant death rate in the city, due primarily to tuberculosis, acute respiratory infections, beri-beri, diarrhoeal diseases, and malaria. Simpson concluded that the covering of land by buildings was excessive; that houses were overcrowded; and that conditions were 'adverse' with respect to light, air and drainage. He was particularly critical of houses built back-to-back without proper provision for drainage or the removal of refuse or nightsoil; in some cases three buildings of two, three or four storeys might be so built, with light and air available to the middle building only through narrow airwells or spaces between the buildings.[79] Houses were often subdivided into airless cubicles for rent, with renters sharing facilities; as many as 200 residents might share two or three kitchens and latrines. In all cases, too, wet waste was carried through the centre of the house along a common open drain, as was the case in Kuala Lumpur. All refuse was removed through the front of the house; from upper storeys, by the front stairs. A four-storey tenement on Sago Street provides an example:

> The shop is tenanted by a barber on one side of the street and by a tailor on the other side. Behind the shop is a central and badly-lighted passage, having on either side of it cubicles which are so pitch dark in their interior that a lamp is necessary for their inspection. The first cubicle is occupied by the tailor and a food hawker, the second by a general goods hawker or haberdasher. His cubicle is crowded with stores of all kinds, such as boots, shoes, pipes, whistles, soap, towels, lamps, tooth powder, and such like. The bench, on which he sleeps, is 22 inches wide and 5½ feet long, and there is only 18 inches between it and an upper shelf, containing some of his goods ... The third cubicle is occupied by two food hawkers, one sleeps on a bench below, and the other on a bench above ... In the cubicle is a stove with dishes, which is carried by (the) Chinese hawker, selling food; there are also stores of salt, rice, vermicelli and such like. The fourth cubicle contains three beds; it is occupied by two hawkers, one of whom is suffering from a cough and is spitting on the floor ... The fifth is occupied by one man ... He sells ducks, which he keeps in baskets in the air well, and prepares them for food in the kitchen behind the cubicles ...[80]

And so on: twelve cubicles which shared a common kitchen and latrine area. Malay houses were better lit and ventilated, Simpson argued, but also dark, unhealthy and haphazardly built.

Other reports provide further evidence of crowding and congestion. Middleton's description of No 5, Hokkien Street, dated 30 May 1908, is typical. Part of this house was a bakery, and 'through the Bakery in front runs the open drain from the back premises ... and along which flows the bath and sullage water, urine and the washing of nightsoil pails. Here also the sugar is boiled and cakes are baked'.[81] The front upstairs area was divided into two sections, with eight sleeping benches in each, occupied when Middleton visited by '19 men of the cooly class smoking opium or sleeping off the effects. The available cubic space is largely taken up with boxes placed under the beds and along the floor and with bundles of clothing, bedding etc., deposited on the floor and sleeping benches or hung on the walls'.[82] The house, like virtually all those that accommodated labourers, rickshaw pullers and street vendors, lacked adequate bathing, cooking and latrine facilities, the ground floor lacked light and air; food risked contamination from the latrines and flies.

Water storage pots stood by the latrine, and in this and other houses without taps, people carried water from standpipes in the street to store in jars and tanks. Since leases were short, property owners and landlords invested little in maintenance. Tiles on floors were often broken and the ground beneath water-logged and feculent; the walls decayed and infested with rats, cockroaches and bedbugs.[83]

Simpson also provided a detailed description of sanitary arrangements. A nightsoil pail was positioned in each kitchen/bathing area near the well; people urinated directly into the open interior drains. Nightsoil collection was contracted between the householders and a farmer, who employed coolies to collect it. Usually each morning a coolie would call to collect the contents of the pails, pour off liquid waste, empty the solids into his own bucket, rinse out the house pails and empty that waste water into the kitchen drain. Pails were made of wood and were sometimes broken down, the coolie splashed water and faecal remains around the kitchen area and occasionally spilled his full bucket as he left the house, and drains were often blocked with kitchen waste. The sludge was transported by the open drain through the centre of the house, with contents from the upper floors fed by pipe to the ground floor drain, emptying into a larger open street drain through the front door. Since houses were built back-to-back there was only one exit for effluent as well as people. Sewage consequently posed a real health hazard, especially for servants who slept in the ground floor rooms and for children who played in the area and occasionally came into direct contact with it.[84]

Sewage collected from houses and public buildings such as the hospital, gaol, the barracks and government offices was used as fertiliser on coconut plantations and vegetable gardens and for maggot breeding for duck feed. Simpson estimated that around 40 percent of the pails used to transport nightsoil to the plantations and maggot farm leaked, resulting in further contamination.

Simpson recommended, *inter alia*, the creation of a Sanitary Board for the Straits Settlements to include the Principal Civil Medical Officer of the Colony, other senior officials, an unofficial representative of the Singapore Legislative Council, and representatives of the municipalities of the settlements. To improve sanitation, he recommended that the bucket system be replaced gradually with the Shone system, which used compressed air to pump sewage to a central area for treatment prior to it being dumped at sea. He recommended too that no further houses be built without back lanes and that the number of tenement buildings be increased to meet pressure for cheap housing. Having said this, he listed as priorities for improvement the Lunatic Asylum, General Hospital, prison, police station and offices, barracks and the 'better class houses' in the Fort Canning area, other institutions, and other European quarters. Low priority was therefore accorded to the poor whose health was most compromised.

Amendments to the Municipal Ordinance were introduced and passed by the Legislative Council in July 1907 to enable the demolition of insanitary buildings and provide funds to property owners so that they might alter buildings. However, the proposed establishment of a Sanitary Board was rejected. Schemes put forward by the municipality in 1908 to improve housing were also rejected because of cost, and Simpson's building recommendations were largely discounted as 'impracticable'. A second bill, introduced in August 1911 but then withdrawn, sought to amend the law to enable the Municipality to order property owners to provide back lanes and purchase land and houses to ensure sufficient open space. Another bill was introduced in November 1912, and passed in April 1913, regarding compensation payments for the provision of back lanes. Again cost was a factor: the total to provide back lanes, including compensation payments to owners, alterations to houses and the provision of pavement, was estimated at between six and ten million dollars.

Between Simpson's inquiry and a second one in 1917 little action was taken and things were in a 'hopeless muddle'.[85] The 1917 Commission, established in face of this inactivity and presided over by W. George Maxwell, documents the intransigence of the government and property owners over improving housing, and covers much of the same territory as the previous inquiry. Its report notes, for example, no change in the conditions of the interiors of houses since Simpson's inquiry. Rooms in tenement buildings, sub-divided into cubicles with tea-chests, matting, sacks or other cloth, were grossly crowded; in one sample area in 1917 the population density was 1,304 persons per acre, compared with an estimated density of 547 persons per acre in 1908, then regarded as over-crowded.[86] Poor sanitation was still a problem, and Europeans rather than Chinese had benefited most from any improvements.

Individuals presenting evidence to the commission lay at least some blame on victims rather than property owners and claimed that the high mortality rates of the city had more diverse causes than housing. W. R. C. Middleton, the Municipal Health Officer of Singapore, for example, claimed that the health customs and tastes of Asiatics contributed to the high death rate, including the

employment of unskilled attandance at birth, improper feeding and clothing of infants, carelessness in the disposal of refuse and nightsoil, concealment of infectious disease, evasion of vaccination and revaccination, overcrowding, storage of water, carrying on certain occupations in dwelling-houses, filthy habits of dairymen, adulteration of milk, use of nightsoil as manure, preparation of food under insanitary conditions [by Food Hawkers and Eating-house Keepers], use of polluted wells, and the universal habit of spitting.

He noted too that 'Europeans might also be mentioned owing to their carelessness in inspecting their outhouses and in the disposal of broken bottles, empty tin cans and other receptacles capable of collecting water and breeding mosquitoes'.[87]

Dr Lim Boon Keng, in his evidence to the commission, argued that 'poor people are not adequately paid to enable them to live'.[88] The commission too emphasised the relationship between poverty and overcrowding, arguing also that illness and death were a drain on community resources and that funds needed to be allocated for preventive measures. It also commented on the patterns of settlement and work in the city that favoured the concentration of industries, and flowing from this the lack of residential alternatives for working class men and women: the tendency for pottery dealers to live and work in one street, coffin-makers and tombstone cutters in another; artisans and labourers as close as to their work as possible, usually by the river, the harbour or the wharves; food-hawkers near theatres and other amusements, and so on. Throughout the city, shopkeepers, their families and assistants lived in their shops, for they could not afford a separate residence, and employers or headmen of groups of labourers would rent a house to accommodate large numbers of workers.[89] This was the case, for example, with rickshaw coolies, whose buildings were often especially overcrowded because of high rent. Hooper, Registrar of Vehicles, claimed that the rent was inflated because the coolies were 'notoriously undesirable tenants' who made a 'filthy mess'; but there was clearly extraordinary pressure for cheap accommodation – Hooper claimed that there were 9,000 rickshaws and over 20,000 coolies in Singapore at the time – as rents rose by 25 to 50 percent over a three-year period and as food prices also inflated (see below), while wages remained relatively static (Tables 4.1 and 4.2).[90] For many, too, the cubicles were a happy option. Others were homeless. Drivers of buses, taxis and rickshaw coolies often slept in vehicles at night, or dozed between workshifts, and

Table 4.1   Population, housing and crowding in Singapore 1891–1917

Year	Population	Occupied houses	Vacant houses	Persons per house
1891	155,683	17,732	1,719	8.7
1901	193,089	21,132	1,245	9.1
1911	259,610	26,196	2,406	9.9
1915	289,375	25,806	1,073	12.5
1916	296,951	25,997	860	11.4
1917	304,815	26,811	581	11.3

Source: Singapore, *Report of the Housing Commission 1918*, p. A11.

Table 4.2   Houses occupied by rickshaw coolies, 1917

House address	Rent before war ($)	Rent in 1917 ($)	Occupants per house
41 Mosque St	50	72	85
36 Mosque St	50	75	80
151 New Market Rd	54	60	65
128 New Market Rd	45	52	35
126 New Market Rd	45	65	25
27 Park Rd	40	50	80
24 Park Rd	40	50	85
12 Lim Eng Bee Lane	16	20	24
1 Lim Eng Bee Lane	16	20	28
104 Beach Road	22	26	30
25 Erskine Road	20	30	25
23 Erskine Road	20	30	28
96 Bencoolen St	50	70	110
107 Bencoolen St	35	45	35
106 Bencoolen St	35	45	37
206 Waterloo St	18	24	55
204 Waterloo St	18	24	60
127 Rochore Rd	35	52	60
134 Rochore Rd	30	52	65
96 Queen St	17	24	15
129–132 Queen St	18	32	35
18 Muar Rd	16	18	25
31 Muar Rd	18	25	28
38 Johore Rd	23	25	40
37 Johore Rd	18	26	35
124 Victoria Rd	75	80	175
109 Arab St	14	30	35
114 Arab St	14	22	30
42 Bain St	8	20	20
37 Bain St	17	22	25

Source: Singapore, *Report of the Housing Commission, 1918*, p. C17 (W. E. Hooper to President, Singapore Housing Commission, 14 November 1917).

it was estimated that temporary housing was required for 10,000 labourers to alleviate congestion in central Singapore:

> It is amongst the poorest class that the struggle for existence is keenest … They have to put up with what they can get in the way of a room, or a share of a room, for the only choice is between accepting and giving up the struggle … the persons of the classes, which herd in the Congested Areas, are so situated that they must live there if they are to live at all … that being so, they continue to live there and to endure all the miseries that are entailed thereby.[91]

The 'white plague'

Most residents in crowded housing in the FMS and settlements were Chinese and comments on sanitary conditions and crowding, whilst acknowledging problems of supply, also opted for a measure of cultural determinism. Tuberculosis was seen to spread because 'Chinese' liked living in cramped quarters, spitting and recreational activities were conducive to its spread, and reluctance to seek medical care led to further transmission. A Selangor report from 1907, for instance, claimed that the habits of the Chinese fostered tuberculosis

> ... from their love of dark ill ventilated cubicles, the opium habit with its opportunity for catching the disease, and from the fact that many of their occupations are favourable to its ravages ... nor do the poorer classes, at any rate, seek admission to Hospitals until too late to benefit themselves, and it is from these advanced cases whose sputa are teeming with Tubercle Bacillus that such a large number apparently contract the disease, which is blown about in the dust of streets and houses, and places of public resort, and which the advent of the motor car consequently helps to spread.[92]

The image of tubercle bacilli 'blowing about' in the streets was a recurrent one in official discourse; Dr Finlayson, in giving evidence to the commission in 1917, spoke also of 'the actual baccili [sic] flying around the room'.[93] The concentration of infection and mortality in 'dying houses', the vulnerability of individuals in close contact with cases, and the difficulty of controlling air-borne infection, further influenced arguments for screening, providing quarantine for arrivals and repatriating tubercular patients rather than building sanitoria: 'Singapore is no place for a phthisical patient'.[94]

Despite the attention to nightsoil and sanitation, therefore, both the Simpson and Maxwell reports related poor housing also to the incidence of tuberculosis and other respiratory infections. The Maxwell Commission, in particular, characterising tuberculosis as the 'disease of darkness', drew on research findings from the United Kingdom and Europe (particularly Glasgow and Paris) to argue for the demolition or modification of houses. It recommended also that an expert on tuberculosis be appointed to the Muncipal Health Department to develop appropriate interventions to treat cases and prevent further transmission, and for tuberculosis to be declared a notifiable disease.

Tuberculosis and acute respiratory infections were a major cause of morbidity and mortality in all states (Table 4.3), although the full picture of morbidity was hindered by poor case detection, the limited number of pneumonia and other chest infections presented at clinics or outpatient departments, and lack of data on chest infections and lung disease other

than tuberculosis in summary statistics. Estimates in the FMS for 1910
suggest that around eight percent of all hospital deaths were due to
tuberculosis and perhaps as many as 24 percent to respiratory infections
from all causes, the consequence, the Federal Secretary of the FMS
maintained, of 'primitive habits and ignorance of all hygienic measures'
(i.e. spitting).[95] By contrast, figures for inpatients in all hospitals in the
Straits Settlements in 1920 indicated seven percent of cases with tuberculosis, and the disease accounted for 32 percent of all deaths; in 1924
the number of cases had increased by nearly 20 percent, with tuberculosis accounting for nearly ten percent of them, and for 41 percent
of deaths.[96]

Tuberculosis was believed to be far more prevalent than reported,
masked, it was argued, by other immediate causes of death such as
diarrhoeal disease and other co-infections.[97] Clarke argued that pneumonia deaths particularly often disguised tuberculosis, but pneumonia
was not well diagnosed either and attracted little official commentary.[98]
Again, essentialist notions of race converged with those of immunity and
disease: Indians for example, were believed, to be particularly suscep-
tible due to low 'resisting power' and the insanitary and crowded conditions of coolie lines. While most Chinese transmission occurred in town
cubicles, miners were also at risk due to crowding in mining *bangsals*,
(sheds, 'lines') and transmission was exacerbated owing to delays in presenting to hospital until late in the course of disease; meanwhile diseased
miners would continue to share a room with 'a crowd of other persons
and act as centres of infection'.[99]

Table 4.3 Tuberculosis deaths in government hospitals in the Straits
Settlements and Federated Malay States, 1927–1937

Year	Singapore City	Straits Settlements	FMS
1927	1,523	2,903	1,118
1928	1,411	2,727	1,074
1929	1,500	2,710	1,078
1930	1,622	2,795	1,061
1931	1,377	2,461	975
1932	1,088	2,081	919
1933	1,189	2,027	821
1934	1,253	2,120	894
1935	—[1]	2,077	1,441[2]
1936	—	2,181	1,488[2]
1937	—	2,268	1,413[2]

1 Separate figures for Singapore are not included in reports for 1935–1937.
2 Figures represent all inpatients, not deaths.
Sources: SSAR 1927–1937; FMSAR 1927–1938.

Inpatients with tuberculosis were not isolated, and while this presented a risk of cross-infection, segregation was rejected because it would result for patients in 'intolerable isolation from relatives and friends'. There was concern, however, that there were inadequate beds for patients with tuberculosis in large towns other than Kuala Lumpur and the settlements, where the climate was drier and therefore preferred for tubercular patients.

Early control measures to reduce transmission were somewhat punitive. Under the FMS Sanitary Board Enactment of 1907, people with tuberculosis were barred from using public bath houses or from working in bakeries or dairies, and the Federal Secretary maintained that no person should work or knowingly employ a person suffering from tuberculosis in a broad range of occupations: baker, butcher, gardener, cook, any other trade or occupation involving contact with articles of food or drink, washerman, tailor or any trade involving the manufacture of or contact with wearing apparel, or domestic servant, nurse, *jinrikisha* puller, or hackney carriage driver.[100] Government policy later emphasised the need for active case detection and encouraged voluntary notification, which by the late 1920s had resulted in health education leaflets, posters, public lectures on cleanliness, personal hygiene and the dangers of overcrowding, and films drawing attention to the risks and dangers of tuberculosis and the need for treatment.[101] Personal behaviour also came under scrutiny to reduce the transmission of respiratory infections, hence an anti-spitting campaign and a regulation from the 1920s that coffee shops provide spittoons.[102]

Housing, 1920–1938

The 1917 commission of inquiry into housing recommended that a Singapore Improvement Trust be established and a town planner appointed in order to take active steps to improve the city. The Land Acquisition Ordinance in 1920 and the appointment of a town planner created high expectations but with little immediate effect, and the 1920s were characterised by continued lobbying. The general impression created by contemporary reports, as in the *Straits Times*, is of administrative inertia and the continued misery of the underclass. In 1920, sanitary conditions in Singapore were being described as 'about a century behind the times';[103] the following year the city was referred to as 'perhaps one of the most behindhand ports in the world with regard to sanitation and health'.[104] Public pressure mounted following the release of the report of inquiry on tuberculosis, undertaken in 1923 by Drs Hoops, Finlayson, Hunter and Dawson, which again stressed the link between substandard accommodation and the prevalence of disease. Editorials claimed that people continued to live in 'holes not fit to shelter mere animals',[105] that legislation regarding housing and building standards, including the provision of back lanes, were 'preposterously restrictive' and 'owner-favouring', and that housing improvements benefited the wealthy rather than 'the great inarticulate masses of the poor'.[106] European admini-stration, the paper charged, was apathetic and bowed to local business self-interest from the time of the Simpson Report; administrators were portrayed as cowardly, ineffectual and greedy in their eagerness to fall in line with local pecuniary interests.[107] Statements regarding the acquisition of slum buildings and the establishment of a Housing Improvement Trust fuelled lack of confidence in the government. Legislation to set up the trust followed the example of the fiascos after the Simpson Report: a bill was prepared and rejected in 1919; then again in 1921, in 1923, and in 1924. Further delays occurred through 1925 and 1926 until the appointment of a Board of Trustees; a bill was finally introduced to the Legislative Council on 7 February 1927.[108]

The delay in introducing legislation for housing improvement related in part to the lack of conviction of some that there were any financial gains in public health measures, apparent reluctance to invest in capital improvements, opposition to government involvement in private sector issues, and some dis-ease with changes in social and political rela-tionships that might result. In a letter to the editor of *Straits Times*, W. Campbell argued that it was not possible to improve housing 'while the best interests of Singapore and Malaya have to do with cheap labour ... Cheap labour causes the earnings of the masses to be so low that it is not sufficient to permit them to be tenants of decent and healthy rooms while paying a fair proportion of their earnings as rent'.[109] Campbell and others maintained that it was impossible to build tenements which met ordinance requirements; provided water, sewage disposal, back lanes, light, and air; were located near work places; *and* were affordable:

(T)he tragic truth is that the majority of our working class population live under the conditions they do because they have a low standard of living, a standard to which most of us shut our eyes, since it is the standard of the East, and one which cannot be suddenly raised without revolutionary changes in a social structure which has been built up here in the course of a century.[110]

A new scheme had been announced in 1925 involving government acquisition and demolition of various blocks of shop-houses in the Rochore and Victoria Street area, the provision of drains and lanes, and sale of land for development. A number of blocks were also to be partially demolished to provide back lanes; in the Middle Road/North Bridge Road area houses without street frontage were to be demolished, whilst those facing onto streets would be left standing.[111] Confiscation and demolition of property was, according to Lornie, the Deputy President of the Municipal Commissioners, the only feasible means by which to deal with urban slums.[112] These interventions and related housing schemes were delayed however until the establishment of the Board of Trustees of the Singapore Improvement Trust.

From 1928 various slum clearance schemes were in operation. But changes were too few and introduced too late to have real impact on tuberculosis or other respiratory infections. While in some areas improvements reduced crowding, the tuberculosis rate fluctuated. In Georgetown Municipality in Penang in 1938, for example, deaths from tuberculosis had increased due, it was claimed, to continued congestion and poor housing since 'it is quite impossible for single families to pay the rents';[113] Penang authorities also claimed the rate was somewhat inflated due to the in-migration of people to Penang when sick and unemployed. Here estimations of overcrowding were given as a percentage (that is, of excess over estimated optimum occupancy), but the story, in the end, was the same. In 1938, 599 common lodging houses were licensed; according to municipal reports, 72 were overcrowded by at least ten percent, eight by more than 100 percent and one by more than 288 percent: 'It is inconceivable that human beings would live under conditions endured by the sub-tenants unless it was forced on them by economic necessity'.[114] For this accommodation, men might pay $5 per month, half their salary, to live near their workplace. In the FMS, authorities claimed in the late 1930s that there had been 'radical improvement' of conditions which was 'one of the most potent measures' against communicable diseases,[115] effectively reducing the high mortality in towns. But rates remained high, and respiratory infections including tuberculosis still contributed in 1940 to around 25 percent of the death rate and had not yielded to public health interventions. Housing and related infections remained a public health problem post-war.

Surveillance and public space

In general, the state's concern was with domestic matters that spilled, like sewage, into public space, when they constituted a public health hazard. Sleeping arrangements became a state interest in terms of tuberculosis because crowding enhanced transmission and, since tubercle bacilli 'blew about', anyone might be infected. Other public health campaigns and preventive measures were sporadic and were enacted in public spaces; issues within the domestic sphere that might impact upon their spread were largely left alone. So it was with cholera, smallpox, and plague: highly infectious diseases that had a high fatality rate and were easily spread, which required energetic state intervention during epidemics and for prevention. For these diseases, the metaphors of war, clichéd in the discourse of medicine, are most appropriate, and in the absence of real wars and battles that stripped the colonists of the need for Pax Britannia, it was politically helpful – and economically fundamental – to fight infectious disease.

Food hygiene and safety was another example of the way in which public health was defined and surveillance extended in its interests. Food hygiene was regarded as important given its contribution of diarrhoeal diseases and typhoid. The focus was on food prepared and cooked in urban public space, for many cubicles were so poorly provided with facilities that people primarily ate food cooked by hawkers.[116] The surveillance of the household, hence domestic issues relating to food safety as well as nutrition, were left to home visitors through the maternal and child health programs (see Chapter 7).

Sanitary Boards were responsible for hygienic standards of the markets and food stalls. Food was often contaminated. In the late nineteenth century meat was frequently described as 'unfit for human food' and there were regular reports of infected fish and other seafood, and worm-infested or maggotty meat, leading to increased pressure on municipal authorities to police the sale of food.[117] Milk caused especial concern to health authorities, because of the risk of bacterial contamination through adulteration from watering down prior to sale (that is to say, through the use of unclean water), and because of the possible risk of the transmission of tuberculosis.

Most tuberculosis was pulmonary (phthisis) and there was little bovine tuberculosis in the colonies, as Simpson had pointed out.[118] Even so, the conditions for the storage and bottling of milk were poor and the risk of microbial infection was certainly high. Simpson's report presented a picture of poorly constructed, dark and dirty cowsheds; milking cans, measures, bottles and lids stored under the beds of the milkmen (though this arguably was as much a question of matter out of place as a hygiene risk); bottles and cans washed in roadside water or from well water contaminated through surface drainage; a dead calf in one cowshed; buffalo teats covered with manure; ground contamination from human faeces as well as animal manure; milk pails used for carrying animal food and well water as well as milk for sale. Simpson argued that the payment of fines for keeping dirty premises would not have great effect, since this would be less expensive than improving the premises, and he recommended instead wider power to enable the municipality to demolish buildings on unsuitable sites, order repairs and alterations to buildings, and ensure that only licensed dairymen and milk sellers operated.[119] Like the recommendations for housing, this was pretty well ignored.

The Singapore dairies were not exceptional. Reports from elsewhere in the colonies drew attention to continuing 'deplorable' sanitary conditions and problems of adulteration.[120] In Perak this was addressed to a degree when in 1907 a government dairy was opened in Ipoh to check the sale of watered milk.[121] A proposal to open a similar dairy in Kuala Lumpur was rejected, and in all other states government intervention was limited to the inspection of premises and the collection of milk samples to check for adulteration or contamination, primarily to prevent typhoid.

Public health regulations and the association between living conditions and disease enabled increased surveillance that included incursions into private space, although police were already empowered in the settlements in the early 1880s to inspect households, and to fine householders whose residences were in 'filthy and unwholesome states'. Household inspections were not necessarily diligent, however, and there were regular requests to government to increase measures to 'accomplish and enforce complete cleansing of street drains' and ensure the 'disinfection and deodorisation of filthy and polluted back yards in the native part of the town'.[122] The task was not easy, and hygiene and sanitation surveillance, in contrast to cholera, for example, lacked a sense of emergency that might have bred compliance. This was keenly felt by public health workers in the late 1920s, during the hookworm campaign, as they sought to convince people to give faecal specimens, take medicine, build (and use) latrines, and wear shoes.[123]

On occasion too police and sanitary inspectors were paid bribes by householders and businessmen (milkmen, food vendors) to avoid prosecution and maintain licences, and medical officers constantly complained that there were too few sanitary inspectors, assistants and related public health workers to be effective. In Kuala Lumpur, there were regular rumours about bribes paid to members of the Sanitary Board by stall holders and other food vendors to maintain licences;[124] in places such as Trengganu and Kelantan, accusations were usually of inefficiency rather than corruption, due to the enormous size of the task, inadequate and incompetent staff, and low budget allocations.[125] The chairman of the Sanitary Board in Kota Bharu in 1914, for example, defended the work of the board against accusations of corruption in terms of the difficulty it faced imposing public health measures in an 'overgrown village' where residential and commercial buildings were mixed, where drainage was largely provided by earth drains, and where there were no systems for the removal of nightsoil, no state land for dumping rubbish, no town water supply, no incinerators for rubbish, and too few staff:

> The wonder to me is that the San(itary) Inspector keeps the place as clean as it is ... if I had *carte blanche*, I would simply pull the whole place down and rebuild it with the aid of the Survey and Engineering Departments. That, however, is a utopian dream.[126]

CHAPTER 5

Sickness and the world of work: The men on the estates

The transfer of authority of the Straits Settlements from the India Office to the Colonial Office and the extension of British suzerainty over the Malay States, coincident with industrial expansion and its demand for raw materials, created the preconditions for the rapid growth of extractive industries and plantations, including sugar, tea, coconut and rubber. The rate of development, the amount of land opened up and the acreage under plantation depended very much upon the availability of workers; this became an imperative from the turn of the century with the growth of the rubber industry and its greedy absorption of labour. Tamil men were recruited from south India as estate workers; Chinese, Javanese and local Malays also worked on estates. Their working and living conditions and the impact of these on health and illness are of especial concern here.

Recruitment from India

The Indian Immigration Fund was set up with compulsory payments from planters to facilitate migration to provide estates with sufficient tappers and other labourers. Legislation introduced in 1877 and modified from 1885 allowed the Straits Immigration Agent to register and grant licences to recruiters who were sent to India from Malaya to secure labourers on three-year contracts, after which period of indenture they might return home or continue to work in Malaya as 'free' labourers. A second important means of recruitment was through the *kangany* system, whereby the *kangany*, the labour overseer, was sent by the Malayan estate to recruit workers, often through his own kinship networks or familiarity with particular villages. Contracted workers were transported to special *kangany* camps in Madras or Negapatam,

medically examined, then given passage to Malaya by the Indian
Immigration Fund. Labourers docked at Port Swettenham in Selangor
or Penang, and after a three-week period of quarantine, were transferred to the estate which had recruited them. Their passage and other
advances were not recoverable, and until 1910 they were indentured to
the estate for a specified period. The *kangany* was paid a fee by the estate,
between 5 and 15 rupees per recruited labourer.[1]

The fund also enabled the immigration of free labourers, covering the
expenses of recruitment and passage, maintaining homes for 'decrepit'
and unemployed labourers, their children, and orphans of labourers,
assisting labourers in need, and meeting the costs of repatriation.[2] Since
unemployment was relatively uncommon until the 1920s, the need for
homes was limited, and the primary purpose of the fund was to recruit
labourers rather than provide for their welfare. Under the conditions of
recruitment, labourers were employed either for 300 days or one year,
working 9-hour days and – under the terms of the Labour Enactment of
1904 – were required to work no more than 26 days per calendar month.
By contrast, contracts for Indian coolies sent to Sumatran rubber estates
were indebted to their employers for five or six years before their debt of
passage and cash advance were repaid. Labourers were to receive mosquito nets, a sun hat, coat, other basic items of clothing, a blanket, food,
medical treatment and accommodation. Chinese agricultural labourers
were also indentured under the terms of an agreement between the
United Kingdom and China in effect from 1904–1914;[3] they were usually
contracted to work for 360 days per annum, not necessarily consecu-
tively, for $30 annual salary, and their recruitment included a repayable
advance of $19.50 for passage and the free provision of food, a mosquito
net and clothes.[4]

From 1890, the Indian Immigration Fund agent or his officers were
empowered to inspect estates and to make inquiries regarding the treatment of labourers, their housing, food, and the provision of medical
care, hospitals and sanitation. As a result the documentation of conditions on estates is extensive, far more complete than that available for
other worksites in the colonies. As I explore in this chapter, there was
considerable transgression of the contractual obligations to labourers,
which resulted in a series of inquiries into conditions of employment
and alleged ill-treatment.[5]

Death, disease and Indian dispositions

From the late nineteenth century, the rubber estates sustained exceedingly high death rates; in some areas, half the workforce would die
within a year of arrival in Malaya. Officials attributed this primarily to

malaria but also to diseases of poor hygiene, and they occasionally temporarily closed estates to prevent further infection. Until the turn of the century, however, the relative contribution of malaria and other infections to the death rate was contested. Many planters argued that it reflected the poor selection of labourers rather than the unhealthy conditions of the estates, and estate managers and government officials together argued that, whilst the health of labourers deteriorated on the estates for various proximate reasons, all labourers, both free and inden-tured or 'statute' coolies, looked 'equally wretched' on arrival in Penang, and their poor prior physical condition and purported cultural practices regarding diet and hygiene contributed to their illness and death.[6]

European understandings of Tamil cultural practices and national characteristics permeated explanations of the incidence of death and disease. The disproportionately high rate of hospitalisation and death among Tamil labourers in Negri Sembilan in 1899, for example, relative to other residents of the state, was attributed to poor physique and low resistance to disease, the result, according to one commentator, of 'wholesale inbreeding'.[7] The Commission of Inquiry into the conditions on estates in 1890 argued that '(t)he cooly cares little or nothing about cleanliness or ordinary sanitary precautions',[8] and Tamil labourers were reputed to be poorly nourished because of strict dietary regulations, preference for toddy (distilled palm wine or other alcohol) over food, 'stinting' on food, and the alleged disinclination of unmarried men to cook for themselves or employ a cook.[9] Further, the selection of labourers was not well supervised. While emigration officers denied that selection procedures were remiss, immigrant workers were often sick on arrival. There was some criticism, too, particularly to the 1890 inquiry, that men were recruited without appropriate experience: they were characterised as 'bad material ... beggars, weavers, dhobies, diseased persons and children, instead of agricultural labourers accustomed to out of door work'.[10] Labourers substantiated this in their own repre-sentations and complaints of inappropriate recruitment:

> Men flung themselves on the ground, and numbers endeavoured to make complaints. Making every allowance for the circumstances, there could be no doubt that discontent prevailed. Many of the men appeared strong and well grown, but as a whole the coolies were far from presenting an appearance of happiness ... the initial grievance was nearly always the same – that the man had followed some other trade in his own country, expected to follow it here, and could not do the work now required of him.[11]

A 1900 account also described arriving labourers as emaciated, 'famine stricken', and 'old decrepit men who should never have been allowed through the depot in India',[12] and as late as December 1938, the

Deputy Controller of Labour maintained that the ages of newly immigrant labourers were often inappropriate, that their health was poor, and that free immigrants were not subject to medical examination before embarkation.[13] Neither the settlements' nor states' governments had specific authority over ordinary shipboard passengers travelling from India to Malaya, although all intending immigrants were placed in quarantine on arrival and a small proportion were repatriated. Others were treated while in quarantine – this was the case for those with hookworm, although recruited labourers were also given anti-helminths prior to departure.[14]

Deaths were supposed to be registered, usually through the local police post, but this was not always so and record-keeping of sickness and death was somewhat casual. In consequence, the good health of estates, or its absence, was often 'a matter of rumour'. Planters resented being required to report to government on conditions, minimised local factors that might have contributed to morbidity and mortality, and painted an image of labour that fitted poorly with the scant statistics.[15] Hence the comment of the District Surgeon of Perak in 1901 that 'if they (estate labourers) are really cheerful, contented, well-fed and well-clothed and if the hospitals are really in excellent order, the death rate does not receive, but requires more explanation. It is to be hoped more care will be taken in future selection and supervision.'[16]

Estate life

Conditions on the estates varied. Usually, labourers lived in 'lines', rows of crudely built huts or dormitories which lacked proper provisions for cooking and storing food. They were often in a 'disgraceful state', 'very smelly in places'.[17] Household waste was dumped around the grounds; without latrines, adults defecated in neighbouring fields, children indiscriminately around the huts. A nearby river or stream provided water for cooking, drinking, bathing and clothes' washing; and huts were often located in areas proximate to those ideal for mosquito breeding (Figures 5.1 and 5.2). Overcrowding was also common:

> On one estate the building is divided into a number of rooms about 10 feet square, in which six people are usually put. Other rooms in the same building are 20 feet by 14 feet, and in one of these eighteen people were living, men and women indiscriminately. Sometimes three married couples are together in one small room; in other cases one or two couples, as well as several single men.[18]

In some places conditions were far worse. At Malaka Pindah Estate, Malacca, for example, in 1890, one of the two buildings used for accommodation for labourers was a converted cow shed, its sides

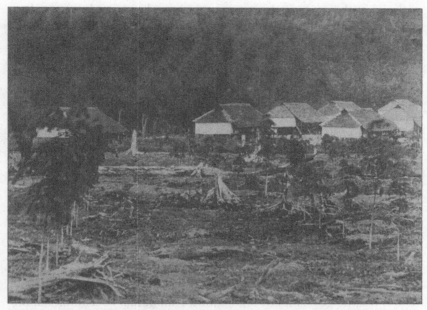

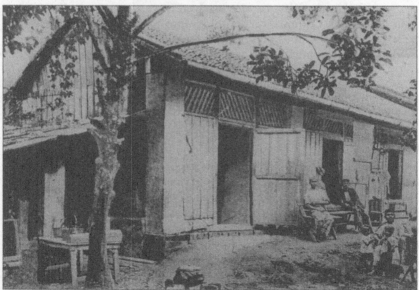

Figure 5.1 Coolie lines on Bukit Ijok Estate, showing their position at the foot of the hills and the mouth of a ravine. Printed with permission of Arkib Negara Malaysia, Kuala Lumpur, N 217/82, p. 66.

Figure 5.2 Coolie lines on a Singapore plantation. Printed with permission of National Archives, Singapore. Photograph No. 29439, NA 25/5.

enclosed 'with rags or sticks or any rubbish, and with no drainage what-ever'.[19] Reports of estates over the next 30 or more years provide a con-tinuing bleak picture. Rubana Estate, Seremban, in 1904, for example, lacked potable water, its labour lines were poorly built and damp, and while hospital facilities and a dispensary were provided, the building and its grounds were dirty enough to warrant an order from the Protector of Labour to build a new hospital.[20] On Damansara Estate in 1911, accord-ing to A. S. Haynes, 'the drains round certain lines are stinking and awfully bad, many were poorly kept, and some lines lacked drains at all'.[21] The lines on Lye Whatt's Estate, consisting of three buildings of mud walls and attap roofs, were dank. The huts were divided into small rooms for two to four people each, and either lacked benches for sleeping or had only benches in ill repair. On Batu Kawan Estate, Province Wellesley, the men's barracks were attap dormitories with earthen floors, with 45 men each allocated their own sleeping platform. Several women slept in the barracks with their husbands too, in the absence of suffcient one-room huts for couples. In some barracks, men slept on a continuous platform to gain storage space, ventilation was poor, and overcrowding must have resulted in the rapid spread of viral infections. On many estates, despite government regulations, rudimentary accommodation was provided by the labourers themselves.[22]

In 1910, a new Commission of Inquiry into conditions for Chinese and Javanese labourers on Chinese estates looked in greater detail at accom-modation and sanitation. Its summary was, on the whole, uncritical:

> As a rule the labourer is fairly well-housed in lines raised some feet from the ground. The lines of most of the estates visited were satisfactory in type, airy and fairly clean. In several cases cooking was done in the covered verandah of the lines. This is not desirable, as much refuse and dirty water are thrown into the drains.[23]

The Health Officer for Perak in his report to the commission gave a less generous account, however, and described the Chinese estate lines in Krian as 'scandalous', 'mere hovels (where) sanitation is conspicuous by its absence', 'hotbed(s) of contagion'.[24] Later reports (from the 1920s) indicate that substantial improvements were made, often concomitantly with preventive health measures for the control of hookworm or malaria and as a result of increased pressure by government officers on estates.

Disease on the lines

Poor hygiene and sanitation led to high rates of diarrhoeal disease and helminthic infections, particularly ankylostomiasis (hookworm). Although some contemporary commentators argued that coolies were reluctant to use the latrines because of 'terrors of darkness ... sickness-producing odors and ... restrictions of caste',[25] lines usually lacked latrines and as a result soil pollution was pervasive, the grounds around the lines and beyond were dirty and infected. Poor drainage systems, the disruption of undergrowth, and swampy ground favoured the breeding of *Anopheles* mosquitoes, the vector of malaria, and hence the incidence of malaria was also typically high despite considerable variation with respect to both the vector and endemicity.

It was (and is) difficult to assess with any precision rates of morbidity and mortality, however, or to evaluate their putative causes. Death returns were required only of estates greater than one hundred acres, representing a fraction of the total estates: in 1924 it was estimated that 1,340 estates were this large, 1,700 were between 25 and 100 acres, and some 100,000 to 110,000 were less than 25 acres. Returns often excluded Chinese contract labour, and included days in hospital rather than days sick, leading to gross underestimates in morbidity. 'Native-owned' (Malay) estates typically sent in nil sickness and death returns; and a death was excluded where it occurred after the labourer had left the estate. Finally, the skewed demographic structure of the estate population by age and sex depressed the death rate, and estate returns to the District Officer did not always include information on dependents. Official estimates set the estate death rate at around 25–30 per thousand for much of this period, but it may have been higher; in Selangor in 1912, for instance, among 61 estates employing at least 200 labourers, 43 had a mortality rate of greater than 75 per thousand, two mortality rates of 222, and one, 274.5.[26]

As noted earlier, epidemics of infectious diseases such as smallpox and cholera accounted for sporadic peaks in the death rate, but they were far less important than endemic disease.[27] For example, in 1906 the highest death rates on estates in the FMS in Selangor (300) and Negri Sembilan (214) were due to the high incidence of malaria.[28] The death rate at Sungei Krudda Estate, Kuala Kangsar, Perak, was 220 per thousand the same year due to dysentery and diarrhoea. On Kuala Pergau Estate in Kelantan, 32 *sinkeh* (Chinese labourers) of a total workforce of 247 died between 12 September 1912 and January 1913 from 'bowel disease', leading to recommendations for improved sanitation, an improved estate hospital and the establishment of a small mortuary, and statewide the death rate of Indian labourers was high (Table 5.1).[29]

Living conditions on the estates – the crude huts, their cramped interior living space, and the lack of latrines, potable water and rubbish disposal – contributed to the transmission and prevalence of disease. Estate workers often took water direct from streams, and wells were rarely protected from seepage and pollution. Latrines – 'dark, dirty and

Table 5.1 Death rates of all Indian labourers, Federated Malay States, 1911 and 1914

State	Death rate 1911 (per 1,000)	Death rate 1914 (per 1,000)
Perak	49.8	25.9
Selangor	60.3	28.5
Negri Sembilan	195.6	70.9[1]
Pahang	109.5	24.7

1   However, the death rate had been down to 53.2 in 1913.
Source: Sel. Sec 1313/1915.

at a distance from lines'[30] – were not commonly used, and the 1924 Commission of Inquiry into health conditions on estates in the FMS reported that: 'Some managers are obviously interested in this detail, and succeed by mingling chaff, persuasion and threats in getting their labourers to use latrines, despite the hereditary disinclination of the Tamil labourer to obey the calls of nature anywhere but in an open field. Other managers … neither know or care.'[31]

To reduce the risk of infection of cholera, typhoid, and plague as well as endemic parasitic and microbial infections, and for more aesthetic reasons to improve conditions around the labour lines, estates were required by the early 1930s to construct brick or cement wells fitted with pumps, to provide brick drains around the lines, and to provide pit latrines, including small latrines for children, near the lines: 'Every attempt has been made to interest estate managers in the real economy of preventive medicine … at first it was found (that) the coolie lines on a number of estates were in such an appalling insanitary condition as to require complete demolition and replacement.'[32] Estates were also required to employ a qualified dresser to visit the lines daily to treat minor ailments and to send labourers sick for more than 24 hours to hospital; to enable this a bullock dray or launch was to be available.[33] In addition, labourers were to be examined and treated twice yearly for helminthic infection: hookworm was estimated to be particularly high.[34]

The 1924 Commission of Inquiry into estate health attributed the high death rate to the combined effects of malaria, the size of estates (hence the large areas of land which needed to be controlled to reduce the risk of infection), 'insanitary habits' and 'lack of discipline in personal matters', 'indifference' to medical services on the part of labourers, their free movement and the role of local migration in the spread of infection, and the dependence of estate managers on the government to take action to improve health.[35] Other government sources perceived a less complex epidemiological picture, and primarily blamed concurrent malaria and helminthic infections.

Malaria took the heaviest toll on lives. The ability and willingness of estates to control mosquito breeding by means of oiling and spraying, and variation in local ecological conditions, the predominant vector, and vector behaviour led to considerable variation in malaria morbidity and mortality. Everywhere, though, malaria was endemic and immigrant labourers, apparently immunologically naive to *Plasmodium falciparum* malaria, if not to *P. vivax*, suffered severely.

Immigrants came from regions of India where malaria was endemic and therefore should have had some immunity to both *P. vivax* and *P. falciparum*. However, Curtin's data provides us with some clues to the death rates of immigrants. At around the turn of the century in India hospitalisation of cases was predominantly for vivax malaria. From 1895 to 1904 among British troops the rate of hospital admission for malaria was 291.4 per thousand, but the death rate was only 0.62.[36] Malaria in India therefore was characterised by high morbidity but low mortality; by contrast in Malaya, there was constant recruitment of labour and high mortality on the estates, with *P. falciparum* probably predominating. In Batu Gajah, Perak, in 1933 and 1934, for example, there were around five cases of falciparum to every four of vivax.[37]

Although the impact of malaria on estate health derives from highly suspect statistical information, later figures provide corroboration. Malcolm Watson, whose distinguished career in British Malaya included his appointment as Chief Medical Officer of the FMS, maintained that death rates of 200 per thousand on rubber estates around 1910 were not uncommon (for 1908 and 1909, see Table 5.2); the rate was 185 per thousand for all estates in Negri Sembilan in 1911.[38] Morbidity was extremely high around this period: in 1914, for example, Watson, using figures provided by the Rubber Growers' Association, claimed that 939

Table 5.2 Death rates, Indian labourer on rubber estates, Federated Malay States, 1908 and 1909

State	Indentured 1908	Unindentured 1908	Indentured 1909	Unindentured 1909
Perak	84.8	48.9	77.5	38.5
Selangor	70.1[1]	64.5	38.1[1]	35.0
Negri Sembilan	24.3	117.1	34.1	85.5
Pahang	214.3	—	20.4[1]	58.2

1 Public Works Department. All other figures are for estates.
Source: Parr, *Report of the Commission*, p. 45.

Table 5.3 Malaria cases among workers, British Malaya, 1914–1924

Year	Average labour force	Hospital inpatients	Hospital outpatients	Total no. treated	Percentage of labour force treated
1914	658	815	5,370	6,185	939
1915	804	900	3,235	4,137	513
1916	811	933	1,558	2,491	312
1917	770	719	546	1,265	162
1918	639	718	315	1,063	149
1919	825	614	10	624	75
1920	916	1,236	—	1,236	132
1921	780	609	—	609	77
1922	620	369	—	369	53
1923	577	56	—	56	9
1924	557	6	—	6	1.08

Source: Watson, *Some Pages from the History of the Prevention of Malaria*, p. 18.

percent of the labour force were treated for malaria per annum – that is, each worker averaged nine to ten episodes of fever each year (see Table 5.3). By 1924, following extensive environmental control measures, it was only 1.08 percent, and Watson was euphoric.[39] The figures possibly exaggerate the trend, but they reflect the general pattern.

However, as late as 1932, malaria cases in the FMS comprised over 25 percent of all hospital cases.[40] In the UFMS, malaria emerges as even more important. Figures for Kedah and Perlis for 1927–28 indicate that 37.5 percent of all deaths were due to malaria. State hospital returns for Kelantan for 1927–1931 show the same trend, with malaria by far the most common cause of hospitalisation and with the highest case fatality rate;[41] in 1937 malaria was still responsible for around one-third of all hospitalisations and 25 percent of deaths in the state. Not all malaria was due to environmental disruption following the opening up of forest land for rubber, but the broad environmental and ecological changes that occurred with the establishment of new settlements and changes in mode of production consequent upon colonisation led to the increased incidence of this disease. Hence, as noted, the migration of apparent non-immunes into malaria-endemic areas, and the migration of para-sitaemic labourers to other areas, were both factors which affected trans-mission; the destruction of primary jungle and the maintenance of pools of water in secondary growth (*lalang*), and changes in population density and patterns of settlement, all resulted in increased cases.[42]

Various mechanisms were instituted to control transmission, but estate managers were often reluctant to follow through, as I shall discuss below. Their resistance to innovation and change, and to the regular commit-

m⋯at of funds to maintain anti-malarial activities, led to repeated moves
ag⋯nst estate management by government, including from the 1920s
the⋯emporary closure of estates where the incidence of disease had
ɾea⋯ɾed epidemic proportions.[43]

The economics of illness

Disease carries an economic cost. For this reason, employers shared with
colonial medical and health officers concern about the health risks on
⋯tatɾs. But they were conservative and reluctant to invest in sanitation
or to employ dressers to meet the most immediate needs of those
injured or sick, insisting that the government was responsible for
environmental control:

> I Jntil sites have been found or made healthy, money spent on such things
> as drains etc. will be of no value in reducing sickness ... to ask the estate to
> brick drains and build wells for new lines, which are practically under trial, or
> for old lines which are likely to be abandoned, especially where there is not
> the slightest reason to support [the proposition that] they will influence the
> health of the labour force, seems extraordinary.[44]

In response government spent much time demonstrating rhetorically
the cost of illness, to persuade planters to comply:

> In this country malaria is accountable for ⅓ of all deaths recorded, and
> assuming the death rate to be 2 percent, this means that at least 20,000
> persons are attacked annually ... But the economic aspect of the disease is of
> yet greater import. It is hardly too much to say that nearly every native
> inhabitant of the country is attacked by malaria once or oftener every year.
> The incapacity resulting from the attacks lasts from a few to many days and
> the material losses resulting from the suspension of labour capacity of such
> individuals must amount in the year to enormous sums.[45]

Throughout the colonial period, officials returned to this theme.
Cameron, who chaired the 1890 inquiry, claimed that estate managers
and owners were mindful of the relationship between health expenditure
and profits, between low production costs and a healthy labour force,
hence 'it was an economically sound proposition to spend money on
health measures'.[46] In 1901 the Acting Resident General for the FMS,
W. H. Treacher, argued that 'probably the most important matter in
connection with the treatment of the free coolie ... relat[es] to his health
... Apart from the point of view of humane dealing with the coolie, the
monetary loss to the employer due to death and sickness is very great'.[47]
The British Adviser of Kelantan similarly maintained that two men

without parasitic infection could do the work of three with infection, and quoted published studies of the monetary value of healthy labour to harness his arguments for increased health infrastructure and personnel.[48] Watson, in response to the drop in the incidence of and mortality from malaria from 1910 to 1920, argued that: 'However we look at the matter, it would appear that the whole cost of the subsoil drainage was repaid and probably much more than repaid in the year 1919 ... In other words, apart from the saving of human life and conservation of "bark", the cost of subsoil drainage has probably been repaid several times over in the past five years.'[49]

The politics of health

Immigration policy emphasised the recruitment of workers; given contemporary understandings of the capabilities and roles of men and women, this meant primarily the recruitment of men. But women were also recruited both as workers and as dependants, and children who travelled to Malaya with their parents were also employed as general agricultural labourers. Although the Labour Code of the FMS prohibited the employment of children under the age of ten, detailed regulations were not introduced to control their employment until 1922, when the Children's Enactment specified weights that could be carried by them and tasks potentially injurious to their health.

Estates were liable for all medical expenses incurred by dependants as well as workers, although 'women's health' – that is, maternal and infant health – became important as estates began to look to their own workforce to reproduce itself, as the costs of importing labour rose. Women received little care during pregnancy and confinement, even so. They suffered from anaemia due to malaria, hookworm and poor nutrition, and in general their health status was 'suboptimal', aggravated by frequent childbearing.[50] Maternity allowances provided in the Labour Codes of the colonies from the 1920s allowed for one month's leave before and one month after delivery, paid at a rate determined by the earning power of the woman in the preceding six months. These were introduced to improve women's reproductive health and outcome of pregnancy, although they were later seen as a mechanism to encourage women's migration, family formation and the establishment of a more permanent labour force. Since the allowances were related to the previous six months' work, they were subject to considerable criticism for providing 'additional inducement for the woman to work at a time when she is least fitted to do so and at a period when such work is likely to produce the most deterimental effect on the future health and well-being of two lives, if not to produce death itself'.[51] Women often used the money paid at the time of delivery – around $12 in the 1930s – for 'anything but the care of themselves and the impending infant', raising questions as to whether benefit should not be given in kind instead of money payments.[52] But most families working on estates were dependent upon the wages of both women and men. The additional financial burden of an extra child, it was argued, put pressure on women to return to work as soon as possible, and so to cease breastfeeding early, thereby jeopardising the child's chance of survival.[53] The infant mortality rate became an increasing concern to estate managers as well as government officials, leading in some cases – as on Cauly Estate in Perak – to a bonus payment of $5 to women for every child still alive at three months of age.

Cruelty and violence

Regulations proposed by employers reflected their interest in maintaining labour rather than their sense of responsibility for occupational health. Technically estate responsibility for labourers' health continued to the termination of employment and covered illness immediately following its cessation, a provision intended to prevent estates from firing sick labourers to avoid paying for their medical care. In the FMS and in parts of the UFMS, the Labour Code stipulated that where hospitalisation was required after cessation of employment, estates were to pay for expenses of free labourers within 10 days of departure and for contract coolies within 7 days. But such rules and regulations also served plantation interests and increased control over workers. The Kelantan Planters Association, for instance, in 1913, proposed that coolies wishing to leave an estate should have a medical certificate of fitness for travel; if not fit, the labourer should be 'retained' on the estate to receive medical attention.[54] This imperious treatment reflected the wider propensity of planters and managers to treat labourers simply as estate property, and the Chinese Protectorate saw in this proposal a means by which labourers could be retained against their will, such that the medical certificate served as a leave pass inhibiting further their mobility and freedom.[55]

Plantation managers frequently ignored regulations and recommendations of authorities such as the Protector of Chinese and the state health officers that were designed to reduce sickness and provide for the care of sick workers. Owners and managers were reported to be 'absolutely indifferent to the welfare of their labourers, indentured or otherwise'.[56] But reluctance to treat sick labourers was simply the most subtle abuse. On some estates, labour conditions were exceptionally harsh and brutality and violence common. The 1890 Commission of Inquiry, presided over by Maurice A. Cameron, gathered substantial evidence of abuse and ill-treatment of labourers by the *tyndal* (foremen)

on both European- and Chinese-managed estates, although such abuses
were claimed to occur without the knowledge of the employer. On Tan
Kang Kok Estate, Penang, for example, men were kept for up to nine
years against their will because of indebtedness, and a labourer was
starved to death in a stable at the back of the employer's house. The
hospital on this estate was 'a little shed in the stable yards of the
employer's private house. The dresser was from the neighboring estate
and [was] not always called over if the cooly was dying – the employer
"did not care to run to the expense for nothing" '.[57]

Further reports of poor living conditions, abuse and ill treatment, and
unacceptably high morbidity and mortality rates, led to a second inquiry
into the Conditions of Indentured Labour in the Federated Malay States,
concerned predominantly with Javanese and Chinese labourers, held in
1910 and presided over by C. W. C. Parr. The commission concluded
that, in contrast to the charges of gross abuse that emerged in 1890,
there was 'little actual ill-treatment'.[58] But the evidence brought before
the commission included examples of pay withheld or reduced as
punishment for uncompleted tasks, pay withheld until the end of the
contract period to discourage absconsions, labourers 'encouraged' to
forgo their days of rest, and labourers deprived of medical care or
penalised when sick.

In addition, a number of reports to the inquiry document explicit
cruelty and ill-treatment. W. D. Barnes, the British Resident of Pahang,
claimed that labourers on Chinese estates were 'ill-treated and ill fed',[59]
and 'cruelty and abuses' described as 'severe and ferocious' occurred on
Kurau and Krian River Estates in Perak, both at the hands of headmen
in charge of labour lines and of employers. Ayer Tawan Estate in
Sitiawan, Perak, which employed 83 Javanese including 15 women, at
night locked the labourers into two dirty dormitories, bolted from the
outside and with barbed wire on the roof and the top of walls of buildings. The labourers were routinely beaten and fined. On Saga Estate in
Negri Sembilan, Chinese labourers were confined to a palisade from
6pm to 6am. Confinement of men on estates and mines to prevent
absconsion was common, and it was argued that the differential death
rates between free and contract labourers were due to the absconsion of
the healthiest indentured labourers (see Table 5.2 above).[60] In Parit
Buntar Hospital, seven out of ten labourers from Sama Gagah Estate
had marks on their legs, arms or back from beatings, provoked either
because they allegedly did not work well enough or because they were
too sick to work; all were in hospital with diarrhoeal disease.[61] Sick
labourers from this estate were habitually referred to hospital late; it also
had a high rate of gonorrhoeal ophthalmia due, it was argued, to
infected bathing places. Other examples of cruelty, of men who were

handcuffed, beaten, whipped, kicked, forced to eat excrement, and raped, suggest the extent to which general physical and sexual terror was used to control the workforce. Whilst the source material is silent, it is likely that sexual abuse was extended to women as well as men.[62] For many workers, indentured employment on the estates was akin to slavery, resulting in the local Chinese term for the system, evocative of the conditions, as *kuai* or *mai chu-chai* ('selling young pigs').[63]

Abuses and brutality on European estates were less well documented but also occurred. The general manager of Duff Development, Kelantan, Mr Marriner, was dismissed in 1907 following a report by the Vice-Consul at Senggora, W. R. Wood, into his alleged assault of employees; he was described as a man 'absolutely hated by every person, white and brown, who has any dealings with him', who acted in an 'arbitrary and inconciliatory way', delivered corporal punishment to coolies, and withheld medicine as a further punishment.[64] Elsewhere sick labourers had food costs deducted from their salaries, were subjected to other pay abuses, and their referral to hospital was delayed; despite legal provisions, sick coolies were not infrequently discharged from work and then drifted unemployed, sick and dying to government hospitals. Labourers were often in a weak position to lay charges, since the person most likely to perpetrate ill-treatment, the labour foreman or the estate manager, was usually present when workers met with outside officers, and was likely to deny the abuses at the time and retaliate later.[65] Complaints were therefore most often made in hospital when employment had terminated.

Alcohol and opium

Conditions may have been intolerable for some estate workers, leading to their absconsion, but many more sought temporary retreats in alcohol or opium. Alcohol was readily available on the estates, usually in the form of palm wine ('toddy'), *samsu* (rice spirits) or other stronger liquor. Conventional wisdom held that 'Indian labourers will walk a long way for a drink of an evening', and estates usually provided toddy shops on site, which served a number of purposes, including profiteering and the extension of managerial control over workers' movement and association.[66] Toddy was sold for around ten cents a bottle in 1915, when rubber tappers and weeders on estates were being paid as little as 20 cents a day for their labour; they therefore spent half their cash income on alcohol. On some estates, such as Ayer Tawan Estate in Sitiawan, liquor was given to indentured labourers in lieu of wages, and they were also sold opium on credit. Given their wages, it was virtually impossible for these men to honour their debts.[67]

Government authorities sought to reduce the amount of alcohol consumed by Tamil estate labourers by introducing an import duty and controlling the sale of spirits to labourers,[68] both to reduce indebtedness and because of notions of its immorality. The 'toddy problem' caused further concern following reports of drunkenness on estates and allegations of the adulteration of alcohol and its association with dysentery and diarrhoea. Legislation was introduced enabling the prosecution of toddy shops for selling over-acidic toddy and for keeping dirty premises: premises were supposed to be clean, set back from the road, and provide plenty of seating; ordinary houses, shop-houses, or old coolies lines were regarded as inadequate. At the time of an inquiry into alcohol in 1915 and 1916, a licensing board was operating only in Negri Sembilan, and the government exercised little control over the sale of alcohol other than its basic composition (not more than ten percent alcohol, not more than 0.8 percent acetic acid).[69] A spate of deaths in the Langat Group Hospital, apparently alcohol-related, triggered an official inquiry in Selangor, although the association was, the Senior Health Officer Dr Lucy claimed, 'theatrical and over-stated'.[70] The inquiry established that the deaths were not due to toddy poisoning and that stale and highly acid toddy would not lead to death; but it also revealed the degree of drunkenness and the general poor conditions of health and hygiene on the estates, provoking much discussion about raising the price of toddy to force labourers to save their money 'for a more useful purpose'.[71]

Records of estate inspections for the FMS and settlements provide little documentation of opium use among labourers, and it was regarded primarily as a 'problem' among urban Chinese labourers and miners. But at least in Trengganu, opium was also used by Indian and Chinese estate workers. The British Adviser noted as late as 1938 that, on the basis of records of sales of *chandu* (opium prepared for smoking), 75 percent of opium was consumed by coolies working in isolated areas on mines and estates, where no recreational or social facilities provided an alternative to the use of drugs. International pressure on the Colonial Office, particularly from the United States, was far greater with respect to opium than to alcohol, and a meeting held in 1938 in Bangkok called for 'counter attractions' to reduce its use. Britain had earlier resisted suggestions to forbid opium smoking because of local tax benefits, and the British Adviser in Trengganu regarded the Bangkok recommendations as fanciful for social and cultural reasons: the state of communications and the absence of facilities for socialisation of any kind, anywhere in the state, as well as the belief held by many that opium was an effective anti-malarial.[72]

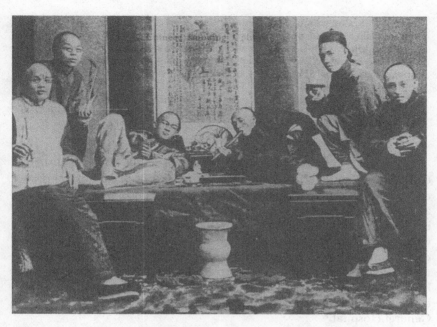

Figure 5.3 Opium smoking, early 1900s, Singapore. Printed with permission of National Archives, Singapore. Photograph No. 29451, NA 25/17.

Estate hospitals

Rules governing employers' responsibilities, covering estates in both the Settlements and FMS from 1886,[73] included the provision of hospital accommodation, medical attendance, and a sufficient quantity of medicines of good quality. These rules distinguished two classes of hospitals, as determined by the distance of an estate from a government hospital: first-class hospitals were to supply one bed to every 25 statute labourers, to employ a dresser with at least apothecary qualifications, and to maintain a substantial list of medicines; second-class hospitals, located within three miles of a government hospital, were to provide one bed for every 50 statute labourers, to employ a medical officer able to dress wounds and dispense simple drugs, and to maintain a restricted supply of medicines and ointments. The rules were poorly enforced where estates were distant from government facilities and surveillance, although everywhere the skills of the attending medical officer were questionable and conditions of buildings poor. For example, in 1890:

> The first ward of the hospital on the Gula Sugar Estate is in good repair and well suited for the purpose, but the partition between the male and female

wards is in an unsatisfactory state, and a middle tier of beds appears undesirable. The second ward is in an unsuitable building. Very few beds [are] supplied with blankets, patients being said to tear up blankets and mosquito nets to clean their persons; ulcer patients get sacks. One coolie stated that he was sick, felt lazy and could not work, and if he was not fed unless he worked, must die ...

On Gading Estate, Malacca, there was a building called a hospital, in reality an indifferent cattle shed. The Manager said it was never used, and indeed it could not be [of] service as a hospital.[74]

There were numerous examples of purpose-built hospitals, usually comprising a single wide room with three rows of beds, but many so-called hospitals were earthen-floored huts. Not all hospitals had latrines and patients were often 'left to wander into the jungle as they please'; buckets were supplied at night but routinely removed during the day.[75] Conditions were poor especially in the Malay States. In 1906, three estates only in Negri Sembilan and Selangor were reported to employ their own dressers; most simply referred sick coolies to the government hospitals. Treatment was provided free by the district hospitals to all labourers, with a charge of 30 cents per day levied at the Kuala Lumpur General Hospital.[76]

The continuing high mortality from malaria led to an approach in 1907 by planters to government to provide hospitals for labourers. The government refused, and instead elaborated the rules in the Labour Enactment regarding the provision of hospitals as a responsibility of the estates. Henceforth all estates were to establish hospitals, or where estates were too small to be able to do this, they were to contribute to a group hospital serving a number of estates. Hospital accommodation was to be provided for two percent of coolies, hence five beds for every 250 coolies employed. Where labourers were referred to a government hospital, the cost of treatment was to be billed to the estate at rates set out in the Labour Code, whilst charges at government outdoor dispensaries generally would be free.[77] Patients were to be fed a special diet, which included vegetable and salt fish curry, but no eggs, fresh fish or meat. A number of estates argued against these provisions, claiming that labour requirements were amply met where there was a dresser and dispensary, relatively close access to district hospitals, transport to hospitals for sick coolies – a boat in some areas, a bullock cart ambulance in others – and a relatively low record of illness.[78]

Ideally estate hospitals were to include a number of isolation wards and a 'reasonable ratio' of dressers to patients,[79] and large companies in the settlements, the FMS and UFMS often provided well for their employees. The Duff Development Company in Kelantan, for instance, provided its estates – 'not the healthiest in the state' – with a main hospital at Kuala Lebir, with a special ward for European managerial staff, and seven other 'native' estate hospitals; it also operated a river launch on a daily basis to ensure all sick persons were treated.[80] There was considerable variation, however. By late 1907, Perak had eight hospitals serving nine estates and a further six were under construction; in Negri Sembilan there was only one group hospital serving three estates and three more were being built. The first hospital in Selangor was still being erected on Bukit Rajah Estates, and a group hospital was under construction at Jugra to serve eight to nine company estates. In Negri Sembilan planters employed their own medical officers to supervise; in Perak and Selangor, the government provided the supervision and charged the estates. Threats of prosecution by the Federal Secretary pushed planters to comply with rules, but whilst the Superintendent of Indian Immigration noted general compliance in Negri Sembilan, in Selangor 'planters were determined not to make any move in the matter unless absolutely compelled',[81] and they remained reluctant to do so.[82]

In the end, health officials in Selangor favoured the establishment of group hospitals rather than individual hospitals in the interest of economies of scale and staffing, although their location was often problematic, and they tended to serve far too many estates and so were overcrowded. The Petaling Rubber Estates Group Hospital, for instance, provided 60 beds for 2,300 labourers employed on Petaling, Ledbury, Kinsara, Castlefield, Puchong, Killinghall and Bukit Itam Estates. The Senior Health Officer recommended an increase of 48 beds, of which twelve were to be reserved for diarrhoea and dysentery; estate representation led to this being reduced.[83]

As already noted, the hospitals were rudimentary and reports of inadequate medical provisions and hospital facilities were routine. Bukit Rotan Hospital, Selangor, for example, was inspected in February 1911 by A. S. Haynes and the Health Officer, Dr Gerrard, and described as 'lamentably deficient'; it served twenty estates and 5,000 coolies with 65 beds, although legally it should have had 250 beds. It had no bathing place for women, no woman in attendance, no assistant surgeon, and lacked an isolation ward for dysentery and diarrhoea cases: 'Nothing short of stopping labour supplies or vigorous prosecution will induce these managers to meet the responsibility of their positions.'[84] The report continued:

> The general condition was what I should call disgraceful; this Hospital is maintained by 16 Estates, and there were the following omissions and insufficiencies, all of which were gone into carefully by the Health Officer:
> Diets utterly insufficient; scale not followed
> Clothing very dirty
> Patients very dirty

No bathing accommodation
Filter not used, out of order
Only one dresser
It seems to me that the law will have to be a good deal more stringent and
much more strictly administered unless these Estate Hospitals are to become
a farce.[85]

According to the medical officer in Krian, Perak, 'sanitation as a rule
[is] nil', and frequently hospitals lacked bathing facilities and latrines.[86]
Some estates had a building but no staff. Many estates failed to employ
dressers, who anyway were sometimes of little use: Bagan Serai Hospital
was closed in September 1909 because of the habitual intoxication of the
dresser in charge, and a report of Rantau Panjang Estate notes that its
dresser was 'unqualified and useless', that brick drains were absent and
the buildings dirty.[87] Unqualified and uninterested dressers resulted in
poor care on the lines, as the following indicates:

Spent a good deal of time enquiring into a supposed case of suicide that had
taken place more than two months before. Saw a number of coolies in the
lines. I made particularly enquiries into the case of 2 or 3 coolies who were
sick in the lines, and found that one had not had anything to eat that day.
This is probably only too common an occurrence.[88]

The number of estate hospitals and the adequacy of their
accommodation and staff was improved following the establishment in
1911 of a health branch of the Medical Department and with the work of
its senior executive officer. His appointment led to an increased number
of inspections and a rapid increase in the number of single and group
hospitals. By 1914, Perak had 59 estate hospitals serving 93 estates,
Selangor 58 estate hospitals for 184 estates, and Negri Sembilan 40
hospitals for 58 estates.[89] Not all were well run nor capably staffed, but
even so they were regarded as contributing to the decline in the death
rate by one-half to one-third what it had been a few years earlier (Table
5.4). Local and international pressure was placed on the Malayan government to intervene further. In particular, a report by the government

Table 5.4   Declining mortality on rubber estates, British Malaya, 1911, 1923
and 1932

Select rubber estates in states settlements	1911	1923	1932
Acreage cultivated	1,632	2,650	6,801
Average Indian labour force	870	450	957
Number of dependants	—	220	575
Crude death rate (per 1,000)	**232**	**3**	**1.1**

Source: Christy, *Notes on the Prevention of Malaria*, p. 46.

of Madras in late 1916, following a visit to Malaya by two Indian commissioners, claimed that the present system was 'indefensible', that only government hospitals were under the charge of registered practitioners, and that 163 estate hospitals, with a total of 6,488 beds, were 'merely visited by a qualified medical practitioner' or provided care by people without any qualifications. In defence, the FMS government claimed that it had considered providing government-run hospitals, but since these had not been an 'unqualified success' in Ceylon and had led to friction between the planters and government, it had opted instead for estates providing services.[90]

The criticism was taken seriously, however, and in January 1918 the government approached the Planters' Association with a proposal to increase government surveillance of existing hospitals and to play an increasing role in their provision. A proposed Enactment prohibited the erection of further estate hospitals, empowered the government to construct new district hospitals at the expense of local estates, and enabled it to take over estate hospitals when asked to do so or when estates did not comply with existing laws related to the provision of medical services. Both the Planters' Association and the Society of Estate Medical Officers, the latter under the presidency of Malcolm Watson, took exception to the proposition. They argued, *inter alia*, that the death rate on rubber estates had fallen significantly (from 62.9 in 1911 to 18.17 per thousand in 1917), proving the effectiveness of the current system; that locally trained dressers, sub-assistant surgeons and hospital assistants were supervised by European medical officers and were adequately trained for the work required of them; and that many were capable and possessed invaluable local knowledge. They further argued that the cost of employing assistant surgeons rather than dressers and sub-assistant surgeons would increase the budget in the FMS by $200,000 per annum, that the proposal would reduce European medical supervision and centralise hospitals, and that 'European and Asiatic women and children would tend to fall into the hands of the Assistant Surgeon' who would have no training in maternal and child health.[91]

At a number of meetings, both the Planters' Association and the Society of Estate Medical Officers upheld the proposed Enactment as an example of excessive government interference and of the lack of cooperation between the estates and government; it was, they said, a 'public scandal'.[92] In the end, the government backed down, and the provision of primary care and basic hospital services on estates remained the responsibility of the planters.

By 1924 when the next inquiry into estate health was conducted, around half the labour force were employed on estates where provisions were 'fair to good'. But of 1,304 estates greater than 100 acres, 1,000 still

Table 5.5 Hospital services and health conditions on estates, British Malaya, 1934

Health variables	SS	FMS	Johore	Kedah	Kelantan
Indian estate pop'n	19,185	105,607	18,802	17,679	1,071
Deaths	113	711	131	153	12
Crude death rate (per 1,000)	5.89	6.73	6.97	8.06	11.20
Number of estate hospitals	26	129	36	11	6
Group hospitals	1	49	4	6	—
Number under charge of a resident MO	1	10	4	—	—

Source: Ahearne, 1935, pp. 31, 36.

lacked hospitals, only 32 percent of these were visited by a medical practitioner at least once per month, 50 percent of dressers in charge of estate hospitals had no qualifications, and only 11 percent had first-grade qualifications. Estates could not attract dressers as competent as those recruited into government service, and a final assessment of the system years later was that health services and medical care for estate workers should be a government responsibility.[93] Further, while the number of hospitals provided on estates in Perak, Selangor and Negri Sembilan had increased, conditions in Pahang were described as a 'scandal': 7,000 labourers on 144 estates over 25 acres were served by eight hospitals, and no visiting or resident medical practitioner had been in Western Pahang during the preceding three years.[94] Diets in estate hospitals in all states were described as 'basic', and according to the Commission, after the First World War had been 'cut down in some estate hospitals very near the margin of safety ... to economise'.[95] Later reports indicated that while some hospitals were in good condition and were well staffed, others offered 'a box of first-aid remedies and a few bottles of mixtures to be administered by anyone who felt competent to undertake the task' (see Table 5.5).[96]

To what extent did labourers take advantage of these facilities? Early reports refer to the reluctance of coolies to go to hospital, but later accounts such as evidence to the 1924 Commission suggest that delayed presentation for treatment was primarily due to the distance of hospitals from family and friends, and access to medical services, rather than to either superstition or 'ignorance of or disbelief in Western Health measures'.[97] Orde-Browne in 1939 noted too that workers preferred to go to local estate hospitals even if the building were 'modest'.[98] A combination of factors – attitudes and beliefs regarding diagnosis and management of sickness and help-seeking behaviour, and accessibility and availability of services, together with poor living conditions – compounded to contribute to the continuing high mortality rate.

Legally, under the orders of the FMS Labour Department, a sick labourer was to be taken to hospital 'without any special reference to his own wishes'.[99] On Chinese estates, however, referral depended largely on the attitude of the labourers – if the labourer wished for Western medical attention, he would inform the estate managers; if he wanted Chinese medicine, he would usually seek care without formal referral.[100] Despite the rules governing Indian labour, too, sick Indian coolies were not always sent to hospital, or were referred late; in consequence, the case fatality rate remained high. This was especially so under epidemic conditions. Stark recalls: 'During the 1918 flu epidemic I was visiting estates in K.Silangor (sic) and I saw a lot of people lying by the roadside, dying I suppose ... there was quite a lot of sickness on the estates.'[101]

Surveillance of the workplace

Until 1910, conditions of employment and living on estates were the responsibility of the Labour Department, although medical officers monitored conditions and collaborated with the Protector of Labour and the Indian Immigration Agent to ensure that certain health and sanitation measures were undertaken. Increasing concern with the health status of labourers, and the continuing demand on new immigrant labour that flowed from a massive number of deaths, led in 1910 to the introduction of a special enactment, the Estate Labourer's (Protection of Health) Enactment, later incorporated into the Labour Code. The following year, as noted already, a separate health branch was established within the FMS Medical Department. Similar provisions operated in the Straits Settlements, codified within the Labour Ordinance of 1920, to enable the Controller of Labour, on the advice of the Health Officer, to deal with the provision of 'sufficient and proper' accommodation, potable water, sanitation, medical attendance, hospital accommodation, patient diets, equipment and medicines. These rules provided health officers with some teeth: estate managers could be subject to severe fines for breaches in hygiene and sanitation (for instance, faeces observed around coolie lines). But there was constant need to monitor conditions and provisions for sick men,[102] and compliance with government regulations was poor in all states; an inspection of rubber estates in Kelantan from 21 February to 6 March 1917, for example, revealed several major problems, including the poor quality of tinned milk available (used for infant food), the lack of adequate measures for the disposal of refuse, and especially the lack of malaria control measures.[103]

Management resistance to provisions under the Indian Immigration Enactment and Labour Codes,[104] and the poor conditions which characterised life on the estates, led to a further inquiry into estate health. As already noted, the first had been the 1890 Commission of Inquiry chaired by Cameron; the second had been held in 1910, concentrating on Javanese and Chinese labourers and presided over by Parr. There was also, as discussed, an inquiry into alcohol on estates from 1915–16, and a Colonial Office committee on Indian emigration to the colonies.[105] In 1924 again, a commission presided over by Arthur Selbourne Jelf was appointed to inquire into the health of estates in the FMS, specifically 'the measures to be taken to improve conditions in regard to health, sanitaton and prevention of disease on estates, the system of estate hospitals and nursing and medical attendance therein, and the system of visiting estates by medical practitioners'.[106] The inquiry was concerned only with agricultural estates, although there was little to distinguish the conditions of labourers on estates and mines, or indeed railway or other labourers employed by the Public Works Department.

The 1924 Commission was interested in the effectiveness of different systems of surveillance. In Perak it was claimed that the strong Department of Chinese Affairs led to relatively good conditions for Chinese compared with those that prevailed for Indian labourers: lines were clean, hospitals reportedly excellent, and labourers treated without charge although 'employers cannot be got to send labourers to hospital as often or as early as necessary'. Elsewhere inspections of conditions of employment of Chinese labourers were uncommon. During the 1910 inquiry, it had been charged that inspections were superficial, and Parr, the Commissioner, and Ridges, the Acting Protector of the Chinese in Perak, took 8–9 hours over two days to inspect one estate, even then not completely; they noted that a hurried inspection could not uncover abuses and labourers would be too afraid to complain.[107]

Under the Labour Code, specified government officers could enter any place of employment to query conditions and enquire into disputes on wages, wrongful detention, misconduct, food, medical attention, sanitation or any other matter related to conditions of labour.[108] All European estates were supposed to be visited at least on an annual basis, although there was some concern that this was too infrequent.[109] As documented in the 1910 inquiry, too, inspections were superficial. Scott, providing evidence to the 1924 Commission, claimed to make 170 estate visits per month – that is, at least six per day – 'giv(ing) each estate I visit value for money' by calling in on the estate hospital to do minor operations and give injections, treating any sick coolies and staff, discussing issues of hygiene and prevention with the manager, visiting the lines if there were any specific infections, and undertaking a mosquito survey and a 'muster' of coolies in the event of an increase of malaria.[110] In Province Wellesley twice-yearly visits were conducted excepting where estate conditions were known to be poor, when visits were more frequent. By the 1930s, visiting frequency had increased: in a number of states, often monthly; in Selangor a large group hospitals was visited twice weekly and small estates once every three months.[111] Ideally, too:

> Once a month all the pregnant women were mustered and examined by the doctor. A monthly urine and haemoglobin examination was carried out and all findings recorded on their maternity card (sent with women to the maternity hospital at the time of delivery). Once a month all the children were mustered and examined for anaemia, splenomegaly, nutrition, skin infections. Any requiring treatment were dealt with at the hospital. Once every three months the complete labour force was examined by the doctor, who noted the spleen rates, etc …'.[112]

The language – the 'mustering' of people – is telling. But this was the ideal, rarely met. In states like Kedah and Perlis, it was impossible to enforce sections of the Labour Code relating to health and medical services because of the lack of qualified medical practitioners, and whilst some estates employed a private doctor, others refused to pay their share of a doctor's salary or to use their services. A Health Board was established in Kedah in 1927, with the Protector of Labour as chairman, the Senior Health Officer as vice-chairman, and the majority of members planters. This moved some way towards rectifying the situation by encouraging estate owners to send workers to hospital, advising them of relevant charges, and preparing schemes to build hospitals, increase the number of medical professionals, and ensure regular visits to estates.[113] Workers on large estates were best served, since these estates either provided their own hospital facilities or belonged to group associations which ran their own hospital; small estates did not have access to these facilities nor were they covered by labour legislation. Nowhere in the colonies could small estates afford their own hospitals, and they evaded or ignored government recommendations and rules. But government officers found it difficult to enforce high standards even on large estates. Inspections of Asian-owned and managed estates were particularly difficult due to 'obstruction' by the owners and their reluctance to discuss recommendations regarding provisions.[114] Colonial officers were also not always well selected to ensure maximum cooperation. W. J. A. Stark, Assistant Controller of Labour in Klang from 1915 to 1920, remarked that:

> When I first went to Klang, labour conditions on estates were very bad. The planters hated any officer from the Labour Department. Smith-Steinmetz was a very peculiar, morose, man: planters disliked him and this dislike was passed

on to anyone who worked under him. So when I went out to estates there was always a feeling of hostility when I met the planters.[115]

Police or sanitary inspectors, or both, were responsible for the investigation of outbreaks of disease, with police primarily concerned with the maintenance of quarantine measures for infectious diseases such as cholera, smallpox and plague. Regular inspections were carried out by district health officers, local sanitary inspectors and staff of the Institute of Medical Research, depending on the specificity of the task – routine inspections of hygiene and sanitation measures were conducted at a local level, and aimed at maintaining the minimum standards necessary to avoid sickness. They were, as indicated above, driven by an appreciation of the economic value of the absence of sickness:

> The economic value of the work of the Health Branch [in Perak] on estates is indicated by the very rapid fall in death-rates during the last 3 years which has occurred progressively as more and more unfit coolies have gone, thereby suggesting that the standards of sanitation achieved are sufficient to maintain in health those coolies who are not already weakened by sickness and debility.[116]

The state ensured compliance for specific preventive health measures, best illustrated by the anti-hookworm campaign of the 1920s. Regular examination and treatment of workers in Malacca, for instance, was regarded as the only means by which, 'owing to the habits of Tamil coolies', estates could be kept free from ankylostomiasis.[117]

Environmental inspections of estates assessed the extent of draining and oiling, that is, the extent to which estate managers adhered to the recommendations of the medical officer, Sanitary Board or the Malaria Advisory Board (MAB) of the Institute of Medical Research (see Chapter 3 above). The MAB was established in response to the increased incidence of malaria, particularly in Kuala Lumpur, but was ineffective during its first decade. Maxwell, Chief Secretary to the Government of the FMS from 1921, found on his arrival that it had not met for some years; under his leadership its role was enhanced with the establishment of Mosquito Destruction Boards, chaired by local health officers and responsible for control measures in major towns.[118] Specifically, the boards were to ensure that every proprietor carried out 'proper and reasonable anti-malarial measures' upon his land, and were to undertake these tasks themselves for small-holdings and town or village areas; whilst the Public Works Department was responsible for railway reservations, the Mosquito Destruction Boards were also responsible for anti-malarial activities on other state land and reservations. To ensure the effectiveness of anti-malarial measures, the boards were also responsible for cooperating with estates and ensuring their cooperation with each other and the health officers.

The 1924 inquiry and the revitalisation of the MAB led in 1926 to the establishment of Health Boards under the Health Board Enactment of the FMS. These boards were granted primary responsibility and authority to supervise health and medical services on estates and the organisation of estate hospitals. A Central Health Board was established which employed its own medical officers and could remunerate private practitioners to undertake preventive and curative work on estates. Local boards were appointed by the British Residents after consultation with the Central Health Board and were in charge of local health areas; they were to make recommendations regarding services; employ health and medical workers to visit estates and other small holdings; and develop and implement anti-malarial work on plantations, mines, and state land. Activities were funded through an annual tax or 'cess' on estates and mines. The government paid the board a similar amount for small-holdings, and was entitled to charge a levy on small-holdings to meet this if needed. It also paid a cess for state land at the same rate as estates and mines.[119]

The development of these mechanisms increased surveillance of the estates, and malaria declined. But the boards ceased operation in 1932 after the depression hit the rubber industry.[120] During the 1930s surveillance was lax and the government did not insist upon estates improving living conditions or maintaining public health measures. In Kedah, this resulted in increases in the incidence of malaria in both central and southern areas of the state, although large and wealthy estates sustained anti-malarial measures as a 'vital necessity' for which 'money is not grudged'.[121] Elsewhere people's health declined, leading to renewed concern by officials that owners and managers should 'fully appreciate the economic advantages of the measures recommended for the improvement of health conditions':[122] 'While it is impossible to expect estates to continue to carry out major sanitary improvements (unless a very vital sanitary service is involved) with the present prices of rubber and copra, nevertheless careful supervision is exercised to ensure that the present sanitary conditions are maintained.'[123]

By the late 1930s, death rates on estates had declined due apparently both to anti-malarial and other public health measures. Yet poor conditions prevailed: Major Orde-Browne, for example, noted continuing bad conditions where no compound manager was employed to deal with hygiene and sanitation, and where the welfare of labourers was in the hands of the general manager whose interests were primarily commercial. Other managers he characterised as 'die-hards', for whom prosecution for non-compliance with regulations would have had little impact.[124]

Malaria control measures

As the preceding discussion suggests, malaria control was the major activity of the health boards, the Mosquito Destruction Boards, the Institute of Medical Research, its Malaria Advisory Board, and government and estate medical officers. The decline in mortality from the early- to mid-twentieth century in Malaya has largely been attributed to the range and scope of interventions undertaken by the estates and by government to reduce the mosquito population to prevent transmission, and to provide appropriate treatment to those presenting with fever.

Ross had advocated behavioural change to reduce human–vector contact from the turn of the century, and in Malaya such public health recommendations were well received and promoted. Health education material, especially pamphlets distributed widely in English, Chinese, Tamil and Malay, emphasised the value of avoidance of bites through the use of repellents and bed nets, the value of quinine to treat fever, and the importance of anti-larval measures for earth drains, ditches, pools, sides of streams, and swamps.[125] The adoption of measures to avoid bites had varied success. Estate labourers were encouraged to use nets but often had to buy their own, few could afford them, and there was insufficient space to use them where three or four adults would have to share a tiny room on the lines. Others found them too hot, or were bitten before retiring to bed while they were resting outdoors in the cool of evening, and in other cases the number of people sleeping under a single net, and rips and tears in the nets, meant that their protective value was poor. Overall, however, neither bed nets nor other mosquito avoidance behaviour (wearing protective clothing, using repellents) were emphasised, other than in advice to Europeans. The use of bed nets was of questionable value in any case where the vector was both exophagic and exophilic.

Although Atebrin and other drugs were alternatives in later years, quinine was the main drug used to treat fever: its value in treating malaria had been discovered in 1820 and it was already standard for the management of malaria among British troops in India by the 1840s.[126] For some time it was also promoted prophylactically. In 1911, for example, 10 gms a day was given to labourers on Highlands (New Division) Estate, where the death rate in 1910 had been 11.03 percent in a total population of 1,114; it was also recommended that quinine be distributed freely by the Sanitary Board for chemoprophylaxis in Kuala Lumpur following the rising incidence of malaria in the town the same year.[127] Quinine was also available free in Perak for the 'poorer classes' through the *penghulu* or other native officials. However, Ross, among others, was sceptical of the prophylactic use of quinine and was concerned that its

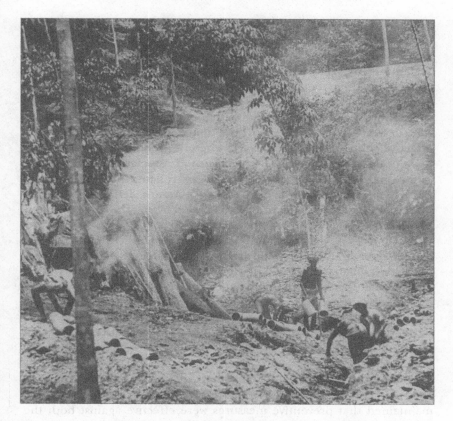

Figure 5.4 Laying subsoil pipes on a hillside, Bukit Ijok Estate, FMS. Printed with permission of Arkib Negara Malaysia, Kuala Lumpur, N 202/82, p. 55.

inappropriate use might weaken its curative power.[128] In the end, it was decided that while the drug was relatively effective therapeutically, it was costly, difficult to introduce for widespread prophylaxis, and caused side-effects that encouraged non-compliance.[129] Chemoprophylaxis in some states, however, continued to provide a back-up to environmental measures during periods of high transmission; in Kedah, for example, many estates either administered Atebrin twice a week or quinine bihydrochloride daily during peak transmission periods, while year round maintaining a weekly program of oiling streams, drains and pools.[130]

As described in Chapter 3, the standard environmental measures for malaria control involved drainage and clearing of undergrowth, in that order, since the reverse – clearing then draining – established ideal microecological niches for increased *Anopheles* breeding, hence a potential increase in malaria (Figure 5.4). There was some seasonal variation in transmission in foothill areas, but in general breeding and transmission was year round.[131] By 1910, the complexity of malaria in Malaya was relatively well understood: different vectors and different ecological settings dictated different control approaches. On estates, the primary vector was *Anopheles maculatus*, which could be controlled through drainage with as little disturbance of undergrowth as possible. A secondary vector, *A. umbrosus*, bred on the forest fringe, and the most effective control to reduce malaria where it predominated was simply to relocate labour lines.[132] *A. sundaicus* was associated with epidemic outbreaks of disease and could be controlled through drainage; *A. barbirostrus*, a diverse inhabitant of open swamps, deep ponds and the margins of paddy fields, could be controlled by clearing and drainage. Environmental control proved successful from 1901, as already recounted; in 1910 Malcolm Watson, then Medical Officer with the FMS, extended the strategy of sub-soil drainage on Seafield Estate, in collaboraton with its manager, H. R. Quartley, to control *A. maculatus*. Watson claimed that there was an immediate improvement in health following drainage around the lines, and by 1915 the entire estate had been drained.[133] Watson continued to promote environmental management strategies in accordance with local vectorial behaviour and ecology, in an effort described as 'an epic in the history of modern preventive sanitation'.[134]

Throughout the States and Settlements, estate managers were encouraged to maintain environmental controls by economic arguments, which maintained that preventive measures were effective against both the direct and indirect costs of morbidity and hospitalisation:

> When examined from the standpoint of economic waste – the cost of hospitalization and treatment, the loss due to incapability during illness, and to partial incapability often over a protracted convalescence – will bring home the magnitude of the tax levied by anopheline mosquitoes on those who dwell in the domain. Nor does this necessarily indicate the total toll, no statistics are available of patients treated in the homes nor of the many thousands of kampung sufferers for whom little treatment is available.[135]

Such explicit statements of the economics of health on plantations, dating from around the turn of the century and recurrent, caught the attention of contemporary observers and critics of colonialism elsewhere in the Empire. Rao, for instance, after a study tour of Malaya in 1939, argued that the political geography of malaria control reflected the intensity of capitalist development and state resources available, and argued that:

It has been made amply clear that the exploitation of the natural resources of Malaya has been mainly dependent on Indian and Chinese labour, neither indigenous. It is well to bear this in mind as it supplies the key to the intense anti-malarial activity in British Malaya. If large sums of money are annually spent for the control of malaria, it is certainly not because the capitalist in Malaya is activated by any philanthropic motives for the welfare of his labourers but because that is the only way by which he can make his investment in Malaya yield.[136]

Nutrition and diet

Infectious diseases were directly responsible for high mortality on the estates, but nutrition was also poor, complicating anaemias due to hookworm and malaria and contributing to the equivocal health status and poor resistance to infection of many workers. From the late nineteenth century, the link between nutrition and health created interest; within the Labour and Medical Departments this was reflected in debate about the ability of workers to feed themselves and the merit of estate managers providing their labourers with cooked food. Nineteenth-century practice had often included the provision of rations, but this was never particularly popular. Most estates moved quickly from this system to one which left labourers to find their own food, although rice or other foodstuffs were subsidised and a provision shop on the estate sold basic foods. Mr C. de Mornay of Malakoff Estate described to the 1890 Commission his experience with cooked rations and his reasons for changing the system; his evidence, quoted at length below, is revealing in terms of the positioning of estate manager and workers, the feudal nature of labour relations at the time, and the way in which food became a vehicle of manipulation and the exercise of power:

The coolies received in 1877 (the first lot under the Ordinance, 238 in number) were a wretched, famine-stricken lot, many almost skeletons. Naturally the death-rate was very heavy, amounting to 17 per cent. However, instead of improving on the ample supply of rice advanced to them (2 gantangs per week), they became worse and worse. I determined to give them cooked rations and commenced to do so in January, 1878.

At one time I had over 300 men being fed in this way. I gave them rice, vegetables and salt fish, curry with a little dholl in it, and charged them seven cents per day. The coolies became as fat as pigs but were very discontented and did little work. I think I could have worked the system better as regards the work, if I had received a little more assistance from the Magistrate in punishing coolies who would not try to work; but instead of that, when I brought a clear case against a strong fat, coolie for not working, he was generally convicted, cautioned and discharged.

The coolies did not like the system at all and tried to force me to give it up, but I continued the system for eleven months, gradually allowing those coolies who seemed willing to work to get their rations of raw rice as usual, but always putting back a coolie who began to look thin onto cooked food.

I thus taught them to see that it was to their advantage to feed themselves properly. The experiment was quite successful as regards the improvement in health of the coolie [but] ... I would not recommend it ... as it is exceedingly troublesome, and the coolies are very discontented and grumble much at the price charged for the food.[137]

Other colonists who presented evidence to the commission shared de Mornay's view that men found it 'distasteful' to have food provided for them, but also argued that the workers consumed poor quality and an inadequate quantity of food even when good nutrition was within their reach financially.

Continuing reports of poor diet led to further interest in providing workers with meals. Treacher, for example, argued in 1901 that all estate labourers should be provided with free rice in the morning:

The Tamil coolie requires as much care and looking after as the draught bullock; he is equally helpless among his new environment and, in addition, is prone to stint himself in the necessaries of life ... [he] is keen on saving every cent of his pay and is therefore prone to stint himself in the matter of food, and in the second place, all the coolies have not the time nor the skill to properly prepare their food, and when improperly fed they become easy prey to fever, diarrhoea and dysentry and are incapable of performing a fair day's work.[138]

The Medical Officer of the FMS, in the departmental annual report in 1911, maintained also that:

It is most essential to build up and strengthen new arrivals who have very little reserve force to call upon either for work or to resist illness ... not only from the human point of view but also from the business aspect it is necessary that this supply [of food] is adequate. Expenditure on prevention of illness is soon repaid with large interest; stupid ignorance or wilful neglect of this important duty means unnecessary wasteful extravagance as well as loss of life.[139]

The Protector of Labour for the FMS, T. S. Hill, also argued that the lowest death rates occurred among those such as Javanese labourers who received rations. He proposed introducing rationing on all estates but this was was rejected by the Resident-General on the grounds that would be too expensive and would lead to discontent.[140] Some estates experimented by providing food to labourers at a charge; the New Amherst Estate, for example, provided cooked food for $4 per month, resulting in an apparent improvement in health. Labourers complained about the monotony of the diet, however, and the scheme was disbanded.[141]

Hill continued to claim that labourers, left to their own devices, would stint on food to save and remit funds to India, and that estate managers had an obligation to feed their workers. The Health and Labour Departments were particularly concerned with the usual practice of workers and their children not eating before noon, hence eating only at the end of their workday; some estates dealt with this by introducing a later 'muster hour' to enable people to eat before work, or by giving women half the normal working day so that they might return home early to prepare food.

Lack of food in terms of quantity and variety was the key issue, but there were also complaints from workers about the quality of the food and the possible links between food contamination and diarrhoea and dysentery. Issues of quality were usually referred back to the labourers and their own presumed poor food hygiene:

> Perhaps the invariable custom of the Tamils of preparing and boiling the rice the night before and after utilizing half of it for their dinner, keeping the remainder in a cold pot and eating it cold the next morning, may be more responsible in causing gastrointestinal disorders ... The dirty habit of eating all kinds of garbage and unwholesome foodstuffs when in the field, e.g. rotten fish from the manure boats, raw tapioca roots, and even dead buffaloes, indulged in by many of the coolies, may I think be largely attributed to these intestinal disorders.[142]

Estates were encouraged to provide vegetable gardens for labourers both to enable dietary diversity and to promote 'more settled labour conditions'.[143] In addition, the commercial potential of estate gardens in the context of food shortages after the First World War led to explorations that estates make land available for food for a wider market.[144] In general, government officers placed the solution back on the plantation sector: it was the responsibility of estates to set apart portions of land for labourers to grow their own food.[145] Some estates allocated land to workers for horticulture, although managers claimed that even when they did so, Tamil workers were 'quite indifferent to [the] quality or variety [of food]', 'too lazy', and did not bother to produce food, or they sold any food produced on allotments rather than use it to supplement their own diet. It was also claimed that Tamil labourers adhered rigidly to a customary diet in which 'rice bulks excessively', and that they 'disliked dietetic innovations'.[146] In contrast, 'the Chinese' were said to spend twice the amount on food and were industrious in its production.[147]

Rice was especially vulnerable to market fluctuations, as discussed in Chapter 3, and was rationed at a fixed price to workers. Fixed pricing was introduced country-wide after the First World War also, in response to severe shortages, unpredictable supplies, and profiteering. Until 1919, maximum food prices were also fixed for meat, fish, onions, potatoes

Table 5.6 Rising food costs, 1914–1920, per unit of sale (weight or piece)

Food stuff	Estimated price January 1914 (SS cents)	Estimated price January 1920 (SS cents)
Beef (local)	30–38	48
Mutton, goat	40	70–80
Pork	26–48	60–104
Prawns	24	30–45
Ikan tenggiri	28	56
Ikan bawal	26–30	48
Large onions	10	35
Small onions	10	32
Cabbage	6	15
Chili peppers	16	25
Coconut	8–10	10–18
Potatoes	7–8	33
Bananas	1.5	1.5–2
Oranges	14	35–40
Pineapple	10	8–10
Chicken eggs	3.5	6.5

Source: ST, select issues 1914, 1920; see also Sel. Sec. 1413/1919; Sel. Sec. 3089/1920; Sel. Sec. G866/1935.

and eggs. The system was later abandoned since the government was unable to control the supply: goods disappeared from the market, were diverted from the FMS and UFMS to Singapore, and were sold above contract prices. In some cases, rationing and price control led to a reduction in the unit cost of foodstuffs: rice available to labourers on the Highlands (New Division) Estate dropped after the war to 29 cents a *gantang*, compared with its 1911 price of 31 cents, while elsewhere it cost around 50 cents a *gantang*. In general the cost of food increased for all but a few local items – onions threefold, chilis nearly double, potatoes fourfold, and so on (Table 5.6).

The unpredictable supply and rising cost of staples caused real hardship among wage labourers and peasants, leading to complaints and deputations to government from individual estate owners, Planters' Associations and labourers. F. W. Douglas, the Acting Director of Food Production for the FMS and SS, in 1920 called for a policy to encourage Malays to plant padi rather than rubber, and urged estates to plant rice in addition to their export crops. While some estates began to produce their own food, there was inadequate local production to meet demand, and the high price of rice caused considerable hardship to the poor and others with little cash flow.

Wages paid to estate workers were low, and this affected their food purchases, diet and nutritional status. Most workers could only buy from a narrow range of foods. Their preference for parboiled rice protected them from the major deficiency disease of the period, beri-beri: this was, as discussed earlier, the disease that was common among Chinese workers. But other nutritional problems caused concern, and by the late 1930s an increasing number of scientific papers were referring to the poor general health and nutritional status of workers.[148] This interest in food, health and nutrition was empire-wide, resulting in detailed reports being submitted to the Colonial Office, a full inquiry into nutrition in the empire, and the first anthropological studies undertaken under the auspices of the Colonial Office.[149] The report of the Commission of Inquiry, tabled in 1939, noted the poor nutritional status of Malayan labourers, the lack of vitamins A and D in diets, 'low physical standards', poor stamina, susceptibility to bacterial infections, and as a result of Vitamin A deficiency, xerophthalmia and night blindness.[150] It offered social explanations for many of these problems. Nutritional deficiency was, for example, partly an artefact of the organisation of labour: since women as well as men worked, food was usually prepared in the afternoon for both the evening and the following midday meal. In addition, while most labourers had been recruited from subsistence villages (in India) and estates were required by law to set aside one-sixteenth of an acre of land for each labourer with dependants for food production, 'these [were] not always taken advantage of owing to the natural disinclination of the labourer to spend a considerable part of his leisure in cultivating gardens'.[151] The report claimed that wages were sufficient for labourers to purchase all food requirements, but that they relied on a limited range of goods available from plantation stores – parboiled rice, dhal, spices and coconut oil with the 'haphazard' addition of tubers, dried fish, and rarely goat meat, eggs, or tinned milk. 'Either from want of facilities or from want of enterprise', they were seen to 'depend far too much on the dried and parched miscellany of the estate shops'.[152] The report also commented on the lack of concern by estate managers regarding nutritional intake and food supply: 'Too often at present the employer is apt to regard his responsibilites as finished when he has paid his wage bill'.[153]

The report refers to the fact that some people reared their own cattle and goats, coastal dwellers fished, and some used local markets to purchase fresh produce. But there is no evidence there or in other unpublished records of the extent to which economic relations existed between plantation labourers or miners, and Malay peasant farmers. It is possible that wage labourers purchased some locally produced food, but it is also possible that alienation of land, the increased dependence of Malays also on wage labour, and the extension of monocultivation affected food prodcution. According to contemporary accounts, Malay peasants also ate from a narrowed range of foods and their nutritional status also declined.

Wages

While lack of availability of varied foodstuffs and culturally based food preferences partly accounted for the nutritional status of the estate labourers, their apparent poor nutrition also related to their lack of cash, and the wage rate was an important health issue. Food prices increased but there was little change in wages from around 1880 to 1940, although there was considerable variation by state and employer (see Table 5.7).[154] In 1881, men in Penang and Province Wellesley were paid

Table 5.7   Select wage rates, Federated Malay States, 1900–1938

Year	State or estate	Daily wage – men	Daily wage – women	Notes
1900	FMS (general)	7–20c (indentured Tamil), 23–35c (free Tamil), 30–40c (free Chinese)	—	Indentured Chinese $4–5 per month (ca. 15c per day)
1906	Negri Sembilan and Selangor	27–35c	20–25c	Children 10–20c; 6-day week with pay on Sundays; rice advanced at cost price.
1910	Ulu Langat district, Selangor	38c	—	55 cents for *mandor*
1911	Bukit Janda Estate, Selangor	27–30c	20c	Rice issued $6 for 18.5 *gantang*
1911	Cauly Estate Perak	25–45c	—	No food supplement
1930	Selangor (coastal)	40c	32c	Chinese on small estates 40–65c
	Pahang (inland)	47c	37c	—
1932/3	FMS (general)	30c (tappers), 20c (weeders)	27c (tappers) 18c (weeders)	—
1938	FMS (general)	45–50c (Tamil) 60–65c (Chinese)	35–40c (Tamil)	Wages dropped from May; rice rose 24–28c per *gantang* July–November

Sources: Sel. Sec. 127, 135, 269; 287; 397; CO273/265; *FMSAR 1938*, pp. 51–2.

20 cents per day of work with free accommodation; in Singapore they received 25 cents per day and in Perak 30 cents; alternative rates of 25 cents for men and 15 cents for women, supplemented by a food ration, were also common. In 1900 in the FMS, Tamil labourers were paid around 17 to 35 cents per day depending on their status as free or indentured workers; Chinese labourers received from about 15 to 40 cents. In 1906 the male wage for an estate worker was around 25 to 35 cents per day, compared with from 40 cents up to as high as 60 to 80 cents per day in the mines.[155] Compared with this, a houseboy or a cook received $10 to 15 per month – around 2 or 3 times the pay of an indentured Chinese estate worker; gardeners and water carriers received around $7 to 10 per month and a syce $9–12. By further contrast, the commencing annual salary of an English woman, posted to a nursing job in the Straits Settlements, was $480 (that is, $40 per month), rising to a final salary of $720 with additional benefits.[156]

Around 1932, it was estimated that labourers' wages on around three-quarters of the estates was low to very low. Women especially were often paid below subsistence, did not always receive due maternity benefits, and their health was especially poor.[157] Wages were affected by fluctuations in the rubber market in the early 1920s and the early 1930s, but labour was vulnerable to other market forces too, and arguments of lower costs of production in competing countries also led to pay cuts.

Illusions of change

The establishment of administrative machinery to monitor estate conditions, the enquiries into the health status and conditions of labourers, the development of guidelines for estate hygiene and sanitation, and the appointment of boards and individual officers to ensure adherence to these guidelines, all led to a sense of confidence among government officials regarding health improvements. Hence the contrast between estate conditions in 1911, following the 1910 inquiries into Indian, Chinese and Javanese labour, and 1923, just before the next inquiry:

1911. – Eight hundred and seventy coolies, practically no dependents, miserable crawling wretches with narrow shoulders, prominent stomachs, bloodless, lifeless, miserable squalor in the lines, no garden or livestock, and no children born alive.
1923. – Four hundred and fifty coolies doing three times the work done in 1911. 220 healthy old people and young children, births have become a chronic habit, the coolies are happy, fat, well set up people, clean and well clothed. There are excellent gardens, over 60 head of cattle the property of coolies, hundreds of goats and thousands of chickens.[158]

The 1924 report argued that health, hygiene and sanitation had not improved universally, but there had been improvement in the provision of health and medical services on estates, the installation of drains and latrines, and anti-malarial measures. Financial stringency with the depression led to a relaxation of hygiene and sanitation provisions and government surveillance of conditions. Estates closed their hospitals and contributed instead to group hospitals, and neither installed water-borne sewerage systems nor were subject to government pressure to do so,[159] although efforts were supposed to continue to ensure safe water at minimum cost. Systems for the collection, burning and burial of rubbish, and the installation of septic tanks, were undertaken on some of the larger estates, but in general health officers recommended simply that anti-malarial measures be maintained, if necessary at the expense of all other health measures. Maintenance work also stopped on lines unless conditions were dangerous, leading to the deterioration and closure of lines on some smaller estates and the issue of orders suspending further recruitment of labourers.[160] Earlier slumps in the commodities' market had led to unemployment, vagrancy and homelessness, and during falls in the price of rubber from around 1914 to the early 1920s many European estates maintained only a skeleton staff while keeping a reserve labour force on call by allowing unemployed coolies to squat and develop vegetable gardens on estate land.[161] From the 1920s there was an increase in the number of paupers, as former coolies were paid off following sickness and hospitalisation, when they were deemed by the estate to be too unhealthy to continue as wage labour. The 1930s depression hit the labour force directly too, as hundreds were stood down and repatriated to India,[162] but its impact was primarily one of scale.

By the end of the 1930s, sanitation conditions and consequently worker health appeared to have improved. There were more bore-hole latrines, safer supplies of drinking and cooking water, and better health services. Housing was reported to have improved; the Medical Department of the Straits Settlements in 1935 reported that on rubber estates '[n]early all of the buildings conform to an approved standard design and frequent inspections by the health authorities and the officers of the Labour Department prevent overcrowding and ensure decent upkeep and cleanliness.'[163]

Certain independent measures reinforced this impression. Most significantly, the death rate had declined. But the infant mortality rate had risen; so had hospital cases of certain diseases. Malaria jumped in 1938, with 34,986 hospital cases compared with 24,776 the previous year. Hospital cases of dysentery, diarrhoea and tuberculosis also increased. Explanations of improved systems of epidemiological surveillance and registration, or of improved use of hospital and outpatient medical facilities, only partly account for the increases in adult morbidity, and do not address changes to the infant mortality rate.

Given this, arguments focusing on the general decline in the standard of living, low salary rates, and inadequate nutrition are the most likely, as advanced at the time. Poor health status was seen less as specific to a vector or microbial agent and more to a system of production that impoverished and exploited its workers. It was at this time – 1939, then the war years – that senior officers of the colonial empire, members of the Department of Colonial Affairs and the Colonial Economic Advisory Committee, began to articulate their concerns and to lend support to the notion of the moral obligations of the empire.

CHAPTER 6

Brothel politics and the bodies of women[1]

Men were brought to Malaya to work in mines, on estates, and on the railways. Women were brought to the brothels. They came from everywhere – Japan, China, Java, India, Thailand, eastern Europe – most recruited by pimps and procurers but others travelling independently to work in brothels in Penang, Ipoh, Singapore, Kuala Lumpur and in the small towns and settlements that grew up as trading posts around the plantations and the mines.

The 'traffic' in women and venereal disease intermittently caused controversy from the 1870s to the 1940s, signalling the contradictions of prostitution in colonial Malaya: the gross disparity of the sexes in the population of Malaya then, on the one hand, and moral issues on the other, in which context questions of health tended to be embedded. Women in the brothels were routinely represented as vectors of venereal disease, 'reeking with infection'. This chapter looks at the material lives of these women, at the role of the state in controlling prostitution, the position of the doctors as gatekeepers of the public's health, their manipulation of the powerlessness and dependence of the brothel women, and the engineering that took place as the colonies moved to suppress prostitution.

The colonies had, as discussed in Chapter 2, an 'enormous preponderance of males',[2] and this was regarded by most colonial officials as predetermining the existence and extent of prostitution. Sexual 'appetite' was portrayed as natural – '(n)ature endows men with desires and impulses without regard to their means of gratifying them'[3] – and satisfaction necessary, in the absence of the possibility of marriage, by prostitution or 'unnatural and abominable vices'. The Reverend W. G. Shellabear held that 'unnatural vice' was the lesser sin: 'it seems to me more horrible for wicked men to ruin innocent young girls than that

166

wicked men should ruin each other'.[4] But this was a minority view. Most argued that prostitution was 'a necessary evil, to save us from something worse',[5] and part of the argument for improving the physical conditions of the brothel buildings and the health of the women who worked there related to allegations that 'intelligent Chinamen descend to forms of unnatural vice' rather than patronise the brothels, which were reputed to be 'centres of loathsome disease'.[6]

Those who argued for legislation to govern its practice, while maintaining that sexual desire was natural, argued also that its institutionalisation was cultural, related therefore not only to the skewed sex ratio but also to matters of 'Chinese character'.[7] Swettenham argued that morality was relative, 'dependent on influences of climate, religious belief, education and the feeling of society',[8] and witnesses to the 1898 Committee of Inquiry held that most brothels were owned by 'well-to-do and respectable Chinese', that both Straits-born and immigrant Chinese accepted the brothel as a legitimate social institution, that 'chastity as chastity' had no value for Indians, and that even Europeans in Singapore, while they 'would not like their sisters or mothers to be engaged in prostitution', had few objections to it 'in the abstract'.[9] These views were held relatively consistently until the 1920s, when they were modified in the face of growing international agitation.

The traffic in women

From all accounts, there were an extraordinary number of people involved in prostitition, including brothel keepers and brothel prostitutes, 'sly' prostitutes, taxi-girls, singers, dancers, and waitresses, some working only in prostitution, others opportunistically. Most were women, excepting the pimps and the clients, and the discourse around prostitution, legislation, government policies and practices all operated on this understanding despite apparent traffic in boys also.[10]

Figures are most comprehensive for Singapore, where brothels and prostitutes were registered under the Contagious Disease Ordinance. In 1864 there were 349 brothels operating in Singapore, and 2,061 prostitutes were registered; in 1871, according to the census, there were a combined 1,635 brothel keepers and prostitutes. The Ordinance was repealed in 1887 for prostitutes, and in 1894 for the registration of brothels. In this latter year, Hare, Acting Assistant Protector of the Chinese, claimed that there were 192 brothel keepers in Singapore; 62 public houses operated in Sago Lane and Sago, Bugi and Malay Streets alone, employing around 3,000 women, of whom 2,000 to 2,500 would be working on any given night. Five years later, police estimated that there were 298 public houses exclusively set aside for prostitution and located in known brothel areas of the town, of which 228 were Chinese, 26 Japanese, 22 European, 10 Indian and 12 Malay. In addition, it was estimated that there were some 131 private houses – 80 were Chinese, 29 Malay, nine Tamil, and four Thai – and from each of these two or three women worked on their own account. In total police estimated that around 2,106 women were working from known public and private houses. Private houses were located disparately; public brothels were geographically concentrated and clustered according to the ethnicity of the workers and their clientele. European women, for example, including German, Hungarian, Austrian and Russian women (many Jewish, part of the eastern European 'slave trade'), worked in the Malay Street-North Bridge Road area and attracted a clientele of mainly European men. Cantonese women, said to 'cater' exclusively for Chinese men, operated out of the public houses in Chinese Street, Hong Kong Street and Smith Street; other brothels for non-Chinese operated in Sago Street, Sago Lane and Bugi Street. Additional brothels were located in Tanglin near the barracks. Women also worked out of coffee and tea shops, eating houses and opium houses.

In Penang, including both Penang Island and Province Wellesley, there were in 1871 281 prostitutes and brothel keepers, running both Cantonese and Japanese brothels; the 1881 census refers to 197 women in Province Wellesley alone, primarily operating and working out of Cantonese brothels in Bukit Mertajam and Nebong Tebal. In Malacca the 1871 census estimates 151 brothel keepers and prostitutes; in 1881 this had risen to 173; and in 1900 the police probably underestimated that 69 Cantonese were women working for 14 public houses, with Japanese women employed in three Japanese brothels, and an additional unknown number of women working as own account workers from private houses: a total of around 100 women.[11]

Although many other women worked as prostitutes, the majority in the Settlements were Chinese, recruited in south China or Hong Kong. Many were 'sempstresses (sic), tea-pickers, boat-girls, weavers and spinners' who had been recruited as nurses, seamstresses, hairdressers, or servants, and who with the promise of relatively good pay on arrival, would take on a loan of $50 to $100 to cover their passage and were then forced into prostitution to repay their debts.[12] Others were promised marriage in the colonies, or were widows or concubines in search of a new life; many came from impoverished families. Migration offered a woman the opportunity to earn money to remit back to China, 'doing her duty', as Hare described it, 'according to her lights in obedience to the principles of Chinese filial piety'.[13] Other women were recruited as prostitutes, or sold to Straits Settlements agents by their relatives or husbands for between $100 and $300, and were held captive by the

brothel keeper while they remained indebted for their 'original purchase price', the subsequent costs of their passage, food, lodging, loans
for medicine and clothing, and 'everything else that the ingenuity of
their masters could think of'.[14] Local women were sometimes also
purchased or born in the brothels, or brought to them as the adopted
infants, daughters or younger sisters of the brothel keepers in Malaya or
procurers in Hong Kong. Importers would often claim at least one child
and an infant as their own, 'settling the matter' with the inspecting
government officer if questioned on arrival.[15] In addition, however,
according to one brothel keeper, June McBreen, 'many companies in
Singapore and China brought women, girls and babies down (to Singapore) for sale every six weeks, and these are sold like goods'. Mrs
McBreen, a Eurasian woman of Chinese descent who reputedly controlled the majority of brothels in Singapore and had been long involved
in the overseas recruitment of women, gave the following account of the
immigration of infants:

> A lot of low class women who have a little money, continually go to China and
> buy young babies and bring them over – these women do not take much care
> of the babies and just give them some diluted condensed milk, and being on
> board ship, the consequence is that a great many of them die, thus a great
> many lives are lost; but if they don't die on board, they are sold like cattle
> when brought ashore.[16]

Societies for the 'protection of women and girls' were established
from the mid-1880s because of kidnapping and child prostitution.[17]
Adult women as well as children came to the colonies under the guise of
kinship, as suggested, for instance, by the following letter from 'AA' in
Sitiawan, Perak, to 'BB' in Foochow, China, dated 31 March 1941 and
intercepted by the Assistant Protector of Chinese:

> Please ask CC's aunt to bring the girl over here. If questioned by the
> Government Officers, she must say that the girl was purchased by us. You
> should remined (sic) the Aunt about this. The best way is for the girl to call
> Aunt as her mother or to declare that her parents are at Sitiawan and the
> girl's surname is A. The girl should be taught to say her name, age, etc.
> properly before she comes ... Please get the Hotel people to notify me about
> the arrival so I can meet them at the wharf and bring them to Sitiawan by
> train. She should avoid coming via Penang as the Government examination
> is very tiresome.[18]

The differences in recruitment to some extent shaped access to
resources. Women reared as 'daughters' by the brothel keeper had no
access to money earned. Those who had come on assisted passages, for
whom freedom was technically a possibility, worked to discharge their

debts; others paid room rent to the brothel keeper and had control over some of their earnings. Other women worked privately, handing over much of their earnings to their 'pocket-mothers' (older women who bought and reared them from infancy); others were able to keep what they earned.[19]

The scale of prostitution was less clear for the Malay States, where there was no Contagious Disease Ordinance nor provisions for the compulsory medical examination. A system of registration operated until 1894, when it was replaced by a Women and Girls Protection Enactment; this was far less effective in keeping track of women and in ensuring their welfare.[20] Estimates of the numbers of prostitutes was always rough, and it was near impossible to monitor population movements where states lacked the portal entries that facilitated surveillance in Penang and Singapore. Swettenham estimated that in Perak in 1891 there were around 863 Cantonese prostitutes living in registered brothels each employing from four to 18 women; 21 Tamil prostitutes 'in various parts of the State' worked in brothels or alone, and 24 Japanese women were living in organised public houses. A further unspecified number of Malay prostitutes worked as 'sly' prostitutes; a few also worked out of established houses.[21] At the end of 1894, the Chinese Protectorate had registered 1,038 Chinese prostitutes working in 92 brothels in Perak. In Kuala Lumpur at the end of 1892, 815 Chinese, 34 Japanese, one Malay and three Tamil prostitutes were registered and placed under the care of the Secretary for Chinese Affairs; in December 1894 there were 705 Chinese and 53 Japanese prostitutes registered, none of other nationalities.[22] As in Singapore, Chinese women were allegedly patronised by Chinese men, the Tamil women by Indian men, and the Malay and Japanese women by Malay, Eurasian and European men. In other towns of Selangor, 'large numbers' of Chinese, Indian and Malay women solicited openly.[23] Working only from these estimates, there were around five-and-a-half-thousand women working in prostitution in the colonies around the mid-1890s; if Warren is correct about the extent of underestimation, the number was perhaps nearer ten thousand.[24]

These figures are substantiated by those from the early twentieth century. The latter, of course, must also have been underestimates, given the propensity of brothel keepers to 'baffle the domiciliary visitations and most effectively thwart the Protector by means of concealment, substitution, bribery and other ingenious devices'.[25] Capper, Acting Protector of the Chinese in the FMS in 1900, claimed that staff within the office of the Protector would forewarn brothel keepers of impending inspections, so that both in the main towns and in outstations, brothels were rarely surprised and the Protector, in turn, rarely saw all women and certainly not the 'worst cases' of abuse or ill-treatment.[26] He maintained that very few women in the FMS came direct from China, since the 'slave owners naturally take their goods to the better market at Singapore or Penang first'; he argued that most were women who, 'for one base reason or another', moved from Singapore or Penang after two or three years' work there first.[27]

In 1906, the Secretary for Chinese Affairs knew of 440 brothels and 3,647 prostitutes in the FMS, two-thirds of whom were Chinese, located in twenty towns in the four states (see Tables 6.1 and 6.2) and numbers remained relatively constant until the 1920s. An additional unknown number of women worked in the UFMS; the Protectorate estimated that 103 women were working in Johore in 1913.[28] Many women moved between cities, travelling from Singapore and Penang to Kuala Lumpur, for example. Of 59 Malay prostitutes known to the *penghulus* in Kuala Lumpur in 1928, for example, 13 came from Kedah, eight from Penang, 21 from Perak, two from Selangor, one each from Malacca, Pahang and Deli (Sumatra); 12 were Javanese and had come direct from Java to Kuala Lumpur.[29]

The number of women known to be working declined only in the 1930s, when pressure from the League of Nations and from voluntary associations within Britain led to the 'abolition' of prostitution and the disappearance from state records of 'prostitute' as a category. Brothel-keeping, soliciting and prostitution continued even so, and hospitals and private doctors continued to treat women sex workers as well as others for venereal diseases. However abolition technically stripped the women in this underworld of their identity, and they fade as historical figures. Until this time, they were important actors in colonial urban life and medical history, subject to scrutiny and surveillance that cuts across the administrative interests of both the Chinese Protectorate and the Medical Department.

Table 6.1 Brothels and prostitutes in the Federated Malay States, by state and ethnicity, 1906 (B = brothels, P = prostitutes)

State	Chinese		Japanese		Indian		Malay		Total	
	B	P	B	P	B	P	B	P	B	P
Perak	107	1,063	90	533	3	8	17	60	217	1,684
Selangor	52	1,022	65	338	—	2	6	32	123	1,394
Negri Sembilan	22	167	35	183	1	12	3	13	61	375
Pahang	8	71	22	107	4	4	5	12	39	194
Total	**189**	**2,323**	**212**	**1,161**	**8**	**26**	**31**	**117**	**440**	**3,647**

Source: Sel. Sec. 2111/1907, f. 2.

Table 6.2   Location of brothels in the Federated Malay States, 1906

State	Town/District	Number of brothels	Number of prostitutes
Perak	Larut	40	249
	Krian	14	40
	Kuala Kangsar	10	43
	Kinta	116	1,162
	Batang Padang	24	120
	Lower Perak	13	70
Selangor	Kuala Lumpur	53	972
	Ulu Selangor	43	274
	Klang	18	96
	Kuala Langat	2	5
	Kuala Klang	1	3
	Ulu Langat	6	64
Negri Sembilan	Seremban	31	242
	Coast	3	10
	Jelebu	8	37
	Kuala Pilah	11	64
	Tampin	8	22
Pahang	Kuala Lapis	2	10
	Raub	31	123
	Kuantan	6	61

Source: Sel. Sec. 2111/1907, f. 9.

Inside the brothels

Physical conditions within the brothels were poor. Floors were usually
divided by a narrow passage providing access to a double row of small
and airless rooms, within which the women lived. Floor plans of brothels
in Sultan and Petaling Streets in Kuala Lumpur in 1893, for instance,
described by government officers as manifestly overcrowded, show
rooms to be as small as 7 ft 7 ins by 7 ft 9 ins, although some reports refer
to cubicles of six by four feet;[30] larger rooms, which may have accommodated more than one woman, were twice this size, with passages around
4 ft wide.[31] Dr E. A. O. Travers, State Surgeon in Selangor, wrote in 1892
of brothels in this area:

> Houses occupied by Chinese prostitutes are of one description, consisting of
> two or three storied buildings, with narrow passages running the whole
> length of the house; doors at intervals along passages open into small oblong
> boxes, which are pitch dark even in the middle of the day, and are lighted
> with a small lamp. The air in the rooms is foul and stagnant. It seems
> incredible ... that women can exist in such a horrible, and in many cases,
> foetid atmosphere.[32]

Reports describe the brothels as dirty and dilapidated. An inspection of brothels in Pudu Road, Petaling and High Streets, Kuala Lumpur, in 1885, for example, noted the 'horribly filthy state of the drains, wells, habitations and outhouses', and noted of one block of houses containing around 200 inhabitants, subsequently demolished, that

> the faecal matter ... is never removed, and what escapes passes into the drains which ultimately empty themselves into the low mud ponds in front of the joss house and the late Captain China's houses, and should it escape into the river, it does so in a concentrated form, teeming with septic germs.[33]

The Acting Residency Surgeon, John Welch, described conditions in 1889 as 'evil'. Like other buildings, the brothels were overcrowded. Water for cooking and drinking was usually drawn from a brick well in the middle of the kitchen, around 15 to 20 feet deep, and surrounded by sewage matter, 'in every case the latrine is in close proximity to the mouth of the well'.[34] Latrines lacked proper buckets and were often located 'not more than two yards' from the well, and the inadequate number of buckets overflowed early in the day; sometimes they leaked too, 'allowing urine to percolate through the floor and sides and reappear in the passage', and also permitted 'pools of urine' to collect 'among broken tiles of the kitchen floor'.[35] Drains were full of stagnant water, seeping into the domestic water supply. Stairs were too steep and passages too narrow for their purpose; rooms too small; walls dirty; ventilation and lighting poor in both bedrooms and the kitchen. Downstairs earthen floors were rank and turbid.

The reports were repetitive and depressing, although those of the 1890s tended to distinguish between Japanese and Chinese brothels, the former on the whole in better condition and cleaner; the latter 'not over-clean', with 'privy arrangements ... filthy and primitive in the extreme'.[36] The reports were coloured by the aesthetic values of the inspectors who wrote them, who failed to note that the interiors were, in fact, little different from those of other workers' residences at the time. Still the cramped, dark, hot cubicles of Petaling Street in Kuala Lumpur or Sago Lane in Singapore appear to have been particularly nasty, hundreds in buildings 'no longer fit for human habitation',[37] and the official descriptions are remarkable in terms of their constraint. The primary concern in the reports was the house, an incubator of infectious disease and moral contagion – hence the concern with the proximity of brothels to shops and other business houses. There is little expressed interest in the welfare of the women who worked within them, who were often described in memoranda as 'inferior animals'.[38]

In late nineteenth-century Singapore, police were responsible for the cleanliness of the brothels and for ensuring that all women who worked in them were licensed; a medical officer inspected brothels once or twice a year as well.[39] In Kuala Lumpur they were visited by the chairman or an inspector employed by the Sanitary Board, and the board periodically recommended improvements which were expensive, impractical and ignored.[40] Regulations passed in 1893 increased the power of the Chinese Secretary to enforce improvements in living conditions within the brothels. However brothel owners tended not to comply unless under threat.[41] In 1894, brothel owners, including merchants Seow Chong and Loke Yew, petitioned the government for leniency to enable the women to continue to work in old brothels whilst new accommodation was being built, so that they might not be 'deprived of a livelihood'. The Resident was unsympathetic and suggested that given the sex ratio, the women would now have a chance to marry and live 'virtuous lives'.[42]

Swettenham, writing in 1898, argued that 'the condition of prostitutes in the Malay States now is probably worse than it has ever been', and that women were 'dealt with by their owners without the smallest reference to the health, comfort or wishes of the women whom they hold in vilest form of slavery'.[43] Hare, then Secretary for Chinese Affairs in the FMS, claimed that this was due to the repeal of the compulsory registration of prostitutes, and that since 1894, the brothels had fallen into a 'disgraceful state' and that 'their sanitary conditions have immensely deteriorated, and the women and girls in them are absolute slaves, are ill-treated, passed from district to district and from State to State, and are sold to the highest bidder'.[44]

In 1902, it was proposed to relocate a number of brothels in Taiping, Ipoh and Kuala Lumpur to ensure their geographic concentration. This, it was argued, would improve access to the brothels by the police and officers of the Chinese Protectorate, and so facilitate surveillance and control, and improve the hygiene and sanitary standards of the buildings and the 'protection' of brothel workers. It would also increase separation between the brothels and 'family houses and shops of respectable people' and improve the appearance of the towns.[45] The concern here related in part to the street life that concentrated around the brothels, and the tensions that erupted among men of different clans; a decade earlier Swettenham had written of mining towns in Perak where 'hundreds and sometimes thousands of Chinese coolies of the lowest class' would mill around the brothels, fighting at 'the smallest provocation'.[46] In Kuala Lumpur, a number of brothels were located near the chapels and the golf links, and it was these which in 1902 were to be closed and moved to side lanes near Petaling Street. There were objections also to the brothels in High Street and Sultan Street near the Victoria Institution, and it was estimated that some 25 houses, each to accommodate 25 women, would be required for relocation.[47] Even when new housing was provided, conditions remained poor and the brothels were always crowded.

In addition to the established and geographically concentrated brothels, 'sly' prostitutes, often allegedly Malay or Eurasian women, worked with rickshaw drivers, hotel employees or pimps to solicit customers:

> (A) prostitute would be riding about in a rikisha, and if she saw a person who looked likely to be a client she smiled at him, and if he seemed to be interested in the proposition and smiled back or turned around to look at her then she would probably just wave her hand or show a handkerchief out of the back of the rikisha, and her puller would slow down until she saw whether the prospective client followed her or not. If he did she either went back to her abode and let him follow, or else went to a quiet place where her rikisha would stop until the follower came up and arrangements for a meeting could be made ... in the F.M.S. generally speaking promiscuous intercourse with prostitutes who are not members of known brothels is arranged through employees of hotels, eating houses, etc.[48]

As already noted, the conditions for those in the brothels were no different from those of other poor urban dwellers; labourers, rickshaw drivers and artisans all lived in conditions of extreme privation, overcrowding, and insanitation, in buildings that lacked ventilation and water and were vulnerable to fire. But living in the brothels was a different experience. Women employed in the Cantonese houses especially had the status of slaves, were confined or allowed to leave only in the company of a 'brothel bully', and tortured and beaten to comply with the brothel keeper's wishes.

Children were born in and grew up in the premises. Police were occasionally alerted to underage workers and would search the houses, although usually minors (that is, those under 16) would be concealed and young prostitutes were substituted with women from other brothels.[49] Most women registered as prostitutes with the Chinese Protectorate claimed to be aged around 16 to 24, but the majority taken into custody by the Protectorate were in their teens.[50] Both underage and older women, as noted, were often held under conditions of virtual slavery and with little recourse for help, particularly where police and brothel owners were in consort. In Singapore in 1901, for example, allegations were made by H. Carus that a brothel owner named Laurence or Laura Maksama lived with the Chief Inspector of the Detectives' Office, that the Inspector 'stops as might at her place so she not be got', that she paid a monthly sum to the Superintendent of Police also for protection, and that any prostitute who ran away was returned to her by the police. Carus also referred to police protection which enabled the sale of women from pimps to brothel owners at the Club House Hotel and Bellevue Hotel.[51] The Inspector-General and the Protector of Chinese, Evans, investigated the brothels in Hylam and Malabar Streets, implicated in Carus' letters, but uncovered neither minors nor 'other irregularities', the Inspector-General being 'entirely satisfied that all of them (prostitutes) are not merely content with their lot but are actually cheerful and lighthearted'. Carus' allegations were dismissed as the work of a crank.[52] If this were true, Carus' letters had led police to those few brothels where conditions were good. Other fragmentary documents and Warren's evidence of the lives of prostitutes in Singapore around this time suggest that this was extremely unusual.[53]

According to Hare, women were often well treated at the time of recruitment by the procurers to ensure that they would leave China, but once they reached Malaya they were subject to systematic violence and cruelty – beatings with rattan, confinement, having their fingers squeezed in boards, and so on.[54] Mrs McBreen claimed that women who ran away were, if caught, 'buried alive or tortured to death', and in a letter written in June 1900, maintained that

> [t]here are a great many prostitutes in the colony and most of them were kidnapped from China, some had men even say that they are husbands and wives; but when they arrive here they are sold to Brothel Keepers for a certain amount of money and for that sum of money they have to be prostitutes for the brothel keeper for a long period. The usual time is 5 years but some of them who are stupid are kept longer. Some of them follow men but even then they suffer the same fate, for after being husbands and wives for some time they are sold again. If the Brothel Keeper has the least suspicion of the prostitutes trying to run away they are sold; if the prostitute is smart, she is drugged first and then sold, and so these also lead a miserable life.[55]

Under the provisions for the registration of brothels, revoked in 1894, women were to be informed of their status as free agents and their right to leave their place of employment at will. This did not always occur, and alternative legislation – the Women and Girls Protection Ordinance (1896) with its various amendments – failed to prevent their bondage.

Venereal infection and the law

Women working in the brothels were infected constantly with syphilis, gonorrhoea, genital ulcers, abscesses and warts, and were forced to work in spite of these infections. Their health was undoubtedly equivocal otherwise: they were vulnerable to cystitis and other urinary tract infections, fungal and bacterial genital infections, gonorrhoea and other pelvic infections. Some of these diseases literally ate away their bodies, causing pain and disfigurement. Galloway's description of lymph node infection in the groin, caused by various venereal infections, illustrates this well: internal and external ulceration, 'sloughy sore(s) with (a) hard base ... creeping on at one part while healing at another'; a woman with her urethral canal eroded by an ulcer; others with 'exquisite pelvic tenderness', fevers, swollen glands, badly inflamed cervix, rigid vaginal walls.[56] Although infertility from infection was common, some women conceived, then sought illegal and dangerous abortions, miscarried, or worked throughout pregnancy and gave birth under conditions of extreme privation. No less than any other women in the community, they would have sustained perineal and vaginal tears during labour, suffering as they were forced back to work as soon as possible after delivery. A number must also have died from post-partum haemorrhages or septicaemia, and many would have watched their infants die from jaundice or neonatal tetanus.

Despite recurrent illness and infection, the women worked long hours, their lives dominated by poverty and fear. They were routinely beaten by brothel keepers, raped and abused by their clients, threatened and bullied by police, shunned by pious onlookers. Their only friends were probably other women subject to the same frightful conditions, their one chance of escape the promises of a pimp or fantasies with favourite customers. Some were murdered; others committed suicide; many sought lesser escape through alcohol. Some kept opium in their rooms for customers, but brothel keepers could keep chandu and pipes for their own use, and the occasional death of a prostitute from opium suggests its wider use. The Anti-Opium Society took exception to the practice, but others were rather more liberal: the High Commissioner's view was that 'the main objection to opium smoking in brothels is the vitiation of the atmosphere in the cubicles'.[57]

The scandal was the silence. Details of the women's health is fragmentary, and even for sexually transmitted diseases, much of the information is indirect or by inference only, since it refers to men's infections, not women's. The Colonial Surgeon, Dr Mugliston, estimated that all of the three thousand prostitutes then working in Singapore were or had been infected, that they were 'chief disseminators of disease',[58] and that the majority at any time were unfit to work but were coerced to continue. Others shared his view that all women had been infected at some time, those worst affected bought 'secondhand' from Singapore to work in the FMS.[59] But doctors were far better positioned to speak of infections among men – prisoners, troops, coolies, and Pauper hospital inmates – than they were about women.

The incidence of venereal disease among ground troops in the Tanglin district of Singapore, for instance, rose steeply once the compulsory

178 SICKNESS AND THE STATE

medical examination of prostitutes ceased with the repeal of the Contagious Disease Ordinance in 1888. During the final five-year period of the operation of the Contagious Diseases Act, from 1884 to 1888, the ratio of admissions to hospital with VD per thousand men averaged 144.28; over 50 percent of admissions had gonorrhoea. From 1892 to 1896, without legislation, the average rate of admissions rose to 434.17 per thousand men, two-thirds with syphilis. In 1895, the rate was 617.53.[60] Statistics for the navy are not available, but ships' captains estimated an increased incidence of around 50 percent per annum once compulsory examinations and treatment ceased. Prison reports illustrate a similar trend. In 1890, 202 of 4,856 prisoners admitted to the Criminal Prison in Singapore were currently or had previously suffered a venereal infection; in 1896 some 1,732 of 3,497 were then or had been afflicted: that is, 50 percent of prisoners in the latter year, compared with only around four percent six years earlier.[61] Hare estimated in 1898 that the prevalence of gonorrhoea and syphilis among Hailam house servants was around 20 percent, the incidence 60 percent;[62] Galloway 20 years later maintained that venereal diseases were so prevalent among men that they 'must appear in the anamnesis of nearly every illness'.[63]

Evidence is that disease escalated following the repeal of the Contagious Diseases Ordinance. In Penang in 1895, approximately 15 percent of convicts had signs of having had venereal disease; in 1897 nearly 25 percent did so, and these rates were lower than those for Singapore only because of the higher rate of marriage in Penang as a consequence of the established Straits-born Chinese community and thus a favourable sex ratio. Estimates of venereal disease in the FMS also increased.[64] Available figures were considered to be underestimates; this was certainly the case for men other than troops or those in gaol. For colonial officers a diagnosis of venereal disease might affect leave or retirement benefits and, in consequence, medical officers completing their health certificates were elusive or ambiguous, or used technical language to ensure confidentiality from non-medical officers.[65]

The increased incidence of and mortality from sexually transmitted diseases was general, and although the brothels were regarded as a reservoir for reinfection, it was certainly not true that brothel workers were the only source. Transmission among men as well as between men and women was not uncommon, and there was an increase in the incidence of anal syphilis among servants after the repeal of the Ordinance.[66] According to Adamson, Chair of the Straits Settlement Association, the Hailamese sex ratio of 70:1 led to 'a large recourse by these men to low brothels', and to 'the common practice of unnatural vice'; Hare also drew attention to the incidence of gonorrhoea and syphilis among servants, largely motivated by a concern that European employers and their dependents were at risk through non-sexual contact:

I allude to the frightful dangers that innocent Europeans and Chinese, with their families and children, are daily incurring of contracting syphilitic and gonorrhoeal diseases at the hands of their Chinese Hailam servants. If a medical inspection were ordered tomorrow morning of all the Hailam servants (valets, cooks, coolies, rickshaw pullers, water carriers, &c) now in service in European and Chinese private houses in Kuala Lumpur, I am confident that at the very least twenty percent of them would be found to be actually suffering from gonorrhoeal or syphilitic affections in one form or another, and that practically sixty percent would be found to have suffered at one time or another from such diseases. If one remembers that these contagious diseases can be conveyed to innocent persons, men, women, and children, through the medium of eating and drinking vessels, clothes, blankets, bathroom towels, and so forth ... it is not necessary to point out what dangers from contracting these contagious diseases, Europeans and Chinese living here run.[67]

Domestic servants and urban labourers, however, were never a target for the application of a (new) Contagious Disease Ordinance, partly perhaps because it was easier to ignore the implications of reputed widespread homosexual activity, and partly because of the assumption that a fellow worker was a poor alternative to a female sexual partner unless the deterrents were great. Hence government control of venereal infection focused on the inspection of women to assure clients that they had a 'clean' bill of health. This was a relatively simple strategy given access to women in public brothels.

Under the ordinance, the government had the right to examine and treat, and operated a Lock Hospital for the isolation of infectious diseases. Repeal had resulted, it was claimed, in untreated infection among prostitutes. Welch, a District Surgeon based at the Selangor Pauper Hospital, reported that a number of women in Petaling Street were forced to work despite advanced infection. Women tended to delay seeking medical attention, often because they were prevented from so doing by the brothel keepers, and would finally be admitted to hospitals in 'an almost dying state' with 'strong evidence of ill treatment and neglect' as well as disease.[68]

The argument for the reintroduction of the compulsory medical examination of prostitutes was premised on the belief that any voluntary system would fail, because the women would not seek medical help, because of their 'innate aversion' to examination and reluctance to go to hospital. The committee appointed by the Governor of the Straits Settlements in 1898 to consider measures to check the spread of venereal diseases argued that Chinese women were indifferent rather than averse to examination, and found that 'Chinese women have no objection, beyond that occasionally shewn by a little childish outbreak of petulance, which is over in half an hour, to being detained in hospital, and absolutely no objections to examination'.[69] The committee recommended a formal system of examination and care, since this would most effectively work around the restraints placed upon them: 'the largest proportion of women (had) absolutely no voice in any matter in connection with their own lives and thus any attempt to reach them as individuals whilst they remain working in a brothel would be useless'.[70] In reaching this decision, they drew on evidence of the systematic refusal of brothel keepers to provide medical care, citing examples of women in tears because they were working through illness, and arguing that on any night, 2,000 to 2,500 women working in Singapore should be in the Lock Hospital.[71] Dr Rogers and Dr Mugliston, the Colonial Surgeon, also argued that the major reason for delayed treatment was that brothel keepers prevented the prostitutes from going to hospital and failed to bring their employees for medical attention, forcing them instead 'to go on plying their trade' to avoid loss of profit.[72]

Medical examinations tended, in any case, to be perfunctory. Prostitutes were registered and examined regularly, generally once a month. A doctor would examine up to 110 or 120 women per hour, primarily by checking whether their glands were enlarged as an indication of venereal infection. Many believed that the inspections were a 'farce', and that no doctor could possibly tell 'whether a woman is suffering from venereal disease or not by looking at her face or feeling her pulse'.[73]

Support for the reintroduction of legislation to allow the compulsory examination and treatment of women with venereal disease received limited support. Some, mainly churchmen such as the Reverend Shellabear, argued against this as an invasion of the privacy of women, 'an indecent outrage'.[74] Non-legislative means to increase women's access to treatment were explored instead. The employment of 'lady doctors' (as they were termed by the Medical Department) to work with prostitutes was rejected on the grounds that visiting Chinese brothels in the hot summer months would be too trying for English women; their health would not stand it; patients would not have the same confidence in women doctors as in men; and a woman doctor 'fond of her profession' would be unable to deal with the monotony of the work, especially since she would be able to persuade only a few women to accept medical treatment.[75]

However, the majority of doctors and other officers argued that legislation had been effective and supported its reintroduction from a stance of cultural relativism: the repeal of the Ordinance had occurred in the context of an inappropriate English morality that failed to account for the realities of the social and sexual life of people in the region. There was additionally a growing feeling, shared by prominent Chinese members of the community as well as European officials, that only legislative measures would overcome the resistance of the brothel keepers to securing medical care for their employees.[76]

The Women and Girls' Protection Ordinance, introduced in 1896, replaced the early ordinance. It aimed to prevent the procuring, receipt, harbouring or use for prostitution of women under the age of sixteen, and to provide state protection for women held against their wishes in brothels or imported without their agreement or foreknowledge of their work as prostitutes. The Ordinance was amended in 1899 to make it illegal too for a brothel keeper to employ a prostitute with venereal disease. Prior to its introduction, officers of the Chinese Protectorate visited all known brothels or summoned together brothel keepers to explain the implications of the legislation and their responsibility under it. W. Evans, Protector of the Chinese in Singapore, interviewed all Chinese and Japanese brothel keepers in the settlements to warn them that they would be held responsible for disease in their brothels. As a consequence, brothel keepers retained the services of qualified medical men to visit the brothels routinely, inspect the women, and arrange for those too badly infected to be treated at the brothel to go to a private hospital or the government Lock Hospital.[77] Although some smaller brothels argued that they could not afford the fees to ensure regular medical attendance,[78] many employed medical practitioners so that women were inspected fortnightly; others arranged for a government practitioner to provide medical care to the brothels in addition to under-taking official duties.[79] Outpatient attendance at government hospitals also increased. Brothel keepers, threatened with the penalties of fines, banishment and the closure of the brothels, cooperated reluctantly.[80]

The brothel clubs

Two small scandals occurred in the early 1900s which reveal the contra-dictions that emerged as a result of the state's medicalisation of prosti-tution. Obsessions with hygiene and sanitation, disease control and treatment, and outrage at the conditions under which women were held and treated in the brothels, provided individuals within the government with an opportunity to provide medical care to sex workers and to profit from so doing.

Brothel keepers generally resisted domiciliary visits and the inspection of their 'girls' where the segregation of those infected was a possibility, and doctors or apothecaries were usually summoned only when disease was advanced and 'mischief may have been done'.[81] However, a number of Japanese and Chinese brothels in Singapore, Penang and the FMS employed doctors in anticipation of new legislation or as a standard procedure,[82] a few private hospitals existed for prostitutes, and a medical club system operated on a small scale. The first was established in

Singapore by the Colonial Surgeon, Dr Mugliston, who in 1888 was contracted to examine Japanese women in Malay Street brothels. The contract was broken after one month because, he said, his 'strict method of giving certificates (of health) did not suit them', but other doctors continued to provide treatment and issue women with certificates of health to display on the brothel walls. In 1893, Mugliston re-established contact with the brothel world and set up four medical clubs for Cantonese prostitutes, with a private hospital maintained nearby for the quick transfer of critically ill women to prevent deaths on brothel premises. Fees were paid to him directly either by the brothel keeper or the prostitute, where her earnings were under her own control; medicine was provided at a reduced rate from the government dispensary.[83] In establishing the brothel medical club and acting as a consulting physician to the brothels, Mugliston exercised his right to private practice. This raised questions of conflict of interest, given the potential difficulty of brothel keepers and prostitutes in distinguishing between Mugliston's roles as a private practitioner and as Colonial Surgeon. However, Mitchell, Governor of the Straits Settlements, upheld his right to private practice, and Mugliston insisted that brothel keepers understood that they were not obliged to employ him rather than any other practitioner.

Other private hospitals also treated prostitutes. Four additional hospitals were established by brothel keepers themselves in September 1899 to accommodate an increasing number of Chinese patients, relieving the government-run Kandang Kerbau Hospital of additional patients that might have followed from the legislation enforcing the treatment of women with venereal disease.[84] Women inpatients primarily suffered from syphilis, but also from buboes or ulcers, abscesses, genital warts, other skin infections, gonorrhoea, fever, burns, tuberculosis and chronic rheumatism.[85]

In Kuala Lumpur a private Lock Hospital opened in 1901 under the auspices of the Federal Dispensary Company.[86] In arguing the need to improve the delivery of medical care to sick brothel workers in the FMS, G. T. Hare, the Secretary of Chinese Affairs, advocated the establishment of brothel medical clubs such as those operating in Singapore, with doctors contracting to treat inmates on a per head per mensem basis, and to keep a small dispensary and private hospital. The pecuniary interests of the practitioner ensured that the system would work well and would protect the prostitutes from 'Chinese quacks' and 'second rate unqualified European practitioners'. Brothel medical fees, Hare argued, 'would be a fairly certain source of income, and there should be a fairly good private practice besides amongst the Chinese upper classes and non-official Europeans and Eurasians'.[87] In the FMS, he suggested that a sole practitioner be responsible for brothels in each of the major towns, while others bore responsibility for brothels dispersed in smaller mining towns. A government officer such as the Protector of the Chinese or the State Surgeon would be responsible for ensuring compliance with the Ordinance, and could refer women to the practitioner for treatment. Hare also proposed that, in the interests of health and hygiene, government medical officers take a lead role in directing if not running the medical clubs through their right to private practice.[88]

Hare also proposed that there be government Lock Hospitals in the larger towns in each state. His proposals rested on the supposition that Cantonese women, who constituted a majority of prostitutes, would not use general hospitals, and the new hospitals would need to take into account their preferences:

> I am quite sure that a Lock Hospital would be a success if it were established unconventionally and conducted primarily on Chinese lines with European supervision and medical attendance ... one large sized private house with an upper storey near a Brothel district could well be converted at little cost into a Lock Hospital ... There would not be the same prejudice to going into such institutions as exists in the minds of the Chinese against going into Hospitals, [and] Lock Hospitals too would be of great assistance to any Doctors looking after inmates of Brothels in their capacity as private practitioners.[89]

The British Resident argued against the use of government buildings as brothel hospitals, however, and was cautious of the extent of government involvement in their running, preferring instead to see private lock hospitals continue with regular medical attendance provided by private practitioners. The State Surgeon's interest would be confined to 'periodical inspections in his official capacity'.[90]

Private hospitals run by government medical practitioners proliferated, however, following the amendments to the Women and Girls Protection Ordinance in the Settlements in 1899 and in the FMS soon after, with brothel keepers in a given street or district sharing the costs of retaining a doctor and renting a house for the examination and hospitalisation of workers. Severely sick women were sent to the government lock hospitals.[91]

In addition, by early 1903 Dr Travers had opened a private hospital in Kuala Lumpur, Dr John Gimlette had established a private hospital in Ipoh, and efforts were under way to rent a house in Taiping, with brothel owners contributing to the rent and the state, through the auspices of the State Surgeon, providing medicine free of charge.[92] The Ipoh hospital was run, as Hare had recommended, with a Chinese matron-in-charge and a Chinese dispenser. The retainer fee was two dollars, and this provided women with two examinations, treatment for any medical condition, and free medicine. 'Taking into consideration the disagreeable work to be performed by the medical men twice a month', this was regarded as a 'very reasonable' charge.[93] The nature of the work, however, was vague.

Gimlette argued against government officers taking a fee for service, given the impossibility of examining thoroughly 400 women twice a month without neglecting their government duties.[94] In this he was prophetic. Within a few years of the introduction of legislation, and the establishment of the medical clubs and hospitals, charges had been laid against doctors for malpractice and conflict of interest. This resulted in an inquiry first into the activities of Travers, the State Surgeon of Selangor, then into the activities of several senior medical officers in Perak.

Travers and the Petaling Street brothels

In early 1902, following discussions with Hare, Secretary of Chinese Affairs, Dr Travers opened a medical club and 12-bed hospital for Cantonese prostitutes in Petaling Street in Kuala Lumpur. Brothel keepers shared the costs of renting a neighbouring house as a private hospital, and prostitutes retained Travers' services through a fee of $1.50 per month, which entitled them to free medical and surgical treatment at the hospital. Travers employed a dresser to visit the subscribing brothels on a regular basis; Travers himself attended only on request. By 1905, some 666 Chinese prostitutes belonged to the medical club, and by 1907 this had expanded considerably to include a number of Japanese women and other Chinese women from 'outstation' brothels (that is, located out of Kuala Lumpur).

In 1907 moves were initiated by the Governor, Sir John Anderson, and the acting Resident-General, Mr E. L. Brockman, to remove from Travers and other government medical officers the right to private practice because of apparent abuses of the system. In Travers' case, this included profiteering. At the time, some 737 women subscribed to the hospital, with around nine inpatients and 4.5 outpatients seen daily.[95] The average monthly net profit from April 1904 to April 1906 was $854; from April 1906 to June 1907 it was $771, lower primarily because the hospital had commenced providing patients with food. The capital investment in the hospital was, it was argued, practically nil, and conditions poor: a dozen plank beds on trestles occupied by sick women, several other women and children were about, and the place was 'dirty and squalid'.[96] Anderson and Brockman claimed that prostitutes subscribed to the club because of Travers' official status, and that 'the profits made by Dr Travers and others were quite out of proportion to

the services rendered by them'. Brockman also raised questions about
the services that outstation brothels received for their subscriptions:
Kuala Lumpur brothels at least were visited sporadically by a dresser and
could call on Travers if necessary, but there was no evidence that
outstation brothels were ever visited.

The second charge against Travers was that his role as a private
practitioner running a brothel hospital was in direct conflict with his
role as State Surgeon. A couple of cases illustrate this. In 1903 a brothel
keeper was summoned by the Protector of Chinese under Section 14(1)
of the enactment for failing to ensure that her workers subscribed to a
club. The principal witness for the prosecution was Travers. The brothel
keeper pleaded guilty and was fined $200, and thus Travers was not
required to give evidence; a month after the case, the defendant's
brothel became a subscriber to Travers' medical club. Anderson did not
question Travers' ability to differentiate his responsibilies, but questioned whether brothel keepers and prostitutes could do so.[97] Brockman
argued that a wider conflict of interest existed too, since Travers was the
person responsible to the government for private hospitals and for
initiating legal proceedings *against* private practitioners, including any
action with respect to substandard care and accommodation.

Travers was criticised further for his treatment of Japanese prostitutes,
who paid $2 a month for a weekly vaginal examination and the sub-
sequent issue of certificates of fitness.[98] Anderson opposed this on moral
grounds, since by issuing certificates of fitness Travers was, in Anderson's
view, encouraging 'immoral purpose'. Brockman's argument was also
one of ethics: 'There is no doubt that what they (Japanese prostitutes)
subscribed for was not medical attendance but certificates of health,
since some of their clients ask for such certificates, which if signed by
a medical officer of the rank of State Surgeon are valuable to them in
their profession'.[99]

The Kinta scandal

Private brothel practice was highly lucrative. 'It was', the Resident-
General argued, 'the knowledge of the fortunes that were being made
out of this practice that caused the scramble for a share of it among the
Kinta doctors resulting in a scandal that reflected upon the whole
medical service of the Federated Malay States and it has led to quarrels
between medical officers in the Government Service'.[100]

The Kinta scandal involved a series of related legal–ethical cases,
including charges against Drs Fox, Cooper and Brown, the 'Connolly
Campaign' – wherein state doctors vied to prevent the brothel practice
of a medical practitioner *not* in government employ – and the

involvement in the affair by the Perak State Resident. These are described briefly here, to explore the extent to which public health measures, initially introduced to protect women, could be abused.

In Perak, the association of doctors and prostitutes evolved in response to the provisions of the Women and Girls Protection Ordinance (Enactment No. 7 of 1902). In January 1903, Dr Gimlette, the District Surgeon for Kinta, instituted a fortnightly inspection of prostitutes in brothels in the state, and in Ipoh, the state capital, established the Magdalene Hospital to which prostitutes were admitted and where they remained on a voluntary basis. In June 1903 Gimlette left the state medical service, and handed over $500 as a donation to the hospital to allow its expansion for the benefit of its patients. Dr R. M. Connolly, District Surgeon when Gimlette retired, took over management of the Magdalene Hospital; in 1905, his own retirement foreshadowed, he proposed to the government that he remain in the state as a private practitioner with a retaining fee of $800 per month plus allowances to run the brothel medical practice in Kinta where the largest number of prostitutes was concentrated. The battle that ensued over the right of Connolly to the practice was to become known as the 'Connolly Campaign'.

Connolly and W. A. Barnes, Hare's successor as Secretary of Chinese Affairs, recommended that a Magdalene Association be established and that medical care be concentrated at the hospital in Ipoh. The British Resident in Perak, E. W. Birch, opposed the proposition on the grounds that a single hospital would place a number of prostitutes at a logistic disadvantage. Since the District Surgeon, Dr S. C. G. Fox, already also ran a brothel practice in Perak and had done so since 1903, granting Connolly a monopoly practice in the Kinta region would deprive Fox and other state employees of their rights to private practice, and government sanction of the proposed scheme would imply its support of monopolies. Birch appears to have shared the concern of the State Surgeon, Wright, that the Chinese Protectorate's support of Connolly's proposition was vested, since this might facilitate its surveillance and protection of the women. While they had no objection to this, they argued that hospitals should all be under the control of the Medical Department, that a single hospital would not meet community needs, and that instead, a number of small hospitals, geographically dispersed, were required.[101]

Connolly set up practice under a directive by the State Secretariat, sharing the district with Fox. Connolly worked from the Magdalene Hospital in Ipoh and was highly praised by both Dr Wright and Dr Barnes, although there were suggestions of overservicing resulting in women's general avoidance of medical services and subsequent untreated infections.[102] Fox passed his practice on to Dr T. G. D. Cooper.

These two men, together with Dr J. E. M. Brown, the new District Surgeon, pursued their campaign against Connolly and his apparent monopoly resulting in 'a most unbecoming fight for the business' involving direct advertising.[103]

Surgeons throughout the FMS protested that the directive which enabled Connolly to set up practice interfered with the right of prostitutes to the medical practitioner of their choice, constituted a monopoly, and effectively withdrew the right to private practice which had only recently been re-endorsed.[104] In response, the High Commissioner insisted that he did not recognise the vested right to brothel practice of any medical officer and that the matter was the concern of the Secretary for Chinese Affairs. Orders relating to the establishment of a monopoly were cancelled.[105]

Connolly's aim upon retirement, to secure a lucrative private practice, was not in question. What was under scrutiny was the right of state-employed practitioners to counter-tout for the custom of prostitutes, and to be involved in the brothel medical practice while fulfilling official duties satisfactorily. The controversy led to the appointment of a commission of inquiry, chaired by L. M. Woodward, the Judicial Commissioner. The commission drew attention to the involvement of a number of medical officers in brothel practices.[106] In consequence, a triumvirate comprising Woodward, Birch, the Resident of Perak, and L. P. Ebden, Legal Adviser, was established to hear charges against the doctors. The most extensive charges were against Fox: that he regarded his private practice of primary importance and instigated his subordinates to neglect their work to pursue private practice; that he advertised to secure a clientele; that he received fees for medical examinations that were 'most perfunctory' and 'a mere farce'; and that he used government apothecaries and dressers for private practice.[107] He was also investigated for charging fees to examine opium shops and to issue certificates to exhume bodies.

Fox's brothel practice in Kampar had commenced in 1903, with the upper storey of an apothecary's shop serving as a six-bed hospital, barely used and closed after eighteen months. Fearful of losing custom as medical aid societies were set up in the town, Fox then employed an apothecary to attend to prostitutes, contracted women to use his service, and posted notices in the brothels ordering women to go to the government hospital when ill. Fox maintained that the women in these brothels were already his patients, that they were not compelled to see him, and that the notices were posted only in brothels where he had prior contact: 'I emphatically state that the issuing of the notice was an honest intention on my part to try and check venereal disease. Its effect could only be more work for me, and could have no effect on my fees which had already been arranged'.[108] Fox insisted that the notice was not intended to threaten Connolly's practice. The triumvirate in turn found that while it was improperly worded, Fox had no motive 'but to compel the sick women to go to hospital, except he probably thought to bind them to him more firmly by fear of his powers as Government Doctor, and to be able to show that he was really doing something for his fees'.[109] Fox rejected charges of his neglect of official duty and of instigating subordinate officers (Cooper and Brown) also to neglect official duty in favour of brothel practice.

The brothel practice, as already mentioned, was very profitable. Fox was estimated to receive around $719 per month from it, and at the height of his involvement, when he was also District Surgeon, he received a further $150 retainer fee from the mines and an unspecified amount from European patients. When he became Acting State Surgeon, he divided parts of the practice to Cooper and Brown, but retained a significant portion. When he employed an apothecary in Kampar to attend to the brothel workers in his own absence, he was receiving $350 per month. He paid the apothecary $30 per month, and since he was not maintaining a hospital, was making $320 profit per month from this practice alone. Women paid additionally for prescriptions, and obstetrical services attracted a further fee.[110]

The triumvirate described the service given to the women as a 'hurried farce of examination' and 'a totally inadequate return for (their) money'. Examination by Fox and other doctors usually involved a visual check of genitalia, or more often, a cursory glance at the woman's general appearance and a quick feel through her clothes of the glands in her groin. Fox admitted that his examination was cursory but 'the best that could be done under the voluntary method', given women's objections to the use of a speculum. He describes the examination thus:

At the first inspection of the brothels at the beginning of each month I took the interpreter with me. The women were all ready and expecting me, a table and chair were placed before me, each girl came to me separately, bringing her card which I initialled as 'seen'. I felt her glands in her groin, looked at her general appearance, and legs, and felt her pulse. I was a quick worker and it is obvious that in the examination of many of the women who seemed quite well I spent a short time, cases of a suspicious nature were asked to go to the hospital, where an attempt was made to examine with a speculum ... My second visit in the month was paid without an interpreter, it was a sort of surprise visit. I used to go into the brothel and asked to see the keeper who was often absent. I asked the women about if any one was ill or wanted treatment, they nearly always said no ... My examination of the women in Papan, Pusing and Tronoh was conducted on the same lines as in Kampar, only I could not be at these places as frequently as I was in Kampar.[111]

For their part, the brothel keepers were satisfied. A testimony to the Commission of Inquiry from Papan referred to 'admirably good treatments and best remedies of all sorts of diseases', and those of Kampar submitted that:

> We the (undersigned) brothel keepers have engaged Dr Fox to attend the sick amongst us for the last three and a half years. The Doctor has *great ability* and is ever ready to relieve distress. Whenever such people go to him for treatment it is never but that the touch of his hand restores health; the members of those whom he has saved amongst our class is not small.[112]

A 'touch of his hand', however, was not exactly what was required. Japanese prostitutes in Kampar, in contrast, were given vaginal examinations using a speculum twice a month, and received medical and hospital treatment for a charge of $3; they received what they wanted and would have withdrawn their patronage from Fox had he not provided internal examinations.

On other charges, Fox was found guilty but the censure was mild given his contractual entitlement to private practice. Fox himself admitted that he had made use of government apothecaries and dressers for his private practice, but there was no regulation to prevent this and the practice was common.

Charges brought against Cooper were similar to those against Fox: providing inadequate services to the women from whom he collected subscriptions. He made it clear to brothel keepers in Ipoh and Menglembu that he would not visit the brothels to conduct examinations, but that women who were unwell could present as outpatients at the hospital for medication and examination.[113] He visited women in Papan twice a month 'if possible' to supply them with medicine and in the meantime, they were visited on a weekly basis by the Chinese senior dresser in Batu Gajah 'in his spare time'.[114]

Cooper was also charged with touting with the intention of taking patients from Connolly, and with entering into 'a profit-sharing association with two low-class Asiatic practitioners', a Chinese named Wong I Ek, and a Japanese practitioner, Katsuji Matsutaki. Cooper became a joint owner of a hospital for prostitutes with Wong, who had resigned from the Perak Medical Department under suspicion of trafficking in heroin and morphine, and at the time of the partnership was operating a dispensary in Ipoh. Matsutaki had in February 1907 established a hospital for Japanese prostitutes in Ipoh and surrounding areas, and Cooper's profit-sharing arrangement with him, through serving as consulting physician, gave him effective control of the hospital.

Japanese women were given vaginal examinations by Cooper twice a month, in Sungei Siput once a month. A woman named Ouichi died on 29

March 1907 whilst under Cooper's care from an apparent embolism following 'inflammation of the womb', but although neglect was implied, no charges were made nor inquiry held.[115] Japanese women were examined routinely, but this was not so for Chinese women and Cooper visited those in hospital irregularly. Examinations were perfunctory:

> You could not legally make it anything but cursory ... Once a month I used to send round to a particular brothel and say I would like to see the inmates at the private hospital: they would come forward one by one, and I examined the skin of the legs, thighs, abdomen, hands and feet and inguinal glands through the clothes, and the throat if necessary ... About 175 Chinese women per month came to me. I did not have them up all at the same time. To examine a dozen women it would take, as I did it, more or less a half an hour.[116]

Ching Fook Meng, a dresser in the Medical Department, Taiping, claimed that at times the examination was briefer still: 'Some women, he felt their pulse or glands; others, if they complained, he might examine them, or if he suspected anything, he might examine them with a speculum. He might order the woman to be admitted to hospital, or prescribe some medicine for her'.[117]

Cooper was acquitted of all charges. The triumvirate found that he had only entered into a partnership with Wong I Ek when he found out that Wong had gained formal qualifications, that the arrangement between them was solely for the purpose of providing medical and hospital services for Chinese prostitutes, and that he was unaware of any touting by Wong. His arrangement with Matsutaki was similarly solely for the purpose of the treatment of prostitutes. The triumvirate felt that the care delivered was adequate for the fees received, or at least 'of the same standard as those rendered by other Government Medical Officers'.[118] These findings led to an acrimonious report by the High Commissioner, Sir John Anderson, and criticism particularly of the Perak State Resident, Birch, who Anderson felt was implicated in the affair since he had supported Fox's right to brothel practice. Birch in turn was found to be 'an intolerable nuisance' and removed from office soon after.[119]

Not all doctors took advantage of the legislation to profit at the expense of the prostitutes. Gimlette and M. J. Wright, the State Surgeon, were both considered to have been above board. In Taiping Wright had established a hospital for prostitutes with reduced fees, found that the women were willing to attend hospital without any pressure being brought to bear on the brothel keeper, and was in favour of the system continuing to control venereal disease, blackmail and exploitation of women.[120] Gimlette, according to Barnes, displayed 'unfailing tact and genuine interest ... to so win confidence of the women for whom his

Hospital was intended that not only did they cease to object to submit themselves to examination but they readily stayed in the Hospital when ordered to do so and in many instances voluntarily sought admission'.[121]

In most cases, however, brothel medical practice was a lucrative supplement to a state salary and the health of the women and their clients was of secondary concern. The result was a prohibition on medical officers participating in brothel practices from September 1907; thereafter medical officers could only attend women unable to present to hospital if no other private practitioner were available, and government medical officers were to have no financial interests in private hospitals or practices.[122] Brothels were subsequently notified that it was not necessary to retain a medical attendant and that examinations, treatment and drugs were free at government hospitals.[123]

The state as guardian

Profiteering and corruption were, arguably, inevitable appurtenances of a system that tolerated the brothels and the infringements of human rights that they harboured. I have suggested that prostitution was regarded as inevitable, given the population structure of the colonies and the assumed nature of sexual desire; and the brothels that operated in the towns of the colonies were viewed as manageable if not always benign institutions. Local police knew the brothel keepers and the women who worked there, sometimes exceptionally well, and hence were able to keep in touch with (aspects of) the traffic in women. The availability of commercial sex was itself seen to be placatory, a service and an entertainment for the men. At the same time, the state was poorly positioned to deal with the kidnapping, enslavement, torture and extortion that occurred, reported routinely from the 1860s to the early 1900s. The colonists had few skills to tackle these problems institutionally or structurally. Legislative changes had little impact on the operation of prostitution, and so the government opted instead to tackle the 'problem' by protecting men (administrators, troops, and labourers) from venereal disease, and protecting women, through the offices of the Chinese Protectorate, by offering alternative residence and employment.

From around 1910, though, there was a perceptible shift of policy and mood *from* that of protecting men *to* that of protecting women. This coincided with the state's discovery, as it were, of reproduction, and its perceived role in nurturing the family, in monitoring the health of women and children and providing services for them, and in intervening in working-class lives with respect to issues of morality and material well-being. This was a concern within Britain, echoed in the colonies. It was reflected in maternal and child health programs in

Malaya, as discussed in the following chapter, and was picked up in discussions about urban housing in Singapore; for instance, crowding was believed to increase the transmission of venereal disease by encouraging 'promiscuous behaviour', as well as facilitating the spread of airborne infections. At this same time, then, the discourse of prostitution re-oriented to issues of morality and an alternative, contradictory model of sexuality that prescribed women's proper roles. Homes for 'rescued' prostitutes provided an institutional context for some of this work.

Refuges, known as Po Leung Kuk homes, were operating in Kuala Lumpur by the 1890s for women who wished to cease working as prostitutes or needed protection from abuse.[124] But from around 1910, the Chinese Secretariat in Selangor was increasingly active in 'rescuing' women and prosecuting brothel keepers for procuring, kidnapping, and permitting sick women to work. Later the state took a more robust approach and occasionally brothel keepers would be sentenced to gaol for 'retaining diseased girls in their brothels'.[125] The Protectorate largely focused on individuals. But the extent to which brothel practice was controlled by organised crime by the Wa Ka or Broken Coffin Society gave its work an edge; the society, it was claimed, had 'branches in every little out-of-the-way place in the Peninsula and its agents are extremely astute in disposing of women over whom they obtain almost inexplicable control'.[126]

The Protectorate's role was never proactive with respect to mature women and it took action only to protect minors (believed to be under 16 years) or in response to obvious 'suspicious cases' of women held against their will.[127] Its impact, one might argue, was limited. In 1917, for example, when there were an estimated 43 Chinese and 24 Japanese brothels in Kuala Lumpur, and over a thousand women known to be commercial sex workers, around 25 percent of the women left to 'follow' men, found alternative employment or disappeared.[128] But the numbers of brothels and prostitutes changed little from year to year, and there are therefore two interpretations: either the number of women who 'escaped' subsequently returned to the brothels, through their own volition or force, or new women were being imported at a constant rate.[129] Both were probably true. The Po Leung Kuk homes and the Protectorate were important, however, since they at least provided women with the possibility of escape and refuge. They also, as indicated below, pursued an ideological agenda.

The first Po Leung Kuk home established in Singapore in 1888 was a single room with beds for six permanent juvenile residents. In 1896 it was expanded to accommodate 120; new accommodation in 1928 provided for 300 residents. Additional accommodation was provided from 1931 in the Mental Hospital for 'moral imbeciles and feeble-minded girls' unsuitable for accommodation in a Po Leung Kuk home.[130] In Kuala Lumpur the Po Leung Kuk Committee was established in 1895 for 228 women a year, under the immediate charge of a European woman, Mrs Daly, although temporary houses of safety had operated earlier still.[131] A home was also in operation in Perak by 1900. In Penang, women were given refuge in a temporary ward of the General Hospital in Georgetown until a home was established in 1926. The Malacca General Hospital accommodated around eight women and girls at any given time in a Po Leung Kuk ward;[132] in Negri Sembilan, the Seremban Convent was used.[133]

The Po Leung Kuk Committee, which included the Protector, interpreted its custodial right over children to include arranging their adoption into 'proper' families (although some had mothers working in brothels), or providing them with work skills, for example, as seamstresses or domestic servants. There were always some young children in the homes, including those 'found' in brothels and putatively orphaned, and other young children whose mothers were in hospital or gaol.[134] The committee both facilitated adoption and mediated custody. A three-year-old child, found in a Kuala Lumpur brothel, was given to a baker in Malay Street on payment of security of $300; six-year-old Li-Lin-Ming was allowed into the custody of his mother on receipt of security of $3,000 from his uncle and assurance that he would be sent to an English school for his education; Thong-Ah-Moi, a six-year-old girl, was placed in her father's custody after $300 had been paid, because her mother was living with a 'bar-boy' and was regarded as immoral.[135]

Some women used the homes for temporary retreat only, returning at their own will to work in brothels, but the committee also negotiated marriages and found work for residents. In 1931, for instance, of 478 women admitted to the Po Leung Kuk home in Singapore, 11 were adopted, five married, 37 were found employment, and the rest were discharged without assistance.[136]

Appearance before the Po Leung Kuk Committee gave women an opportunity to recount their histories. In April 1912, Phun Lin Kam, aged 19, appeared before the committee and requested that it act on her behalf to arrange a marriage. There is no indication on file of how she came to the home, or of the details of her recruitment and employment, although she must have begun to work as a prostitute at around 16 years of age. Her story is inconsistent, since she refers both to Singapore as her birthplace and to migration from China, but it is informative even so:

I was born in Singapore. My parents are dead. Was a prostitute in Tongkah, and subsequently in Deli (Sumatra) for over a year. I was brought to Kuala Lumpur by a woman named Ah Yee on the 15th of the 1st moon of this year.

We came from Singapore, I was a 'Phi-pha-chai' (singing girl) there. I came to Kuala Lumpur to join Brothel No.105 Petaling Street. Ah Yee paid my passage and other expenses from China. She went to Penang the day after my admission into Brothel No.105 Petaling Street. Have not the slightest idea as to her whereabouts. Have not been registered in the Chinese Protectorate. Have no idea whether any money passed between the keeper and Ah Yee. Do not wish to be a prostitute. I shall be glad if the Protector will secure a husband for me. Am quite happy in the home.[137]

Phun Lin Kam sought the assistance of the Protectorate to leave prostitution. Other women like Wong A. Yan, as revealed in committee minutes, sought protection from being forced into it:

The Protector informed the Committee that the woman complained to the Assistant Protector of Chinese that she had been ill-treated by her husband Chin Sang, a vegetable planter, who had attempted to sell her to be a prostitute. She ran away and lived in the jungle without food. She was sent to the Home with her own consent, pending the appearance of her husband said to have returned to China.[138]

In suggesting that Wong A. Yan would be returned to her husband when he re-appeared, the committee conceded patriarchal authority. This had resonance in committee proceedings when women sought protection from domestic violence. Much of the committee's time was spent not dealing with issues associated with prostitution, but in mediating domestic strife. Kok Yuk Lan, aged 14, for instance, took refuge in the home from her husband Si Yun Siong, a pupil at the Methodist Boys' School, because she was 'grossly ill-treated'.[139] A second woman was given sanctuary from her first husband and allowed to remain in the home until her second husband came for her, because she feared being murdered by the first husband's family if released.[140] Many of the cases appear to relate to separations and remarriages, the legitimacy of unions, and the financial transactions that were involved in them as women were sold by one husband to the next; the men often referred to wives also in China.[141] Members at a committee meeting in January 1914 complained that it had become a 'habit' of young women tired of their husbands to seek committee protection. One of its members, a merchant Khoo Keng Hooi, argued that recalcitrant wives should be placed in solitary confinement as a disciplinary measure. The committee was particularly sympathetic to requests by women to be released into family custody from whom they had earlier sought refuge.[142]

Since it could control a woman's mobility, it did so when it felt it was acting in her best interests, however defined. Yeung Ah Lai, aged 18, had been brought to Malaya from China by an old woman and a man posing as her husband, and she expressed her wish to now stay in Malaya. The committee rejected this request and gave her a month to reconsider, on the grounds that she was 'too young and attractive to be allowed to go to work without security being given'.[143] Women who wished to be repatriated were usually assisted. Those who applied for permission to leave the Po Leung Kuk home and return to prostitution – and there were many – were usually refused, although Chan San Yeng, aged 20, was allowed to return in view of her statement: 'I am determined to be a prostitute of "Yi Lok" brothel, Kuala Lumpur. I was a prostitute at Canton for 3 years. Have no wish to marry'.[144]

The committee also was a marriage broker, often on behalf of tin miners. The arrangements were rather pragmatic, the analogy with prostitution somewhat obvious: men gained company, sex, a housekeeper and a fellow labourer; women gained protection from the abuses of other men. The following extract of proceedings of the Po Leung Kuk Committee, on 13 June 1911, illustrates the contractual basis of such marriages. Chong Hiong, aged 42, and Wong Cheung, aged 26, both proposed before the committee to an 18-year-old, Wong Yam Thai:

> Chong Hiong: I am a 'Thong-thiu' [headman] of the Sin Wing Sang mining kongsi at the 7th mile, Sungei Besi Road. Have been in this country for the last 6 years. Bachelor. Wages $12 per mensem with board and lodging. I also go in for pig-breeding which brings me $20 extra a month. I am able to support a wife.
> Wong Yam Thai: I wish to marry Chong Hiong.
> Wong Cheung: I am agent for Yap Tek Fatt mines at the 7th mile Kanching Road. Salary $20 per month with commission on *chabut* collected by me. I am desirous of marrying Wong Yam Thai.
> Wong Yam Thai: Either of them will suit me.[145]

Politics and the suppression of prostitution

The work of the Po Leung Kuk Committee and the Chinese Protectorate indicates the concern of sections of the government and the community at the extent of prostitution, its associated slavery and the traffic in women. The concern took on an institutional focus; that is, it concentrated on the existence of public brothels in central localities, the cities and large towns of the colonies where traders, planters and miners came to trade, purchase provisions and borrow money, where workers came for recreation, and where merchants, soldiers, sailors and adventurers called for merry-making, gambling, sex and drink. The brothels were an established feature of the ports and larger inland towns, with smaller brothels more widely dispersed. Men from all classes came to the tea shops, dance halls and brothels that sprang up throughout the colonies, and policemen and railway coolies in the least populous states were as likely to visit prostitutes and to contract and spread venereal disease as the men who worked in offices or factories or on the wharfs.[146] Hutchinson's description sets out the geography of prostitution in Kuala Lumpur in the late 1920s:

> The sides of the High St. and Petaling St. were lined with Chinese Brothels, these had open fronts with large wooden bars in front of the 'windows', through which were seated the Chinese prostitutes – painted thick with rouge and powder – these were never patronised by the European batchelors (sic). Down the Batu Road was 'the Malay kip-shop', an huge ramshackle building presided over by 'moma', a very fat jolly Malay woman – here you could get a cold beer or a Malay girl if you wanted one. Nearby was the 'Siamese house' with the Siamese girls ... In the Batu Road and in Petaling St. and further near the Princess Cinema were the more superior Japanese Hotels, wher[e] you could get Beer and almost any race of girl ...[147]

Despite legislation and administrative procedures, the government was relatively casual about the practice of prostitution and interpreted its brief, as already noted, to protect young girls – hence the specific exclusion of children aged six to fourteen from brothels – and to provide the appropriate mechanisms for women to leave. This had the support of the wider community. Complaints about prostitution were relatively rare until late in the colonial period, when external pressure on Britain by the International Labour Organisation, the League of Nations and other international agencies, as well as local activists campaigning against venereal disease and 'immorality', led towards its suppression.[148]

Until the 1920s, the solution to the spread of venereal disease was a biomedical one and the primary intervention therefore was treatment. Now, public health was gaining ground in the colonies, and in this context the control of sexually transmitted diseases also took a new tack. Sex was, it had been argued, 'natural', but now, out of the context of marriage and reproduction, was more likely to be portrayed like opium use as a symptom of boredom that might readily be displaced. The state responded in two different ways: to increase the immigration of women to rectify the sex ratio, therefore to encourage marriage and the family, and to increase recreational activities for single men in order to divert their energies: hence the Singapore Harbour Board's grant in 1921 for the erection of a pavilion, a football ground and other sports facilities.[149]

The first major moves to increase control over prostitution and brothel keeping in colonial Malaya date from the early 1920s, in line with steps taken in other countries also to control sexually transmitted diseases. The period saw a number of international and regional meetings concerned with their control, the introduction of a new international convention relating to the traffic in women and children, the development of an interest in eugenics and social hygiene in the United Kingdom, and the establishment of a network of doctors, administrators and philanthropists who made the control of STDs and the welfare of women their central concern, if not their passion.

In January 1921 Dr Rupert Hailam and Mrs Neville Rolfe of the Social Hygiene Commission visited Singapore; their visit was regarded with some scepticism of their preparedness to come to terms with the 'Asiatic view' of morals or the 'peculiar' local circumstances that affected prostitution.[150] Their report led to the appointment of the Straits Settlements Venereal Diseases Committee in 1923, which recommended to the Singapore Legislative Council the reintroduction of brothel registration and licensing and medical examination of prostitutes to control infection. Legislation was drafted along these lines.

In July 1924, the Colonial Office established an Advisory Committee on Social Hygiene to advise the Secretary of State on issues relating to venereal disease and 'public morality'. The committee was chaired by the Hon. W. Ormsby-Gore, the Parliamentary Under-Secretary of State for the Colonies, and included other members of the British government, the NCCVD (National Council for Combatting Venereal Disease) and the Association for Moral and Social Hygiene.[151] In its report, the committee acknowledged that the situation was a 'difficult and delicate' one, complicated by social, administrative and legal issues, and argued that the earlier Singapore report had failed to take account of the social causes of prostitution, the poor housing that discouraged men from bringing their wives and children to the colonies, and the inadequacies of medical screening and treatment.[152] It recommended the abolition of all known brothels, and the extension of legislation to prevent women and men from living on the earnings of prostitution. As an interim measure, it called for the prohibition of alcohol in brothels, the removal of any lighting that would advertise their existence, and stricter controls over the employment of women in venues such as coffee shops and eating houses. The immediate response of the government of the Straits Settlement was to extend the treatment for venereal disease to the general population by opening VD clinics and extending inpatient accommodation for both men and women.

At this same time, in 1925, in a mood of public health and moral zeal, the British National Council for Combatting Venereal Disease (NCCVD) changed its name to the British Social Hygiene Council and shifted its emphasis from treatment to prevention. The council, involving medical doctors, psychologists, sociologists, biologists and 'muscular Christians',[153] met on a regular basis to discuss issues of prevention and control within and beyond the empire, represented the United

Kingdom and its colonies in international fora, and included in its journal *Health and Empire* extracts from colonial government departmental reports. It established an Imperial Committee concerned with prostitution throughout the colonies. A Joint Standing Committee of the council and the Board of Study for the Preparation of Missionaries was also established; its Far East Committee, concerned with prostitution in east, southeast and south Asia, brought together missionaries, doctors who had served in the colonies, anthropologists and members of the Colonial Office.[154] The Singapore Report was discussed by the British Social Hygiene Council, which had been invited by the Medical Officer of the Straits Settlements to send a trained social hygiene worker to organise 'a year's campaign of public enlightenment among all sections of the community'; Professor Bostock Hill went to Malaya from October to December 1926 on behalf of the council to help initiate the Singapore campaign.[155]

Clinics for the treatment of venereal diseases had already been established. In Singapore the first clinic operated from January 1922 at the Tanjong Pagar Docks. In June an outdoor dispensary for the treatment of VD also opened at North Canal Road, and Bostock Hill was gleeful at their success in terms of outpatient numbers: 6,476 in 1923, 18,994 in 1924, 20,089 in 1925.[156] In 1926 Dr Chambers was appointed Chief Medical Officer (Social Hygiene) and thereafter treatment seeking, clinic attendance and public health education all increased dramatically (see Tables 6.3 and 6.4). Total attendances throughout the Straits Settlements in 1927 was 108,000. The British Social Hygiene Council had distributed some 90,000 pamphlets in Malay, Tamil, Chinese and English; posters and cinema films provided further health education, and from 1 October 1927, a Chinese Lady Visitor was employed in Singapore 'to carry out propaganda amongst women' and ensure that those infected received treatment.[157]

Policies with regard to prostitution were also re-considered in the FMS. The Chinese Protectorate moved to increase its authority in 1925 with a

Table 6.3   Cases of venereal disease treated at government hospitals and clinics, by ethnicity, Federated Malay States, 1929 and 1935

	Chinese		Indians		Malays		Others		
Year	No	%	No	%	No	%	No	%	**Total**
1929	22,615	55.4	11,707	28.7	3,545	8.7	2,935	7.2	**40,802**
1935	7,790	42.3	6,642	36.1	2,602	14.1	1,376	7.5	**18,410**
Decrease	65.5%		43.3%		26.6%		53.1%		**54.9%**

Source: Gebbie, 1939, p. 439.

Table 6.4 Venereal cases treated at government hospitals and clinics, Federated Malay States, 1929 and 1935

Year	Syphilis	Gonorrhoea	Soft sore
1929	24,975	12,366	3,461
1935	10,239	6,653	1,518
Decrease	59%	46.2%	56.1%

Source: Gebbie, 1939, p. 439.

change to the Women and Girls Protection Enactment, which enabled it to increase its power to detain women under the age of sixteen years from two to six months, thus buying time to find them positions as domestic servants or wives.[158] In June 1926 a further amendment gave the Protector authority to require a woman suspected of being infected to be examined by a government medical officer, with non-compliance subject to fine or imprisonment. The British Social Hygiene Council took exception to the amendment, although it recognised that circumstances in the FMS were 'abnormal'.[159] Bostock Hill's assessment of the situation was that the newly appointed Venereal Disease Officer in Kuala Lumpur, Dr E. A. Smith, was 'in full sympathy' with abolition, but needed to proceed along lines that would carry the support of the 'native' (i.e. Chinese) community and avoid unnecessary hardship to the women. Smith also held that general dispensaries should be 'properly staffed racially', and that dressers and other dispensary staff act 'as propagandists in the medical, moral and social aspects' of prostitution.[160]

In the FMS clinics for VD commenced operating in 1923. In 1925 a total of 3,688 people were treated; in 1927 this had increased to 20,508 cases treated in clinics and special treatment centres (Table 6.3).[161] A program to extend clinic services and public health activities was submitted to the government in mid-1925; this program included the education of subordinate staff of the Medical Department, public lectures, pamphlets and posters, and clinic-based education designed to encourage treatment and avoidance of infection or re-infection.[162] In the UFMS, treatment was provided at government hospitals and dispensaries. In states such as Trengganu syphilis cases were low, particularly among Malays, due – according to its Chief Medical Officer, Dr N. H. Harrison – to 'the fact that the population is saturated with yaws'; he claimed however that perhaps 50 percent of the population in larger kampungs and towns were infected with gonorrhoea, with 'its ravages' evident among young adults, older adults, and infants.[163]

Reformists and social hygienists in the colonies and in Britain noted with pleasure progress to close the Singapore brothels. In 1926, there were 2,211 known prostitutes in the city; in 1929, this had dropped to 519. Many of the women had left for other employment, but others moved into 'sly' prostitution.[164] Virtually all European and Japanese brothels had closed by mid-decade; the last 'known' Chinese brothel closed early in 1930.[165] On 14 October 1930 a new Women and Girl's Protection Ordinance was introduced which made procuring and brothel-keeping illegal; prior legislation prohibited women's employment in other areas, for instance, as singing girls in hotels, where prostitution was also known to occur.[166]

In the FMS, however, legislation against brothel-keeping was deferred until a visit of the League of Nations' Committee of Experts, and was introduced in January 1931 after unofficial members of the Legislative Council had withdrawn their objections. The immediate effect was an alleged increase in 'sly' prostitution and venereal disease.[167] Brothel keepers in Kuala Lumpur sought an extension of operations too as the Depression affected their business:

> We have all been established in this town for some time and we have a lot of outstanding debts due by prostitutes to keepers, and the keepers are anxious that the prostitutes should repay the debts for board and lodging and the prostitutes are prepared to pay off all their debts ... The prostitutes are anxious of giving up their trade and to turn into a new leave (sic) and to lead a respectable life, and they require time to do so.[168]

The request was regarded by senior government officers as admission to debt slavery, 'reason to close them (the brothels) in the first place'.[169] Meanwhile prostitutes themselves began to work with women in the brothels, establishing unions and collaborating with other voluntary associations to support working women and those wishing to leave the brothels.[170] The unions received little official support; it was claimed that active members were 'of the Bolshevik type and ... trying to disseminate Communist ideas among all the other fellow prostitutes' as well as being 'of the lowest and meanest class and ... very rude and disrespectable'.[171]

CHAPTER 7

Domestic lives:
Reproduction, the mother and the child

To this point, I have concentrated on the conditions of health and sickness that were created, in some way or other, by colonial capitalism, whereby the health of individuals and the medical services provided were shaped by economic and political considerations. The subjects of the colonial gaze were those people most insinuated into the colonial economy – miners, plantation workers, urban labourers and sex workers. Colonial medical discourse vacillated between an essentialism that absolved the state of responsibility for people's health, and the combined concerns of industry and moral responsibility which, despite certain tensions between these two, established a basis for medical and public health interventions.

Women and children entered the colonial imagination when the emphasis shifted from production to reproduction, or rather, as the relationship between these two became clear. This had a number of implications. First, examination of the immediate causes of maternal and infant mortality led to the development of programs which, whilst they increased state surveillance over women's lives, were effective in reducing mortality. Second, whilst the proximate causes of death were often specific to reproductive health, the attention on women and children documented also morbidity from other causes and provided a basis for the development of public health (for instance, water and sanitation programs). The inclusion of women and children within colonial medical discourse therefore led to a stronger population-based approach to health, in contrast to the prior sectoral, individualised and victim-blaming gaze: from the health problems of 'prostitutes' and 'estate workers', for example, to problems that might be loosely glossed as 'urban' or 'rural'. This shift from individual to population was a fundamental one that whilst differentiating medical and public health perspectives, also discriminated between clinical and epidemiological understandings of health and illness. Finally, the ethnic artefact of colonial immigration policy was, as discussed, the skewed sex ratios of the Chinese and Tamil communities; this was not the case among Malays. Attention to women and children led also to increased attention being paid to the Malay community, and for the first time the government began to address the health status of that population as well as that of the immigrant communities.

The discovery of the child

Until the early 1900s, as I have suggested, the health of women and children received relatively little attention from the colonial government and few medical services catered to their needs. The welfare of individual children was the subject of state attention, however. Children were portrayed as victims, abandoned or raised in 'unsuitable' surroundings, victims of neglect and wilfulness, and the state's role was to intervene to protect their physical and moral wellbeing and sometimes their lives. Some of these children, as recounted in the previous chapter, had been kidnapped in mainland China and given to bogus 'mothers' to be reared in the brothels of Singapore, Kuala Lumpur and Ipoh; others were sold to 'pocket mothers' with the same future in store, or as *mui tsai* or domestic servants; others, baby girls usually, were left abandoned in the streets by mothers too poor to keep them. These were Chinese babies. The Malay child emerged, occasionally, as a subject of the state, primarily as a seven or eight-year-old providing an arm for the carriage of live smallpox vaccine.[1] In general, neither women nor children were of great interest to the state, since they played no obvious economic role in the colony. This lack of interest led to poor accounting, and we therefore know little of their health, welfare and living conditions.[2]

By the early twentieth century, however, the child had been discovered. Rather, a series of political events drew attention to high infant death rates, which led to a new focus on infants and children in Britain, and the development of strategies to increase live deliveries, reduce the neonatal and infant mortality rates and improve the health of older children. The local context was the poor health of working-class men recruited to fight in the Boer War, their poor military performance, and the results of the 1901 Census which indicated a declining birth rate and increasing infant mortality rate. These facts in turn led to scrutiny of and concern with conditions of urban and industrial life, infant and child health and welfare, and midwifery practice. In response, from around 1902–1908 laws were passed to ensure that births were attended by trained midwives and were registered, that school meals were provided, and children inspected.[3]

These events emerged in the context of a new awareness of the links between the child and empire: between infant health, child survival, physical wellbeing, and the politics and economics of the state. As Anna Davin describes, the early concern for infant mortality occurred parallel to an enthusiasm for empire – an expanding British population filling in the spaces of the margins of the empire. In an era when imperial power depended upon *man*power; and when Britain was seen to be competing with other European states for control, power, and prestige, the high infant mortality rate stripped the country of a commodity and a 'national asset', and eugenicists, politicians and doctors argued for health interventions to ensure 'stalwart sons to people the colonies and to uphold the prestige of the nation'.[4] On the periphery of the empire, there were other reasons for acting upon the high infant mortality rate.

In Britain, population expansion and the relationship between population growth and control over its colonial outposts was supplemented by the need for an able-bodied workforce to produce food and provide the labour power for an expanding industrial base. In the colonies the need for labour was paramount. In Malaya until around 1900 labour force needs were met through immigration, but the high death rate of adult immigrants on the plantations, railways and mines led to an evaluation of the economics of immigration, as opposed to the local reproduction of the workforce. Put bluntly, it seemed cheaper to nurture childen to adulthood than to import adult workers. Independently, yet much influenced by changing ideas about population and labour in Britain and in other parts of the empire, in the Malayan colonies too the child was discovered.[5]

This chapter documents government policies and programs implemented to reduce infant mortality and improve the health of women and their children. Government interventions were aimed initially at midwifery and childrearing practices. Infant mortality was associated with poor mothering, and accordingly, colonial doctors were again much influenced by ideas in the United Kingdom. Health and medical officers from the colonies attended national conferences in Britain, such as those of the National Association for the Prevention of Infant Mortality, and submitted detailed reports of papers 'intended to show how the ignorance [of mothers] could be frustrated by means of instructed midwives, district nurses, and health visitors'.[6] Colonial doctors shared with their colleagues in London a belief in the need to educate women to become competent, 'good' mothers. By the 1930s, however, lack of success in controlling midwifery and extending state control over mothers led to an alternative strategy – to educate mothers of the future – hence an increased interest in domestic science education. In this chapter, I examine both direct interventions into midwifery, mothering and infant health, and the introduction of child health and welfare into the school system.[7]

As noted in Chapter 2, the infant mortality rate in early twentieth-century Malaya was high, around 250 per 1,000 births. Both the maternal mortality rate and rate of stillbirths were also high. Pregnancy, delivery and early life were fraught with risk. There was, however, considerable variation by year, state and ethnicity, and fluctuations within states due to local conditions and season (Tables 2.11 and 7.1). Variations also occurred due to the reliability of the data, however, and while the settlements had a high infant mortality rate due to poor urban conditions, surveillance was also greater and reporting of births and deaths nearer to accurate in these relatively small and dense administrative units. By contrast, in the FMS and especially the UFMS, a substantial number of infant deaths were never recorded.

Most infant deaths, as discussed earlier, were uncertified and reported as due to *sawan* (convulsions), a broad term that might have included several causes, including neonatal tetanus. In older infants, malaria and venereal disease contributed to the death rate, and Sansom, the Principal Medical Officer in the FMS, was to write in 1914 of parts of the colony that were 'childless' as a result.[8] Deaths were frequently also caused by pneumonia and diarrhoeal disease, suggesting a pattern not dissimilar from that found in most poor countries in the late twentieth century; in 1909, for example, 65 percent of infant deaths were listed as due to neonatal tetanus, malaria, and deaths from 'dietetic errors'.[9]

Concern about the infant mortality rate occurred concurrently with general government and public concern with morbidity and mortality rates. As we have seen, there was growing concern with the health of immigrant labourers, resulting in various commissions of inquiry into matters of public health. Again, the influence of public health thinking in Britain was not far removed: the inquiry into housing conducted in Singapore in 1907 occurred at around the same time as inquiries and debates in Britain on the relative contribution of environment and heredity to British working-class infant health. In both cases the desparate images of crowding and insanitation gave considerable strength to the arguments of public health workers, who attributed the high infant mortality rate to broader social factors rather than simply to the proximate medical causes of death.[10] That is, they argued that illness was produced under specific sets of social and economic conditions, which in Malaya included environmental conditions, poor maternal and infant nutrition, lack of trained midwives and women's reliance on *bidan* (village midwives) for obstetric help, the prevalence of syphilis and malaria, and childrearing practices. On the whole, poor infant health in rural areas was attributed to lack of access to medical services, urban

Table 7.1 Infant mortality by ethnicity, Straits Settlements, 1908

Settlement	Variable	European	Eurasian	Chinese	Malay	Indian	Other	Total
Singapore	Deaths SS[1]	11	46	1,195	702	133	29	2,116
	Deaths elsewhere[2]	—	—	103	53	9	2	167
	IMR[3]	83.33	30.65	292.60	411.54	31.56	293.48	320.35 (mean)
Penang	Death SS	2	4	564	220	72	14	876
	Deaths elsewhere	—	—	95	15	6	6	122
	IMR	66.67	78.43	421.38	158.05	154.57	333.33	256.29 (mean)
Province Wellesley	Death SS	1	2	10	455	137	2	607
	Deaths elsewhere	—	—	—	10	—	—	10
	IMR	500.00	166.67	144.14	138.76	252.30	222.2	154.11 (mean)
Dindings	Deaths SS	—	—	8	26	—	—	34
	Deaths elsewhere	—	—	1	—	—	—	1
	IMR	—	—	291.67	168.83	—	—	178.37 (mean)
Malacca	Deaths SS	—	26	210	1,149	—	—	1,385
	Deaths elsewhere	—	1	4	2	16	6	29
	IMR	—	308.64	341.63	305.87	2	—	308.27 (mean)
Total	**Deaths SS**	**14**	**78**	**2,057**	**2,552**	**358**	**51**	**5,110**
	Deaths elsewhere	**—**	**1**	**203**	**80**	**17**	**8**	**309**
	IMR mean	**2.55**	**259.26**	**307.62**	**247.57**	**239.47**	**245.71**	**265.63 (mean)**

1 Deaths of infants born in SS.
2 Deaths of infants born elsewhere.
3 Infant mortality rate, per 1,000 live births.
Source: SSAR 1908, p. 10.

deaths to environmental and sanitary conditions, and in both, to 'ignorance or to indifference ... as to the proper management of children'.[11]
The British Resident of Pahang, for example, argued that many children
died from 'improper feeding during the first year' and that many were
'killed by their filthy dwellings' and 'inherited disease from their
parents'.[12] Government interventions initially set aside the contextual
factors contributing to mortality, however, and focused instead on
midwifery and infant feeding, aiming to bring midwifery under state
control and to increase women's use of medical services.

Control of midwifery

The government focused first on midwifery practice for two reasons:
because the immediate risks to women and infants were associated with
pregnancy and delivery, and because midwives were best positioned to
educate mothers.

A maternity hospital was built in Singapore in 1888, and by 1907 provided 16 beds for 'native' and 13 beds for European women.[13] Elsewhere
women were able to deliver in general hospitals. However, there were
too few beds, an inadequate number of nurses, and all doctors, hospital
assistants and native dressers were male. This was not acceptable to local
or immigrant women, and in consequence virtually all Malay women and
most women of all races received their only professional antenatal care
and were attended at delivery by *bidan* (traditional birth attendants). In
addition, women were wary of hospitals as places for the dying, and the
occasional closure of wards because of infection or the need to renovate
or repair the building reinforced their views.[14]

Malay birth practice changed little while it remained a village event.
The ritual demands of pregnancy were managed by the *bidan*, who
provided the expectant mother with dietary advice and massage as well
as ceremonial supervision. Women usually gave birth in their natal
home. Once the child was delivered, the midwife would concentrate on
the placenta; the umbilicus would be cut with bamboo, scissors or a
household knife, the stump dusted with wood ash or a paste of pepper,
ginger and turmeric. The *bidan*'s obligations continued post-partum in
terms of conducting specific rites one and six weeks after delivery,
ensuring the new mother's observation of dietary prescriptions, bathing,
and roasting, and massage.[15]

Lack of knowledge of antiseptic procedures resulted in neonatal
tetanus. A first target for government, therefore, was to reduce the
infant mortality rate by reducing tetanus through encouraging antiseptic
practices by training and supervising the *bidan*. It was also anticipated
that this would lead to reductions in maternal mortality through

increased recognition of complications of pregnancy and referral to doctors. Since, as noted, the *bidan* provided antenatal and postnatal care, she was therefore regarded also as the person closest to mothers, and in theory best able to convey information about infant health and care to them. This approach was also manageable, a clearly defined first step to bring reproduction under state control. Thus maternal and child health programs were introduced in 1905 and consisted of three parts: the registration and in-service training of traditional midwives or *bidan*; the recruitment and training in basic biomedicine, midwifery and nursing of local women who might replace the *bidan*; and home visiting and infant welfare centres to monitor infant health and intervene where necessary. While temporarily the government planned to work with *bidan*, the employment of trained midwives was regarded as a key to women's acceptance of antenatal and infant welfare services, determining community acceptance and compliance and an 'excellent method of furthering acquaintance of the *kampung* Malay with Western medicine'.[16]

The registration of practising *bidan* and the provision for training of local women as nurses/midwives was a relatively pragmatic move given the preferred context of pregnancy and labour, influenced by prevailing understandings of the most effective interventions to reduce neonatal and maternal mortality. With the growing power, prestige and specialisation of the medical profession, there was a trend towards the medicalisation of childbirth, as documented for Britain by authors such as Lewis and Oakley.[17] However, medical opinion in the late nineteenth and early twentieth centuries tended to represent childbirth itself as a normal rather than a pathological process, and while doctors argued the value to women of hospital deliveries, they primarily emphasised improved domiciliary midwifery services and a general nursing education to all wives and mothers in the home care of sick, pregnant and parturient women as the most effective short-term strategies to reduce mortality.[18] In colonial Malaya, the intention was not, by and large, to encourage women to deliver in hospitals, but rather to encourage women to use trained midwives who could refer women with obstetric problems to hospital. Given limited bed space and the lack of 'lady doctors' in the colonies, this was a practical approach.

Moves to regulate midwifery practice and to train local Malay women commenced in Singapore in 1910, under the direction of Dr Middleton, Municipal Health Officer in Singapore, although they were anticipated by Dr Fowlie, Honorary Visiting Surgeon in the colony in 1905, around the time that such moves were being undertaken in the United Kingdom.[19] In the short term, however, in Singapore from 1911 and Malacca from 1912, lecture courses were introduced for practising *bidan*, which covered such topics as the importance of aseptic birth conditions,

symptoms associated with complications of pregnancy and labour, and
the management of complications. Their primary aim was to encourage
the use of aseptic instruments to cut the umbilicus, to ensure no subsequent infection of the cord, and to increase referrals for complications
and obstructed labour – strategies demonstrated to reduce neonatal
deaths and maternal deaths from 'accidents of childbirth'.[20] At the
conclusion of the in-service training courses, delivered in Malay, women
were registered, issued with a free supply of antiseptic, cotton wool and
lint, and placed under the supervision of 'lady' medical doctors or European nursing sisters. In addition, all midwives who had delivered infants
who had subsequently died from neonatal tetanus were interviewed by
the lady medical officer.[21]

Clarke, the Health Officer for Kinta District, like other doctors
stationed in the colonies, supported these measures. He considered
bidan to be 'ignorant' and 'dirty', however, and favoured as an alternative the recruitment of new young women for biomedical training.
Those recruited to receive Western midwifery training were usually
Malay, although some Chinese women were also trained. The allocation
of roles according to race, with superordinate positions held by European or occasionally Eurasian women, reflected contemporary views
about race; these were reflected too in the stratification of health posts
and in other areas of health and health care. Conventional wisdom held
that Malays, Chinese or Indians, or all of them could not understand
basic notions of health and hygiene; with training, they were still liable to
slip without constant surveillance; and even Eurasian women could
'never be expected be the equal of the European trained woman ... to
expect a native woman to do anything in this direction is to hope for the
impossible'.[22]

Under the first scheme, the colonial government paid for tuition and
the Singapore Municipal Government met the cost of uniforms and
subsistence for the trainees. Training was provided at Government
Maternity Hospitals in the settlements. By 1914, plans were also in place
in the FMS to train Malay women as nurse/midwives, in light of the
unavailability of trained Eurasian women, the perceived inadequacy of
women recruited from India, and the unsuitability of midwives from the
United Kingdom.[23] Government medical officers argued for the preferability of training Malay (rather than Chinese and Indian women)
because of the reluctance of Malay women to use non-Malay birth
attendants, and the popularity of Malay *bidan* among other women also.
In Selangor, the British Resident approached and secured the support
of the Sultan for a scheme whereby district officers were to identify local
Malay women prepared to undertake a minimum of one year's training
at Kuala Lumpur General Hospital. During this time they were expected

to witness and assist in a number of maternity cases in order to qualify as midwives.[24] Response was poor. Most *penghulu* were not interested in encouraging women to enrol and reports from district officers suggest that women were discouraged by the residential requirements.[25] Occasionally, too, women would commence training, then abscond. For instance, two women, Fatimah binti Rapok (Rapah) and Mai binti Udin, began training in Kuala Lumpur in September 1915, but did not complete the course: Fatimah 'succumbed to the attractions of a Malay youth' and wished to marry; Mai found life 'unbearable' as a result of the courtship and her exclusion, and wished to return to her *kampung*.[26]

Training was offered to women desiring to become midwives throughout the colonies by the 1920s.[27] In the Malay States, recruits often proved unsuitable because of their age (women in their late 30s or early 40s, widowed or divorced, tended to be regarded as 'too old'), because of their lack of formal education or alleged intellectual shortcomings, and because their recruitment was nepotistic rather than because of a genuine interest in midwifery. Training was sometimes offered to women already working as traditional midwives, but this was not common because of their mean age, their reluctance to modify midwifery practice to accommodate biomedical principles of hygiene and its accoutrements, and their 'stupidity' and 'ignorance'.[28] However, stories of *bidan* malpractice and the prevalence of gynecological problems were emblematic, serving to marginalise the practitioners:

> To the Outpatient Department also, come many cases of Uterine displacement. Most of these women have at some period employed 'Kampung Bidans' with their treatment of fire baths and massage with heavy irons; these usually come for advice about dysmenorrhoea, due to infections and unrepaired tears of the cervix and Vagina as well as uterine displacements and their resultant complications and symptoms.[29]

By the 1930s, accreditation had been regularised throughout the states and settlements, with qualifications graded: one year formal training at the hospital, then practical training in English, with examination and diploma awarded (Class A); six to nine months' practical training in Malay, examined (Class B); and midwives who had been in regular practice for a year before the ordinance (Class C), who might subsequently receive some formal training to be rescheduled as Class B midwives.[30] However, recruitment and retention of women was poor. In Penang in 1925, 22 midwives were reported to have been trained at the King Edward Hospital, but five years later, only fourteen were still working;[31] in 1931, still only six women in Perak had completed their training.[32] In consequence, most women continued to be delivered by *bidan*, and weekly lecture classes for traditional midwives continued.[33]

In the UFMS, training schemes for local women were set up much later than in the settlements or FMS. In Trengganu the first clinic opened in 1929, and was primarily patronised by Chinese women living in Kuala Trengganu. Women wishing to train as midwives from Trengganu and Kelantan were sent to Singapore for a six-month residential course at the Kandang Kerbau Hospital, but distance acted as a considerable disincentive.[34] Moreover, few women had even basic educational skills to gain from training, due 'not so much upon the amount of money that can be made available as in overcoming the reluctance of the rural population to depart from time-honoured customs and inherited ideas as to the status and functions of women in the life of the community'.[35] In Kelantan, the first maternal and child welfare centre opened in Kota Bharu in 1930, but the government was reluctant to invest further in midwifery services since, it claimed, the 'Malays have very definite ideas concerning midwifery, and it is not expected that Malay women will seek advice concerning pregnancy or be willing to come to hospital for labour'.[36] A second-class ward was established for 'native women', but it was primarily intended for and used by Chinese and Indian women unable to make alternative arrangements for confinement. In Kedah and Perlis, a scheme to provide training at maternity clinics attached to hospitals was introduced in 1936, in order to strike 'a direct blow' at infant mortality in rural areas, and 'to lay a sound foundation for the establishment of welfare work on lines suitable to the specific peculiarities of this state'.[37] Local training was also regarded as most appropriate given the differences in 'local custom'. In Kedah, four women were trained in the first intake and four more the following year; these were married women, 'often quite illiterate and unable to tell the time' and without a background in traditional midwifery. By the end of the decade, around 20 Malay women had been trained and had returned to practice with a small remuneration from the state and, occasionally, a house provided by the villagers.[38] In Perlis, training began modestly in 1937 with one student per annum and lacked local support.[39]

While *bidan* remained important, therefore, Dr Brodie's report of villages providing housing for midwives suggests that there was support for trained health workers. English nurses also reported success where they worked with 'local Asiatic midwives' and had the support of local leaders.[40] The resistance, where it occurred, related particularly to delivering in hospitals, which commentators tended to interpret as a simple problem of health education regarding the value of skilled midwives and the importance of asepsis.[41] In addition, however, Malay women were said not to like the 'publicity' of general wards, were unhappy in wards where few if any nursing staff spoke Malay,[42] and where they were unable to observe the immediate rituals of childbirth. Official commentary on birthing practices fails to explore, however, the extent to which women's resistance related also to the discordance between obstetric and village ways of 'doing' birth. In colonial Malaya as well as later, women delivering in hospitals were stripped of their social identity, control and personal support on admission, and left to labour in an environment that was sterile (literally and metaphorically), lonely, and frightening.

Reluctance to use government midwives in the village related to the inability of trained nurses to incorporate the ritual appurtenances into their own model of 'aseptic' birth. The resistance was also economic, however. In Kuala Langat, Perak, for example, fees charged for attendance at confinements dissuaded women from using trained midwives, and the District Economic Board in 1937 approached the Medical Department to provide a midwife free for a six-month trial period.[43] By contrast, a *bidan* might receive remuneration either in cash or in kind, and her supervision of labour and delivery was a small component of the more complete care of the expectant and parturient woman and new mother.

By 1936, there were 720 registered or trained midwives in Singapore, 574 in Penang, and 224 in Malacca. Legislation for the compulsory registration of midwives had been discussed as early as 1905, and was finally introduced in 1917 in the municipal limits of Singapore, Penang and Malacca, though not in rural areas until 1930. The provisions were extended in 1923 with a new ordinance establishing the Central Midwives Board. In the Malay States, there were far fewer trained midwives. Consequently legislation to control village midwifery practice was delayed until 1954, for this reason and on the grounds that childbirth was a matter of custom (*adat*) rather than of public health, hence legislation might be construed as interference.[44]

The surveillance of mothers

The supervision of village *bidan* and the recruitment and training of younger women remained an important component of the state's strategy to lower the infant mortality rate. Alternative government strategies to reduce infant mortality centred on the mother and presupposed that infant deaths reflected women's inability, through lack of appropriate education, to be good and proper mothers. The first step in the supervision and education of mothers was home visiting.

Again, Britain provided the model for and antecedents of home visiting. Home visits had been undertaken on a voluntary basis from around 1860 in London, Brighton, Manchester, Salford and Newcastle, and from 1890 salaried home visitors were appointed in Manchester to inspect homes and provide advice on the management of common ailments, and, increasingly, on infant care and feeding.[45] Under these schemes, women from similar class and background were preferred as health visitors, supervised by 'a superior woman'.[46] In Malaya, this was rather difficult since no native woman was considered educated enough in infant care and mothercraft to undertake this role; even Eurasian women were regarded as unreliable and would never equal European health visitors. In the colonies therefore health visitors were ideally European. Their role was no different to that of English home visitors, however, to provide women with the minimum knowledge of health and hygiene which it was believed would reduce the number of infant deaths: 'The essential features of child welfare work which carries the knowledge of public healtn ; ito the very life of the family is the utilisation of simple methods which can be understood by the most ignorant of the many nationalities'.[47]

The system worked as follows. Newborns were supposed to be registered at the local police station, and upon registration, the police officer was responsible for notifying the district health office. A health visitor would duly visit the newly-delivered woman, provide her with some immediate advice about infant feeding and encourage her to attend the nearest infant welfare centre to enable the infant's health to be monitored.

Malay, Indian and Chinese women were represented variously as negligent, careless and recalcitrant, and this was the moral basis to the program. While some health workers and medical officers insisted that maternal ignorance was the singular cause of infant deaths, others pointed to the social and economic circumstances of women. For Clarke, a colonial doctor, these included water, sanitation, the quality of milk and domestic food safety as well as 'the ignorance or carelessness of the mother'.[48] Others argued that women from certain races were intrinsically better carers than others. Mrs Hamblin, addressing a meeting of a committee on nursing training for the colonies in 1944, suggested that home visiting was straightforward but its impact questionable:

> (T)he Malays, at any rate, rarely, if ever, acted on the advice given to them; they were distinguished by their lethargy and apathy in health matters. The Chinese took advice more readily than the other elements of the Asiatic population; the Tamils often tried to act on the advice given them but were often handicapped by lack of intelligence.[49]

This, however, was only one version of ethnicity, culture and nature. Sansom's view was that malaria control would have had considerable impact on the infant mortality rate of Indians and Malays and *their* mothering was not problematic, but the Chinese showed 'a curious indifference to the welfare of female children';[50] Dr Galloway, in an interview with the Commission of Inquiry into housing difficulties in Singapore (1917–1918), claimed that the high infant mortality rate among Chinese in Singapore was due to improper feeding, diarrhoeal disease, the sequestering of infants in cubicles, and the 'sheer personal laziness' of these mothers.[51] A submission to the inquiry into estate labour (1924) emphasised the lack of maternal skill of Tamil women, hence the need on estates for supervision after delivery to see 'that the newborn infant is properly attended to, as there is a danger to the life of the baby unless it is properly looked after'.[52]

Home visiting commenced in 1911 when the Singapore Municipal Health Department appointed female health inspectors to visit post-partum women, using a list of births provided by the Office of the Registrar of Births and Deaths. Malacca and Penang also introduced limited programs of home visiting by female inspectors within urban areas from around this time, and in 1914, a trained nurse was visiting new mothers also in Kuala Lumpur.[53] It was extended to rural Malacca and Penang in 1927, and later in other states after infant welfare clinics attached to general hospitals had begun operation. Home visiting was difficult in less developed areas, but where transport was available and settlement dense, it was often the first important contact between a new mother and infant welfare staff.

As already noted, a major purpose of home visiting was to encourage women to attend the infant welfare clinics to enable infants to be monitored, while increasing women's familiarity with the centre, its staff and the hospital service. This it was hoped would encourage women to go to clinics, to present for antenatal care during future pregnancies, and to seek biomedical advice and care when they or their infants were sick.[54] Health staff hypothesised that a proportion of infant deaths were the consequence of a lack of immediate medical attention, and early resort for diagnosis and treatment would save lives. Part of the advice proffered to mothers at home therefore was recognition of, and appropriate action consequent upon, signs and symptoms of infant distress. In addition, home visitors offered new mothers advice on the care and feeding of the well infant, transferring contemporary notions of the scientific routine management of infants – regularised feeding, limited handling and so on, as popularised in Australia and New Zealand by Truby King – ideas best suited to middle-class or elite households where there was the least risk of disturbance or distress caused by a crying infant.[55] The educational role of the home visitor was supplemented too by other means of public health education: the 'friendly talks' of district sanitary inspectors and officers in charge of travelling dispensaries on malaria, hygiene and sanitation, for example.[56]

Home visitors concentrated on infant feeding practice, motivated by an apparent shift from breast to bottle feeding in addition to concern at the tendency of Malay women to discard colostrum and feed newborns with pre-chewed banana or rice water until the let-down of milk. Reasons for the use of cow's milk, condensed milks and infant formula either as a supplement to or in lieu of breast milk are several. Tinned milk, baby formulas and other baby foods and milk products were marketed by Nestlé, Glaxo and other milk companies from 1890, and by the early twentieth century these were available even in remoter, rural areas.[57] Both incidence and duration of breastfeeding declined from the late nineteenth century, with earlier cessation of breastfeeding the more common pattern, especially among Malay women. The Medical Report

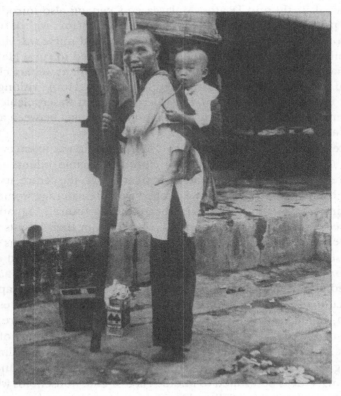

Figure 7.1 Chinese grandmother and child with feeding tube, Singapore, c. 1910. Printed with permission from the Royal Commonwealth Society, London. Files of the British Association of Malaya, BAM/1 – Singapore.

for Selangor for 1904, for instance, noted that many infants were brought to the hospital suffering from diarrhoea caused by 'improper feeding' with tinned milk. In 1907, the Health Officer of Kuala Lumpur attributed the annual infant mortality rate of 313 per thousand to the use of sweetened condensed milk;[58] in Singapore, about one-third of infant deaths were believed due to artificial feeding using adulterated and polluted fresh and imported cows' milk. The Annual Report of the Straits Settlements for 1910 again suggested that a major cause of infant death was the 'faulty feeding of infants'.[59] Further, government medical officers from as early as 1913 argued for the protective value of breast milk and felt that infant health was compromised through changes in feeding.[60] The shift from breast to bottle was consolidated in the 1920s, when powdered and sweetened condensed milk was distributed by infant welfare clinics as part of an attempt to improve infant nutrition; doctors and nursing staff believed that the breast milk of Malay women was 'deficient' due to their restricted post-partum diet.[61] Among wealthy Chinese women, wet-nursing was not uncommon in the nineteenth and twentieth century,[62] and the increased availability of infant milks and bottles simply facilitated an established trend. In addition, numbers of women began to bottle-feed because of the association of bottle-feeding and modernity, reflected by the feeding patterns of expatriate and wealthy local women. Others turned to bottles to resolve the difficulties of childcare and feeding as they moved into wage labour, without nursery facilities or time off for lactation.

The clinics

In urban centres by the 1920s, home visits were the first point of contact between health workers and new mothers. Home visits were uneconomic, however, where populations were dispersed and logistically difficult to reach. In the UFMS especially, home visits had limited effect in encouraging women to attend infant welfare centres; less than 10 percent of the women who were visited in Kedah in 1934, for example, subsequently came to the infant welfare clinic at the Kota Bharu General Hospital.[63] In the UFMS, then, the medical departments concentrated on clinic-based services, and in all states, the clinics provided the main focus of infant welfare activities.

Infant welfare centres had been established by Medical Departments throughout the Settlements and FMS by the late 1920s and in the UFMS by the late 1930s. Singapore and Malacca Municipalities also ran infant welfare clinics, and the Singapore Children's Welfare Society operated two more clinics in areas where women worked in factories; here they conducted home visits to new mothers and provided children in creches

Table 7.2 Home visits and infant welfare clinic attendance, Straits
              Settlements, 1937

Municipalities	Visits to homes		Attendances at clinics	
Singapore	114,700		50,623	
Penang	59,651		11,083	
Malacca	28,391	202,742	5,813	67,519
Rural areas (government centres)				
Singapore	57,577		92,787	
Penang	53,479		43,511	
Province Wellesley	56,490		33,833	
Malacca	51,496		23,926	
Labuan	5,793	224,835	3,361	197,418
Total		**427,577**		**264,937**

Source: SSAR 1937, p. 1026.

with milk, soup, malt, and cod liver oil.[64] In 1936, there were 70 centres
and nine sub-centres in the colonies, and a year later nearly 300,000
infants and their mothers had been in contact with clinic staff in the
settlements alone (Table 7.2). Each had a minimum staff of a health
nurse, midwife and attendant, ran antenatal clinics, infant health services and home-visiting programs, and supervised local midwives.

The centres were microcosms of the cultural world of biomedicine
and spatial representations of the medical hierarchies of knowledge and
control. Each new visitor passed through a reception room, presided
over by a European sister, one at a time, through to the inner room of
the medical doctor. Details of the infant's health, growth, and advice
(instructions) given to mothers were entered onto cards so that the doctor
could 'watch' the progress of the child. In the Kuala Lumpur town clinic
and in some other larger clinics there was a separate weighing room to
weigh the child and 'monitor progress', a 'microscope room' (for limited
pathology tests) and a dispensary. Women proceeded through these
rooms sequentially, by-passing the last two rooms if the child was well.[65]
Infants were weighed, issues arising from any preceding home visit or
clinic session pursued, and advice offered regarding feeding and care,
imparting to new mothers 'the mysteries of child welfare'. The procedures
of the clinics, the treatments offered to women, including the provision
of artificial milk for supplementary feeds despite 'homilies' on breastfeeding, the prescriptions of vitamins, and the admonitions to which
women were subject when their child was sick, too fat, or too thin, or when
the mother's attendance was irregular, all imparted to women contemporary European notions of competent mothering.[66]

Ritual weighing and temperature-taking of the infants and the treatment of minor illness took up most clinic time, despite the rhetoric of preventive medicine and public health. Clinics were represented as 'educational institutions' or 'schools for mothers' to give them basic information regarding health and hygiene, family nutrition and infant feeding, and the value of Western medicine.[67] Health education was given to mothers, theoretically, both in consultations and by displays and exhibitions. Clinics maintained 'museums' of unsuitable midwifery implements confiscated from local midwives; dummies, old feeding bottles and similar items; proper (European-style) baby clothes; and posters of scenes of 'native life'. Lectures by health inspectors dealt with sanitation, 'wholesome food' (the value of eggs, fruit and vegetables), vaccinations, and so on. Displays were also provided at agricultural and horticultural shows and films were screened in schools and to voluntary associations which depicted Malay and Chinese family life, and promoted breastfeeding or warned against enteric infections or tuberculosis. The agricultural and horticultural show in Malacca in 1926, for example, included a health exhibition on hookworm and other helminthic infections, malaria, tuberculosis, yaws, venereal diseases and infant welfare; a permanent display in the health centre at Jasin Hospital included model layettes and methods of feeding.[68]

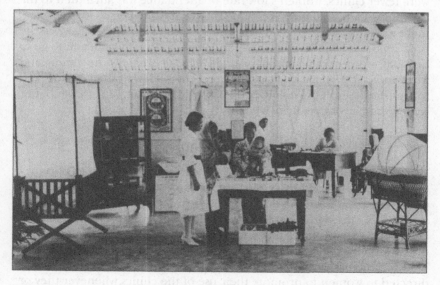

Figure 7.2 Infant Welfare Centre, Balik Pulau, Penang, c. 1933. The Centre's museum is in the cupboard behind the display cot with mosquito net. Printed with permission from Bodleian Library, Oxford. Rhodes House Library, Colonial Records Project, Mss Indian Ocean S134.

Clinics provided transport, distributed free milk, and had baby shows to encourage women and their infants, and in Kuala Lumpur, health officers urged government employees to take their wives and babies to clinics for antenatal care, assessment and surveillance. Program success varied. In the FMS in 1926, it was reported that the infant welfare centres received good support from parents, and the attendance numbers (56,916 in 1925, 61,365 in 1926) reinforced this perspective:

> It is interesting to note the change that has taken place in the attitude of parents towards the aim and object of the centres. They were originally full of fears and prejudices and attended only after much persuasion and in a very hesitating manner; they vouchsafed no signs of approval or otherwise at the instructions given them and appeared completely mystified and far from happy. Today on visiting the centre one can see for oneself that these same people are now thoroughly at home and have lost their fears, their attendance weekly is regular and they bring not only their own babies but persuade their neighbours to do the same.[69]

However, even when clinic sessions were supplemented by an extensive home visiting program, local women presented at the clinics in a sporadic and desultory fashion, depending on the availability of transport and other demands on their time. In the UFMS, where there were fewer clinics, women's low rate of attendance was attributed to the 'chopping and changing' of staff. In Kedah and Perlis, for instance, there were four different 'lady doctors' between 1927 and 1929 when the final appointee went on sick leave, and women, already reluctant to go to hospital, were nervous about seeing a doctor they did not know and would not accept male doctors.[70] There were too few women doctors and nurses throughout the colonies, even though, in fact, Malaya was better served than any other British colony.[71]

Women's health

Women's role in the provision of health care – an integral part of reproductive work – gained increasing importance as preventive health programs expanded, with an emphasis on health centres and other public health fora (the agricultural show displays, for example), on nutrition and preventive measures that could be undertaken domestically against diseases such as malaria, tuberculosis and hookworm. Campaigns were held to encourage the immunisation of children; and education was directed to women to promote their use of the clinics whenever they or their children were sick. The extent to which public health education targeted women reflected their presumed primary role as nurturers and carers of their husbands and children.

In theory, women's own health should have been of no lesser concern to the state, given women's roles in both reproduction *and* production. Yet it attracted limited comment. I have discussed certain health problems in the previous chapter, but sexually transmitted diseases were only one aspect of ill-health. Women suffered from the same infectious diseases as men, and while the disproportionate number of male outpatients and inpatients was partly the result of the skewed sex ratio, differential case fatality rates suggest also that women were less likely to seek medical attention and to have poorer access to it. For example, in the General Hospital in Kuala Lumpur in 1903, 13.73 percent of women admitted died, primarily from diarrhoeal disease and tuberculosis, while only 3.2 percent of men died. The excess mortality was explained in terms of delays in presentation, such that women admitted were 'generally so ill before they seek admission that little can be done for them'.[72]

The only relatively systematic data available is for maternal mortality. Data on causes of deaths in annual departmental reports aggregated infant and maternal deaths as accidents of childbirth, so it is not easy to be accurate. However, women died primarily from post-partum haemorrhage and from eclampsia, fewer from placenta praevia, septicaemia and various fevers; their infants from prematurity, tetanus and convulsions from various causes.[73] Lewis maintains that in the United Kingdom during the First World War, when the associations between foetal and neonatal mortality and maternal health became clear, antenatal care gained importance; certainly from around this time in Malaya there was increased discussion about women's health, foetal outcome and child health.[74] Despite increased antenatal and postnatal care, and the extension of such services throughout the states, the high maternal mortality rate persisted without obvious explanations. In Kedah, 1928–9, the rate was a massive 16.1 maternal deaths per thousand births, attributed to very early age at marriage, early first pregnancy, and dependence on untrained local birth attendants.[75] However, in the mid to late 1930s, the rate was still high in areas despite many qualified and registered midwives and comprehensive maternal health services. Even in the settlements, it varied from 8.4 per thousand population-wide to 22.4 in hospitals, where women with prior known complications or who developed problems during labour were likely to deliver.[76] In the FMS, the population-based rate was around 10.1.

Ethnicity was the one outstanding factor predictive of differences in the rate: Chinese women had the lowest maternal mortality rate, then Malay women, then Indian women, despite significant local variations (Table 7.3). In the Settlements in the mid-1930s it fluctuated geographically from 3.7 in Singapore to 20.65 in Province Wellesley, and was highest among Tamil women working on estates and among Malay women, due to 'numerous customs associated with child-birth that require to be removed' and to 'ignorance and poverty'.[77] In the FMS the 1936 rate was relatively constant between States but varied by ethnicity: 13.2 for Malays, 14.9 for Indians, 4.9 for Chinese;[78] in 1937 it had also improved for Malay women. In general the maternal mortality among Malay women seems to have been associated broadly with health and medical services and general infrastructure, although also it was related to early age at marriage, the presence of a birth attendant and access to hospital. Those living in the UFMS or geographically most isolated were disadvantaged.[79] Among Chinese women rates were relatively low, with patterns similar to those for Malay women. For Indian women, however, declining maternal mortality paralleled an increase in the infant mortality rate from 126 to 169, leading to the conclusion that 'far more attention to the health of Indian women and children' was needed, and provoking recurrent comment by health officers with respect to the effect of anaemia on the health of Tamil women.[80] Additionally, however, as noted in Chapter 5, maternity leave payments were calculated in such a way as to put pressure on women to work as long as possible before, and to return to work as soon as possible after, delivery.[81]

Malaria, anaemia, and poor nutritional status were seen as contributing to poor reproductive health. In particular, the continued high incidence of parasitaemia and clinical cases of malaria in Malaya through this period, des·· te extensive anti-malarial measures, suggests that malaria may have been an important factor in maternal health and pregnancy outcome. Pregnancy increases susceptibility to *P. falciparum* malaria, and increases the risk of cerebral malaria and death; pregnant women are also more likely to develop severe anaemia from malaria-related folate deficiency.[82] Malaria in pregnancy increases miscarriages, stillbirths, pre-term deliveries and low birth-weight babies, whose health outcome also is poorer consequently. Most Chinese and Indian women were non-immune. They were young women newly migrated to the colonies, whose number increased dramatically in the 1930s as a consequence of government policy to encourage family formation and the

Table 7.3   Maternal mortality rates*, select States, 1937

Ethnicity	Kedah (UFMS)	Johore (UFMS)	FMS Total	Singapore municipality
Malay	13.0	10.6	11.1	7.6
Indian	9.5	14.3	15.2	24.35
Chinese	6.7	5.75	4.8	4.56

* Deaths per 1,000
Source: SS/FMSAR 1937, p. 11.

permanent development of a wage labour force. But since immunity is compromised in pregnancy, partially immune Malay women would also have been affected; especially among primigravidae there was (and is) increased risk of malaria and increased intensity of infection.

Among Malay women, as noted, maternal mortality may have been high in some areas also due to poor access to health services and suboptimal birth conditions. Chinese women fared well, in contrast, because of the higher proportion delivering in hospitals. In particular, the Chinese Maternity Hospitals provided women with a relatively safe and acceptable alternative to home delivery, and as indicated in Table 7.4 their admissions and attended births were high and maternal deaths relatively low.

Compared with the infant mortality rate, however, and other health problems, the maternal mortality rate caused little concern. Control over midwifery increased the chances of live delivery, the prevention of neonatal tetanus, and the control of jaundice. Other health problems were regarded as important primarily insofar as these might affect others, and this consideration drove the research agenda. Studies of maternal undernutrition and malnutrition were undertaken because of an interest in the effect of these on foetal development and lactation physiology and the implications for infant welfare. The high infant mortality rate during the first decade, for example, was at times partially explained by 'deficiency in the stamina of infants' due to poor maternal health during pregnancy and confinement, and beri-beri in lactating mothers.[83] 'Maternal and child health', then, was important predominantly because of the role of mothers as carers and nurturers. The extent to which services in the field of primary health care and public health benefited women themselves was largely incidental.

Teaching maternity

As described above, maternal and child health services fell into two parts: control over midwifery practice and the monitoring of mothers

Table 7.4 Kuala Lumpur Chinese Maternity Hospital, 1922–1926

	1922	1923	1924	1925	1926
Number of admissions	679	696	1,200	1,415	1,633
Maternal deaths	4	2	4	7	3
Cases attended elsewhere	168	205	306	350	381
Total births attended by hospital staff	847	901	1,506	1,765	2,015

Source: Sel. Sec. 4170/1927, *Annual Report of the Kuala Lumpur Chinese Maternity Association for 1926.*

Table 7.5 Home visiting and clinic attendance, Straits Settlements, 1931

Authority	Singapore	Penang	Malacca
Municipality			
Home visits	1,112,387	52,070	40,825
Clinic	24,688	—	5,387
Child Welfare Society			
Home visits	43,117	—	—
Clinic	39,579	—	—
Government			
Home visits	38,248	54,204	22,541
Clinic	14,312	38,709	14,385

Source: SSAR 1931, p. 1034.

and their infants. In addition, as discussed later, it covered a third area, school education, wherein the strategy lay in providing an early educational foundation for women in their future roles in reproduction and family health. The first few decades of the operation of maternal and child health services in the colonies witnessed a steady increase in the number of women presenting and continuing to use clinic services. In the Settlements this was particularly the case. In 1931, for example, a total of 363,392 home visits were made, there were 137,060 clinic visits, 5,792 admissions and 5,335 deliveries (see Table 7.4). In all areas and for all states, substantial increases had occurred over the preceding decade, indicating the extent to which state surveillance of reproduction was occurring.

By 1940, it was estimated that approximately 850,000 women received home visits or attended infant welfare centres or women's and children's sessions operating from the outdoor dispensaries, and at least 30,000 women had delivered in hospitals. Yet clinic attendance was unpredictable. The UFMS faced particular problems of acceptance of both outpatient clinic services and hospitals, the departments were unable to respond to community preference for married nursing staff of their own ethnic background and the program was not regarded generally as successful. In light of this, there was a shift in emphasis away from adult women to those for whom motherhood was a future event. Whilst seen as part of a broader health care strategy, domestic science education was a legitimation of female education providing the first premiss – that women needed to be *taught* to be housewives and mothers – was accepted. The side-benefit was that there would be a greater number of educated women with the educational prerequisites for nursing and midwifery training. Mothercraft and 'housecraft' were included within the domestic science curriculum since the general responsibility for health care, particularly preventive measures and primary care, devolved to women.[84] Women were responsible for sustaining good health by providing nutritious food, ensuring clean living quarters and by presenting their children for vaccinations and seeking clinic assistance when the children were ill; they were responsible, that is, for daily as well as biological reproduction. Insofar as the acceptance of Western notions of health and ill-health constituted the incorporation of a particular ideology or logic, women were responsible too for the social reproduction that propped up (part of) the colonial system.

Domestic science subjects had been incorporated into the school curriculum in the colonies from the late nineteenth century, and the relationship between this and the infant mortality rate had been an issue very early in the twentieth century. The Health Officer of Kuala Lumpur in 1907, for example, argued that it was impossibile to 'induce parents to give up their prejudices as to how their infants should be reared' and that 'the only way to endeavour to prevent the waste of life is by means of educating the school children, and thus the prospective parent'.[85] Domestic science skills were incorporated into the curriculum of all-girls schools, and in boys' schools where girls were enrolled and where numbers were sufficiently large to enable the appointment of a special teacher: these included cooking, laundry, sewing, weaving, needlework, housewifery (sweeping, dusting and so on) and specific issues of infant care, including 'how to prepare a layette', how to clothe, bathe and feed babies, and 'how to keep their homes clean and their family free of worm infections and dysentery'.[86] Interest in domestic science education and its function in training young women as wives and mothers coincided also with a wider interest in hygiene and sanitation education. The curriculum included general matters of health, hygiene and sanitation, including environmental measures to reduce the incidence of malaria and helminthic infections; the curriculum for boys focused on these latter extradomestic health matters. A number of schools offered relatively comprehensive instruction on the prevention and treatment of malaria, the importance of vaccination, and first aid. Some colonial officers were particularly committed to hygiene education and saw it in ideological terms that were reminiscent of the debates of health and imperialism in England at the turn of the century. For example, according to Gilbert Brooke:

> [H]ygiene in schools – both as a matter of precept and of practice – is perhaps the most important of all the factors which are concerned in the making of happy individuals, sound citizens and virile nations. Until the teachers themselves grasp this – until they are filled with the enthusiasm of hygiene so that it becomes an integral and subconscious part of their outlook and life, no real progress will be made and the citizens of the future will have as narrow an outlook as their parents. In the hands of the school teachers lies the destiny of the future, and practically the sole control of all the preventable diseases of mankind.[87]

The inclusion, content and frequency of hygiene classes, however, depended upon staff interest and knowledge, the exigencies of time-tabling, and funds where special additional staff were employed from the outside.[88] There were also state differences: Selangor and Perak, for example, had a number of girls' schools and many more girls were attending boys' schools, but in Pahang as well as the UFMS, female education lagged well behind: the first girls' school in Pahang opened only in 1914, and by 1931 still only 272 girls were attending five girls' schools, with a further 730 enrolled at boys' schools.[89] The expansion of female education resulted in increased capacity of schools to provide domestic science teaching in Malay schools by graduates of the Malay Women Teachers Training College (WTTC) in Malacca; elsewhere by a teacher trained in other fields whose primary claim to competence in domestic science and home economics was her own femaleness.

What is significant in this context is, firstly, that through the refinement of the curriculum its authors categorised the roles of women, these in dogmatic terms derived from ideals of English wifehood, motherhood and housewifery. The terms of motherhood were exclusive: the curriculum did not include poultry rearing or rice farming for example (although weaving and sewing were included as proper skills for a Malay housewife). The corollary was the emphasis in the boys' curriculum, at least in textbooks like Blacklock's *Elementary Tropical Hygiene*, on environmental diseases such as malaria, plague, helminthic infections and bowel diseases ('the great preventable maladies of Asia') and on venereal disease, since boys had 'scant knowledge' of the latter and 'not uncommonly infected their homes after marriage'.[90] The commentary on both male and female sexuality within these texts, and the design of the curriculum, is revealing.

Secondly, the inclusion in the school curriculum of hygiene and sanitation acknowledged that public health interests were not sustainable through government intervention and surveillance, but demanded a more complete change in practice through the internalisation of notions of the etiology, prevention and control of disease. Ideas of order, cleanliness, dirt, and disease that shaped contemporary British understandings and methods of disease control were neither ahistoric nor impartial, and their inclusion within the education system functioned, like other subject areas, to legitimise British cultural hegemony, from which flowed social and political control, juridical and administrative actions within the colonies, and their systems of stratification.

In the 1930s there was renewed interest in domestic science teaching concomitant with a growing interest in nutrition as well as the education of girls, and both topics were the subjects of major enquiries and reports for all British colonies. Domestic science education gained support at this time because it was perceived to fulfil two major functions. The first, which provided the rationale for the subject's inclusion in the curriculum, was the importance of teaching young girls fundamental principles of hygiene, nutrition, and housekeeping because of their anticipated future role and responsibilities as wives and mothers. Domestic science addressed issues that pertained specifically to infant feeding and health and generally to the nutrition of all family members; at its simplest, it gave girls a practical education: 'knowledge of cookery is much more useful than a knowledge of geometry'.[91] However, others maintained a wider association between education, the role of women, family health, and medical services, and school classes on hygiene and sanitation supplemented community based health education. The appointment of special teachers also enabled the physical examination of children, their clothing, their heads, and treatment for head-lice. Schools were also inspected – furniture, the classrooms, the compound, the well, latrines, arrangements for the disposal of rubbish and so on. The domestic science mistress was responsible also for the surveillance of fellow teachers.

A primary aim of an expanded domestic science program and the appointment of domestic science mistresses was to improve 'the standard of cleanliness' and 'general alertness'. However the curriculum was sometimes extended to include curative knowledge. The Kedah curriculum, for instance, included the care of the sick and the use of standard medicines,[92] and it was partly because of this wider interpretation of domestic science that a number of officials argued for the promotion of domestic science and the appointment of new teaching and supervisory staff as priority areas for educational funding.

Colonial deliberations

These developments took place in a wider, colonial context, and it is that to which I now turn. In 1935 Dr Mary Blacklock of the Liverpool School of Tropical Medicine undertook a tour of the colonies of Hong Kong, Malaya, Ceylon, Palestine, China, Burma and India, concerned with the welfare of women and children. Drawing on findings from this trip and her experience as a doctor in India and Africa, she argued that progress in the field of the welfare of women and children was poor; that despite various interventions and improved services, infant and maternal mortality rates remained high; women and girls were still exploited; few girls went to school; and little effort had been directed to providing proper medical care for women.[93] Blacklock argued that the poor health and welfare of women and children was due to government failure to allocate adequate resources to train local nurses, or provide sufficient female staff in hospitals. At the same time, she noted the broad economic and social context of ill-health in the colonies:

> The health of women and, even more, the health of small children depends very much on economic conditions, and much of the sickness seen at welfare clinics, both among women and children, can be attributed solely to poverty. I have heard a health sister beg to be excused from visiting among a particularly poor section of a people, because she felt it was ironical to talk of a balanced diet to people who had practically nothing to eat but rice, or to advocate cleanliness when water and fuel were only obtainable with great difficulty.[94]

Blacklock's approach – descriptive of the developments that had occurred in colonial Malaya – was to strengthen clinical services with special services for women and children, and to improve education for women to meet their own and their family's health needs and long-term health workforce requirements. Hence she called for a greater number of maternity centres and wards, more women doctors to be recruited from Britain to the colonies, 'native' women to be trained as medical assistants and doctors, better education for hospital nurses, health visitors (community nurses) and midwives, and better educational opportunities to ensure there were women available for training in medicine and nursing. She also stressed the need for all schools to teach women domestic science and mothercraft to improve family health; her curriculum included sanitation, ventilation, vector control, safe food and water storage, and dietetics.

In a subsequent memorandum, Blacklock proposed joint post-primary education for women in the colonies wanting to be nurses or teachers, the curriculum of which would cover the broad areas of domestic science, health and social welfare and would include literacy and numeracy, natural and social sciences, elementary physiology, nutrition, hygiene, first aid, mothercraft, child care, housewifery and domestic economics (cleaning, laundry and budgeting), and 'social and preventive elements of nursing'. The curriculum, she argued, would provide for women not only as wives and mothers, but also as institutional housekeepers, domestic science instructors, health workers, social workers, clerks, typists, dressmakers and milliners.[95]

The views of Mary Blacklock were not particularly new. Others shared her views with regard to the need for more women doctors, for the appointment of women as health workers at a district and provincial level and for women to be educated.[96] A Memorandum on Education Policy in British Tropical Africa in 1925, for example, had already drawn attention to the association between women's education and children's health, and its points were easily generalisable: 'The high rate of infant mortality ... and the unhygienic conditions which are widely prevalent make instruction in hygiene and public health, in the case of the sick and the treatment of simple diseases, among the first essentials, and these wherever possible, should be taught by well-qualified women teachers.'[97] The Committee on Nutrition in the Colonial Empire in 1936 had made a similar argument for increased training in agriculture, health and domestic science,[98] and Blacklock's work in the mid-1930s thus reflected a growing concern and provided a catalyst for further action. Her article was distributed to colonial administrations with a recommendation for increased training and employment of women, from the Advisory Medical Education Com-mittee of the Colonial Office, and a letter from the Secretary of State recommending increased expenditure on and the expansion of female education.[99] Responses to this letter and subsequent mem-oranda by Dr Esdaile drew further attention to the 'serious lag in the education of girls as compared with boys both in content and degree' and to the fact that 'lack of money has deterred many governments from seriously tackling the problem of girls' education'.[100]

Continued pressure on the Colonial Office relating to the health, education and welfare of women and girls led the Education Advisory Committee in September 1939 to set up a sub-committee 'to report on the means of accelerating social progress in the Colonial Empire by the increased education of women and girls and by welfare work among them'. Much of the work of the sub-committee took place during the war years. To a large extent its deliberations anticipate post-war policy and program changes as much as they provide commentary on the interwar years. Given this, its work falls outside of the scope of this volume. Its general brief and debates do pertain, however. The sub-committee spent much time debating the merits of female education – usually in the context of woman's role as homemaker and mother, 'by nature much more the "pillar of society" than the man'[101] – and discussing the ideal mix of practical and theoretical subjects in the curriculum. Its report advocated special marriage training and nurse/midwifery schools. It also proposed a general curriculum for both girls and boys to meet health and educational workforce needs, with special subjects for girls in domestic science, personal hygiene and physical education:

> Care must also be taken that the interests of the girls are not subordinated to those of the boys, especially when they are in a minority, and that they do not suffer from any feeling of inferiority. The best means of achieving this is probably to have an adequate number of women on the staff of the

Departments of Education in the teaching, inspecting and administrative
branches.[102]

With the 'discovery' of the child and increasing attention to infant
mortality, preventive medical services and health education programs
were directed towards women, including those who were themselves
health practitioners (*bidan*), those who were informally responsible for
family health on an everyday basis, and those in whose hands (or, more
accurately, bodies) lay the responsibility of the reproduction of future
generations. As noted, developments in colonial Malaya in education,
health and medicine, and social welfare reflected ideological changes
and practical developments in England as well as local exigencies. The
surveillance of village midwifery practice and the incorporation of
pregnancy and birth into hospital-based medicine, the establishment of
home visiting, the development of maternal and child clinics, and the
expansion of domestic science education all closely followed developments in the United Kingdom. Maternal and child health care programs
were erected on the basis of understandings of the role of women in
reproduction (with respect to biological, social and daily reproduction),
and they assumed that some women, by virtue of class and race, were
able to undertake these roles 'naturally'.[103] Davies has suggested with
respect to home visiting in the United Kingdom that women were
presumed to contribute to public health *as women*, independent of
special training and as an artefact of 'their natural womanly qualities
which came first – qualities which as middle-class women they brought
from the private sphere; qualities which gave them regard and esteem
but not pecuniary rewards'.[104]

In Malaya, with a local twist, European women, or certainly the
middle-class wives of colonial officers, were seen as natural mothers, but
Indian, Malay and Chinese women were considered less capable,
needing to be taught to feed, care, nurture and treat their infants and
children. There was further irony and confused reasoning as culture and
climate were collapsed: hence conditions in the tropics were believed to
'react with particular severity upon the health of mothers and children',
thus the high infant and maternal mortality rates which warranted
'adequate supervision' by European health workers.[105] Training women
to become mothers, it was hoped, would be the most effective intervention against the high infant mortality rate and this was, in Mary
Blacklock's mind, the *primary* function of the clinics.[106].The approach
stepped around the economic and structural factors that had already
been identified as contributing to poor health outcomes. It provided
government with 'an easy way out', as Anna Davin has argued:

It was cheaper to blame them [mothers] and to organize a few classes than to
expand social and medical services, and it avoided the political problem of
provoking rate- and taxpayers by requiring extensive new finance. And there
seemed more chance of educating individuals, future or present mothers,
than of banishing poverty. So even those who recognized – or paid lip-service
to – the importance of environment were liable to fall back on such measures
as more domestic science in schools, and education for motherhood, and
banning the employment of mothers.[107]

Moves to bring reproduction under the purview of the state, through
controlling the conditions of childbirth and childrearing, had been
initiated early in the twentieth century, as described above. Despite
criticism of their impact, they expanded. Given this, Colonial Office
discussions in the late 1930s are remarkable for their lack of reflection
on the prior four decades of these services either in colonial or domestic
settings. More remarkable again was the lack of sense of history post-war.
P. F. de Souza wrote to the Advisory Committee on Education within the
Colonial Office of Malaya that 'before the war, no local girl could aspire
to become a nursing sister';[108] and later commentaries on maternal and
child welfare rewrote history to date the development of midwifery and
infant health services from independence, after ideas of primary health
care had gained general currency and official support.[109]

CHAPTER 8

Conclusion:
The moral logic of colonial medicine

The shift from curative medicine and disease control to public health was set in place in colonial Malaya with the transfer of governance from the East India Company to the Colonial Office. As an outcome, the tactical response to threats of disease, affecting the lives of those most insinuated into imperialism, was displaced by a more complicated, extensive and invasive project. But while the state functioned to create the preconditions for capitalist expansion, in so doing it created also the conditions for increased illness. In a way, this made it increasingly difficult to 'segment' economic development and its dysfunctional effects (social, medical and political), or to neutralise these in relation to the state.[1] Now, whilst the state was still responsible for disease prevention, its wider brief was to improve health status, as measured imperfectly by changes in morbidity and mortality rates. In addition, because of the association between the prevalence of disease and social conditions, the state was also charged with addressing the moral and economic costs of colonialism. The paradox was this: the state was at the one time both 'reproducer of relations of production and division of labour *and* guarantor of opportunity and advancement'.[2] The contradictions between these goals were as evident in medicine and health as they were in other colonial policies and programs.

I have noted that medical services in colonial Malaya were originally urban-based, hospital-centred and elitist, serving first British officers and other colonists, then, in a concentric order of distance from colonial capitalism, others whose diseases threatened the operation of colonial enterprises. The expansion of preventive medicine and sanitation occurred concomitantly with the penetration of the colonial economy into the hinterland, and rural health programs were developed with this in mind. Thus a major function of and rationale for rural health programs was instrumental: the establishment of the preconditions and maintenance of the labour force for economic development. To the extent that state and capital shared one goal, this served political, ideological and economic functions that are difficult to separate. It is important to note also, however, that there were immediate political benefits of public health, as they both justified the extension of control – embodied by the doctors, judges, district officers, police and sanitary workers – over the population, and took these authoritarian figures into people's homes. Private lives and private acts became matters for public scrutiny and state intervention, and health risks were defined in the course of this incursion. This had the political consequence of providing the moral and intellectual basis of colonial rule. It was not possible, in this interpretation of the role of the state, to rule indirectly as originally negotiated with some of the States (that is, the UFMS).

Following MacLeod,[3] I would argue that medicine, as a cultural agent or force, is an agent of Western expansion. The introduction of bio-medical institutions, practitioners, treatments and cures were part of the colonising project that, by introducing Western cultural values to the empire, insisted on the moral authority of the imperialising power. While early colonialism seemed not to require such moral authority, the extension of state intervention required acquiescence to a particular knowledge base, acceptance of the theoretical basis of biomedicine, and the appropriateness of its institutions. This proved somewhat self-serving: the intellectual incorporation of the biomedical paradigm implied acceptance and accommodation of its organisational structures; these structures (clinics, hospitals, research departments and so on) were available because of colonialism.

As noted, the first hospitals were built to serve the needs of the British officers and their troops. Those at a distance from European settlement, whose illnesses were least likely to affect colonial economic life or the health of others, had little access to medical and hospital services, and the geographical and cultural distance between the hospitals and *kampungs* was not insignificant. However, by the late nineteenth century travelling and floating dispensaries provided some clinical care and referred those who were seriously ill to town hospitals or private doctors, and campaigns against malaria, hookworm, cholera and yaws also brought Malays in touch with Western medicine. It is hard to get a sense of how they perceived medical services or experienced their interactions with hospital staff. The hospitals were both icons of biomedicine and microcosms of British and medical social organisation, reflected in the stratified relationships between doctors, hospital dressers, apothecaries, assistant surgeons, nurses and midwives, British professionals and locally trained doctors and assistants, men and women, and staff and patients.

At any level of appointment, the differences were important both on an everyday basis, since acknowledgement of and adherence to the lines of authority were fundamental to the smooth operation of the institution, and on a symbolic level: hence the density of meaning in the titles 'lady doctor' and 'native dresser'. The stratification of the hospital included patient care: types of hospitals (general, women's, mental), classes of wards, diets, and so on, differentiating people first in terms of race (European and native wards) and then income. It was also represented by the uniforms that distinguished staff from each other and from their patients, by the differential allocation of space (as illustrated with respect to infant welfare centres in Chapter 7), its designated purposes, and access to knowledge of and the right to use the mystifying, technological accoutrements of the hospital.

The employment of local staff came at a price. For the most part, as noted in Chapter 1, traditional healers were ignored and the services that they offered occurred parallel to and had little to do with Western medicine. Midwives primarily were subject to state scrutiny. From 1880 apothecaries and hospital dressers were recruited from India and Ceylon, and they were therefore people who had been subjected to the socialising experiences of an English-based education system in India, a sometimes brutal apprenticeship.[4] There was some interest in recruiting and training people locally also, since without doing so the provision of adequate services was problematic; hence medical department interest in school education.

In recruiting and training, various contradictions emerged. On the one hand the aim was to train people in biomedical theory and practice, thereby providing the knowledge base and frames of reference that legitimised clinical and colonial authority. On the other hand, the curriculum of English medical schools was not considered suitable for the local environment and 'local needs', raising questions of the universal applicability of medical science. Difficulties in recruitment, retention and employment raised a third question about people's 'readiness' for such training and therefore, by implication, their ability to move beyond the paternalism of colonialism. This question was initially side-stepped through the conduit of 'bright youths' from the Victoria Institution to the Institute of Medical Research, then to Hong Kong or Madras for training as physicians and surgeons. From 1905 training took place at the King Edward VII College of Medicine in Singapore. Post-training, these local doctors, and nurses and midwives, were given the role of cultural broker as well as healer, to 'not only to care for the sick but to promote health education and help people to improve their conditions of living'.[5]

The output of both hospitals and clinics is there for the public record, for medical administrations were obsessed with accounts and record-keeping – numbers of outpatients and inpatients, injections given, blood slides taken, stools collected and so on. The obsession, on the other hand, was with the implementation and evaluation of public health interventions, and the interpretation of failures, as indicated by lack of expected or sufficient changes in the mortality rate, in terms of the social pathology of colonialism, development, industrialisation, or 'culture'.

For Malaya, as for Africa, colonial medical departments were concerned with prevention rather than cure.[6] The discussions of the control of cholera (Chapter 2) and prevention of plague (Chapter 4) illustrate the way that epidemic crises enabled the state to impose itself in extraordinary ways, moving populations, interfering with burial rites, and searching and burning housing and personal effects. The 'heroism' of these interventions legitimised the state's role and advanced its proselytisation of medicine. In the case of plague, control procedures finally focused on screening and quarantine procedures, and the flamboyant collection of rats and rats' tails, and there were few cases that required police action. Cholera, on the other hand, demanded quick intervention by medical officers and police, with the co-option of local healers providing a useful means to legitimise colonial authority. The interventions worked in the face of frightening and deadly illness; the approach, the military-like mobilisation of the population, worked also where a simple intervention was required, as in yaws. These campaigns did not require the co-operation of capitalists and they did not interfere with production; they either had neutral effects on economic activities or were positive insofar as they removed the threat of disease also for wage labourers and their managers.

Concurrently, in response to health problems that affected both immigrant labour and Malays, women and children as well as adult men, health services were extended and redefined to include preventive medicine and what might now be referred to as primary health care programs. Concern with the high infant mortality rate and poor maternal health was related, as discussed in the preceding chapter, to the 'discovery' of the economics of reproduction, infant mortality representing the loss of future generations of labour, women's ill-health depleting the human resources available for daily, generational and social reproduction. Adult male mortality, on the other hand, was represented as having far more immediate economic impact: 'All the wealth in the world will not profit a man broken down in health', wrote Gerrard in 1913, and 'a dead or broken down coolie is of no practical use on any estate'.[7] Orde-Browne argued along the same lines in 1937, when he wrote that the capitalist's 'most valuable asset was the labour on which his enterprises depended'.[8] The relative weight that should be accorded to preventive as opposed to curative medicine was to remain a subject of debate throughout the period; enquiries into public health revealed the social and economic context of illness and forced officials to take a broader perspective of death, disease, and the degree to which colonialism was implicated. Within the Colonial Office during the Second World War, the architects of an anticipated reinstated empire struggled to come to terms with 'co-ordinated development' for the colonies, in which context, whilst acknowledging the need for curative services and palliative care, the importance of disease prevention was stressed.[9] In time it was expected that prevention would lead to a reduction in the numbers requiring hospitalisation. In the short term, as was already the case, the effectiveness of public health campaigns might be measured by the increased use of hospital services and out-patients' clinics. This was important with regard to the ideological work of public health, of course, since increased patient numbers were seen to reflect the growing acceptance of biomedicine.

The yardsticks of success were numerical; the annual reports of the medical departments are replete with comparative, incremental successes. This accounting derives from the earlier earnestness of the 'science of social investigation and statistics' to collect data and codify, to build up knowledge of the population and identify demographic trends in order then to regulate and control.[10] The hookworm campaign was a nice example of this – campaign staff travelled 120,000 miles, delivered 1,500 lectures to 80,000 people on sanitary practice and intestinal infection, treated 56,000 people, examined 40,440 stools, identified and determined the intensity of infection in these samples of hookworm, roundworm and whipworm, and showed people their worms since, it was argued, worms from one's own bowel movement 'stirred the imagination of even the most sceptical person' to spend money and provide his household with a latrine. The final report was self-acclamatory and concluded that the Straits Settlements and 'her' neighbours, the Federated Malay States, would become a model colony in public health.[11]

Or take another example from the same period (the 1920s), when both the states and settlements were interpreting public health in a particularly energetic light. Whilst there is much that one could say about sickness and death in the FMS in 1926, the annual report draws our attention to the sheer number of medical institutions and the volume of patients that moved through them: 48 hospitals (district, women's, gaol and dedicated European hospitals), 37 primary care posts including dispensaries, infant welfare clinics and venereal disease clinics – the other club, the planter Hutchinson called it – in addition to nine special residential institutions (asylums, quarantine stations, vagrancy wards, leper colonies) and the Pasteur Institute. In that year, 127,332 patients were admitted and 9,128 died; a further 630,052 were treated as outpatients including 156,652 by travelling dispensaries and 16,817 by dispensary boats operating along the Pahang River. Success was measured arithmetically: the comparative 1925 figures were 103,762 inpatients, 6,969 deaths, 621,793 outpatients. The point that I am making here is the power of these figures to represent success in disease control, although they might be interpreted either as an improvement or a decline in the service or in people's health. Does an increase in inpatients, for example, reflect increased prevalence of serious disease, increased case detection resulting in hospitalisation, changing case management affecting inpatient rates, or increased presentation of sick people to hospital?

The extension of health and medical services was important, however, both materially (more sick people were treated and fewer people died) and, as discussed above, in terms of the ideological functions of medical services, by establishing and maintaining political authority and control. The annual tabulations provided evidence of the colonial state's fulfilment of a social contract, hence its legitimacy: I am arguing here that the colonial state as much as the 'modern state' must necessarily minimise the 'dysfunctional side effects' of capitalism in order to maintain its authority.[12]

The establishment of order within the colonies – controlling disease and extending medical services were part of this exercise – was demonstrated not only by the quantification of activities but also through systems of classification that were imposed on both social and biological landscapes. The obsession of colonial officials to categorise was reflected in their efforts to establish order where there was, if not chaos, *terrain vague*, the imposition of order onto colonial space was part of the exercise to know, claim and control. Hence at a mundane level the zealousness of those who collected stools and organised their laboratory analysis, or at a grander level (in terms of scholarship rather than public health) the composition of compendia of agricultural products, plants, medicines and so on, or the social and biological taxonomies in medical articles that arranged the sick as they defined the disease.[13] One example is a lengthy report on beri-beri prepared by the FMS government for the Secretary of State of the Colonies in 1904. 'Chinese' are divided into *baba*, or Straits-born Chinese, including merchants, shopkeepers and 'retired wealthy', and China-born Chinese; the latter then subdivided into free coolies, contract or indentured coolies, and master-workmen; indentured coolies are further differentiated as *lau-kheh* ('old arrivals') and *sin-kheh* ('newcomers'), the master-workmen as *tukang* (tradesmen), *kepala* (headmen) and *towkay* (merchants), and so on. The risk of beri-beri for each of these groups differed, it was argued, on the basis of wealth and difference in diet. Although the micronutrients implicated in beri-beri were not known, the significance of the consumption of decorticated rice had been established, and here, food preferences, dietary habits, the availability of different foodstuffs, class and recency of migration lined up in a neat early example of social epidemiology.[14] Articles concerned with tuberculosis, venereal disease, malaria, and enteric infections, as well as those describing the social environment of disease (housing, estate work, prostitution), took a similar approach in an effort to tease out the social and cultural from the biological. Colonialism provided these embryonic epidemiologists (state medical officers and their colleagues) with a field laboratory to test out the differences between racial groups and associated with, if not caused by, race.

Race and class were socially constructed according to understandings of the time, but it is interesting to note bureaucratic insistence on the social, economic and political basis of illness and its concern to identify social fields where state intervention was possible. Inaction consequent upon this designation was a separate issue. Vaughan has observed of Africa that 'what is so striking about much of the medical knowledge ... is its explicit concern with finding social and cultural "origins" for disease patterns', and this was also characteristic of Malaya.[15] Notwithstanding the fact that in this context biomedical knowledge defined the cultural and natural, social and biological, it was also true that the colonists (planters and government officers) were acutely aware of the need to reduce morbidity for economic and domestic political reasons.

In referring to the taxonomic obsessions of those writing about sickness and death, I have argued that the colonial state sought to replace chaos with order in line with contemporary notions of the world, evolution and development (see Chapters 1 and 3). At the micro level this occurred, I suggest, with the incorporation of nature into culture through inscription, categorisation, cataloguing and labelling, a task that drove laboratory scientists employed at the Institute of Medical Research, for example, in their efforts to 'know' about tropical diseases.[16] At the macro level, it was the role of the state to replace anarchy with government, shape plantations and farms from primeval jungle, and through educational, judicial and medical systems establish institutional and ideological order. This was presumptuous in the Malay peninsula, of course, given the prior claims of the Malay States, Islam and *adat* (Malay custom), hence the arrangements for indirect rule in the UFMS, the presence of advisers, acknowledgements of the authority of *adat* in matters of Malay culture, and requests for support from Malay royalty. The state was not able to displace Malay authority and at times acceded to its prior rights with respect to Malays (but not Chinese or Indian immigrants), but it did insist on the primacy of biomedicine and largely ignored sacerdotal and secular alternatives. Since medical policies and programs were not threatened by traditional practice, there was little need to intrude on public health grounds except, as described, to circumscribe village midwifery, or, when their support was needed in times of crisis, to co-opt the *bomoh.*

Medicine's project was to bring under control the pathological body, the body out-of-control; colonial health programs were more modest, perhaps, and aimed to influence individuals and their human environments rather than biology. The establishment of order in public health occurred in a different domain, with the state inserting itself into private lives. Malay, Indian and Chinese behaviours and practices were, depending on the context, defined as 'innate' if not 'natural'; the role of the sanitary officer, home visitor, or hospital dresser was to introduce change or displace cultural practice with 'proper' hygienic behaviour (represented as culturally neutral). Public health campaigns dealt not with biological pathogens or the 'natural' environment, but with domestic and personal domains. The major campaigns were concerned with food, sex, and their by-products, or – in terms of actions – with eating, defecating, urinating, coughing, sleeping, cooking, love-making, birthing, lactating and childrearing. The need to intervene in personal matters took the state into the home, into domestic space, into both women's and men's lives, and away from the workplace where government's role was well-defined and in respects legitimate. The incursion into people's homes was partly for descriptive purposes – sanitary officers measured floor space, estimated cubic area, counted beds, latrines, buckets and so on. But the state also entered the home to search for vermin, to whitewash walls, and to disinfect premises where there were outbreaks of diarrhoea, dysentery, enteritis, diphtheria, chicken pox, cholera, smallpox and plague. In addition, householders were sometimes prosecuted for having 'filthy premises'; 'filth', like 'crowding', was of course culturally defined as well as circumstantially determined.[17]

In an effort to collapse the issues of ingestion and excretion into manageable components, in terms of the development and delivery of programs, the state then essentialised through the substitution of the individual with the group: hence published reports wrote of 'the Malay', 'the European', 'the Chinese' and so on. Again, data related to the hookworm campaign illustrates this well. European elimination was by its exclusion sanitary; 'the Malay is more or less subject to the conservancy regulations of his religion ... (and) prefers to use the jungle near a little stream or near a rice field', although he is not averse to using latrines; the Chinese 'in his conservancy habits is influenced by the economic value of night-soil'; the 'Tamil coolie ... has many superstitutions about the terrors of darkness, about sickness-producing odors and about the restrictions of caste'. The child was positioned in these texts as closer to nature – even European children were responsible for 'soil pollution … under the direction of their Chinese, Indian or Malay nurses, and in other cases most peridomestic pollution is attributed to the child, not yet socialised in terms of culturally appropriate ways of defaecating'.[18]

The colonial record is dense with these commentaries that imbricate race, class and personal behaviour in accounts of what people do with their bodies, the extent to which their actions were risks for the transmission of disease, and the interventions that were proposed and implemented to reduce transmission. These were often injunctive ('Don't Spit!'). But what is remarkable here is the extent of the invasions into people's lives as a consequence of various formal inquiries and investigations, as a result of routine annual reporting and the programs themselves. The official record offers no clues as to how the people subjected to this scrutiny viewed the Europeans who investigated where they slept and shat.

Exudations were manageable from a public health point of view since they concerned the individual rather than, for instance, structure or biology. Not all public health and medical problems were so easily collapsed into sanitary laws, however. The policy towards people with health problems that could not be managed was isolation. This occurred in the case of both physical and mental health problems, where the manifestations of illness and the physical or behavioural pathologies were dramatic. Those on the margins – criminals, vagrants, lepers and lunatics – were sequestered in asylums, leper colonies, gaols and vagrancy wards. The treatment of inmates, their ailments and deaths, is beyond the brief of this book. However, there are a few points to note that are salient and contrast with the public health programs.

Leprosy is of interest in terms of the limitations of government policy and programs, given that the disease caused such fear within the population and was so charged with metaphor. Lunacy too was a health problem, a manifestation of disordered inner states, to which the government had a limited response. Here were bodies out-of-control, whose presence within the community threatened wellbeing in often rather ill-defined ways. Colonial medical policy was, as discussed, concerned with prevention, hence the community rather than clinic focus. In the absence of means of preventing leprosy or lunacy, the state incarcerated those who threatened moral order, challenged in unconventional ways social and political structure, and lived beyond the boundaries of culture (although the constitution of madness in other cultures, and the recognition of it by colonial doctors, was a problem). Each category of people threatened the state, symbolically more than literally: the criminal by undermining the institutional provisions for authority, order and control, for flaunting the codes of behaviour that challenged stability and continuity; the 'leper' for carrying a history of stigma, signifying corporeal and moral decay; the 'lunatic' for uncontrolled slips into chaos, again threatening wider social order and stability. The colonial imagination was particularly captured by Malay excursions into madness, as evidenced by the way in which cases of 'amok' were recounted in the courts and reported in the press and government minutes in terms of danger, threat and uncontrollable violence.[19] Sick people intercepted at ports on entry to Malaya posed a more immediate threat to social order as well as people's health, and were also incarcerated; the location of quarantine stations and leprosariums offshore was intentional.

The living conditions in these asylums and the gaols were frequently described as 'deplorable'. The medical report for the FMS in 1900, for example, commented wryly that the death rate of 683 per thousand within the lunatic asylum 'may be partly accounted for by the bad state of persons admitted, but if the rate continues, lunacy should soon cease to exist in the Straits'.[20] Since this did not occur, the Medical Department instead allowed that it was 'preferable that such patients should from time to time escape' to relieve population pressure within the institutions and to release Malay patients to kinsfolk in order to reduce the risk of infections in those crowded conditions.[21]

Others whose behaviour was unorthodox or who for a variety of personal or circumstantial reasons were marginalised – the pauper, the beggar and the vagrant – were also accommodated by the state when necessary. Pauper hospitals and vagrant wards provided clinical care to those brought in from the streets. Their homelessness and indigence revealed the fault lines of colonialism. Reports on vagrancy and routine arrests and admissions suggest the desperation of those who, immigrant and without kinship and village-based support, fell on their wits to survive when they lost work through illness or economic exigency. The number of people dying on the streets was small, though, as the coroner remarked, 'due to the majority of them being taken to one of the Hospitals by the Police when found to be ill'.[22]

Institutionalisation enabled the state to contain those most acutely affected by poor living conditions and disease, as well as those it was least able to help and heal. However, as described in this book, others, Malays and immigrants, suffered less obviously under colonialism, as capital penetration, the decline of subsistence production, growing dependence on the wage and fluctuations in the international economy led to changes in the distribution and incidence of disease, destitution, and declining health and nutrition. Inquiries into health, nutrition, prostitution, housing, labour conditions, welfare and education illustrate the scope of suffering under colonialism.

In the 1930s, a series of new inquiries into health, welfare and education were conducted within Malaya, and, with respect to all colonies, by the Colonial Office. League of Nations' interest in the impact of colonialism, particularly from its Health Organisation and its conferences, reinforced this reflexivity.[23] The inquiries questioned the changes in economic status of people under colonialism, and the extent to which social interventions, including health and medical programs, improved people's wellbeing even as expressed in terms of simple demography. They also anticipated the end of the empire, despite some optimistic planning within the Colonial Office. The outcome was a series of clear statements of the moral obligations of the colonial state.

The Depression accelerated a decline in health and welfare in the early 1930s, according to contemporary reports. Unemployment resulted in an increase in vagrancy and a reduction in public health measures by both government and private companies (Chapter 5). This led to an increase in various parasitic and microbial infections and nutritional problems as the quantity and range of foods were reduced. There appears also to have been a decrease in the numbers of medical staff available, which in turn affected case mortality from diarrhoeal diseases and malaria.[24] There was some evidence too that despite government injunctions that estates should maintain environmental measures to control malaria, permanent measures requiring substantial capital outlay had yielded to cheaper recurrent measures like oiling, particularly in poorer areas.[25] The effect of the Depression was uneven, however, contributing to contradictory reports that coolies were living 'hand to mouth' whilst the health status of Malays had improved with dietary change due to their reversion to subsistence production.[26] Alternatively, those on estates were to some degree sheltered from the worst of economic exigencies, while Malay and Chinese day labourers were said to be living on the 'verge of safety'. Drummond, the former Under-Secretary of State for the Colonies, argued in 1933 that 'in the last few years it has been realised that the problem of nutrition is one of the most important we have to face'.[27]

Discussions of health conditions in Malaya coincided with a wider concern of the impact of colonial development and the wellbeing of subjects, triggered by labour 'troubles' in the West Indies and reports of serious health and nutritional problems in African colonies. In an effort to analyse these questions, governments veered from infectious disease to nutritional status as indexical of health status. In October 1936, a committee was appointed to survey nutrition in the empire and to advise on measures to improve health and nutritional status. The Malayan report drew on five major sources: a review by Professor Rosedale on health and nutrition, a paper on dental caries, a summary of reports of deficiency diseases among prisoners, and two field surveys – by Vickers and Strahan on dietary standards in Kedah, and Burgess on nutrition among coastal Malays.[28] In their report, Vickers and Strahan argued that problems of anaemia were the result of the synergism of malaria, helminthic infestations, bowel diseases and 'dietary defects', and noted too that 'any crisis or abnormal endeavour' caused nutritional stress and health problems.[29] Subsequent reports provided collaboration. De Moubray, British Adviser to Trengganu, writing at the end of the decade, again argued that health status was poor among peasants and fisherfolk as well as wage labourers, and that the emphasis on infant mortality over the preceding 20 years had diverted attention from the major problems conributing to morbidity and mortality – malaria, yaws, worms, and poor nutrition.[30] Others maintained that poor nutrition was far more important than malaria and hookworm in contributing to anaemia and the equivocal health status of peasants and labourers.[31] Many also explained the decline in health status in terms of social and economic factors, specifically that wage rates were too low to allow people to purchase sufficient food. The Committee on Nutrition concluded that 'the problem of malnutrition (was) a problem of economic development' which would only be resolved by an increase in real wages.[32] In this context, it was later conceded that medical services alone were of limited value, since health problems arose from 'faulty hygiene, ignorance and harmful social conditions on which hospital treatment can have only slight effect'.[33]

The evidence of declining health and nutritional status, while contradictory at times, led to considerable reflection regarding the state's responsibility to its subjects. Depending on individual politics, it was argued that the social progress of the empire was 'necessarily bound up with its economic progress', there was a need for increased expenditure in the areas of social welfare and that it was 'essential to get away from the old principle that colonies can only have what they themselves can afford to pay for'.[34] Within the Colonial Office in London it was suggested that continued economic gains from colonial possessions depended on maintaining a healthy population (and one compliant to colonial rule), that – after the outbreak of war – the war effort would benefit from continued production in the colonies so that expenditure within them was justified, that there were long-term political gains in improving living conditions in the colonies, and, finally, that the continuation of the empire was itself contingent upon such improvements. Consider two examples:

> Politically the whole point is that we should be able to make a big thing of the 'welfare' side. If it is just going to be 'development' on the old lines it will look merely as if we are going to exploit the colonies in order to get money to pay for the war.[35]

> For my only comment is that if we are not now going to do something fairly good for the Colonial Empire, and something which helps them [the

colonies] to get proper social services, we shall deserve to lose the colonies
and it will only be a matter of time before we get what we deserve.[36]

In justifying the maintenance of the colonies and explaining health
and social welfare expenditure, the Colonial Office turned to the
economic rationalism that had characterised turn-of-the-century
debates. In so doing, social welfare programs were situated also in terms
of the legitimation of the polity. As I have explored, there were shifts in
ideology and practice over time, from the Taylorism of the late nineteenth century to the moralism (of individual behaviour and government policy) voiced in the late 1930s. These were theoretical debates
among those exercising power, but ideologies and politics had their
resonance in state programs and projects, and in the everyday experiences of sickness and health, disease and dying. The polity and economy
had a major part in determining morbidity and mortality and structur-
ing response, but these were underpinned by cultural ideas, values and
theories. Health care and medical services, sanitation measures and
their enforcement, immunisation programs and public health education
were developed and implemented in ways that were influenced by the
forces of the political economy and the moral logic of colonialism, in
turn informed by understandings of race, sex, health and disease.

The tensions between political economic and social–moral goals were
played out in all fields in the colony. As the end of empire approached,
these contradictions became explicit. On precarious political scales, the
figures of morbidity and mortality were weighed up against those of
development and production. Issues of science and knowledge, the
privileges of medicine and its institutions, were not in question, however,
and colonial self-reflexivity did not extend to the relationship between
knowledge and power. But ideology – in its expansive sense including
scientific knowledge and practice – buttressed colonialism. It provided
intellectual legitimacy to the domination of one people over others and
it institutionalised this in its education and medical systems. This logic,
the rationalisation of control, was arguably most explicit when the state
turned its attention from production – the colonisation of the interior
and the opening up of mines and plantations – to reproduction, thence
to the lives of those who in the nineteenth century had remained outside the colonial economy. Sickness provided a field for cultural
colonialism: the political economy exposed, and often caused, health
problems; the state had the knowledge, institutions and technologies to
prevent or cure them. The incorporation that occurred here with the
extension of medical and health services was both intellectual and
institutional; sanitation programs, public health acts, rural extension
work and health education all served to legitimise the state and to give
to it a moral authority that derived from the valorisation of its science.

Notes

Preface

1 For the region as a whole, see N. Owen (ed.), *Death and Disease in Southeast Asia: Explorations in social, medical and demographic history* (Singapore: Oxford University Press for the Asian Studies Association of Australia, 1987); P. Cohen and J. Purcall (eds), *The Political Economy of Primary Health Care in Southeast Asia* (Bangkok: Australian Development Studies Network and the ASEAN Training Centre for Primary Health Care Development, 1989); G. M. van Heteren, A. de Knecht-van Eekelen and M. J. D. Poulissen (eds), *Dutch Medicine in the Malay Archipelago 1816–1942* (Amsterdam and Atlanta: Rodopi, 1989); P. J. Rimmer and L. M. Allen (eds), *The Underside of Malaysian History. Pullers, prostitutes, plantation workers ...* (Singapore: Singapore University Press, 1990).

2 P. L. Rosenfield, The potential of transdisciplinary research for sustaining and extending linkages between the health and social sciences, *SSM* 35 (1992): 1343–1358; L. Manderson, Social science research and tropical disease, *MJA* 160 (1994): 289–292.

3 The exception is the pioneer work of Vicente Navarro and colleagues publishing in the *International Journal of Health Services*.

4 F. B. Smith, *The People's Health, 1830–1910* (London: Croom Helm, 1979) is a notable and relatively early exception.

5 See A. Knight, Tan Tock Seng's Hospital, Singapore, (1st pub. 1913) *JMBRAS* 42, 1 (1969): 252–255.

6 H. C. Chai, *The Development of British Malaya, 1896–1909* (Kuala Lumpur: Oxford University Press, 1964), chapter 6.

7 Published primarily in the *Singapore Medical Journal* and the *Journal of the Malay Branch of the Royal Asiatic Society*, but also in *Medical History*, the *British Journal of Anaesthesia* and the *British Dental Journal*. See entries for Y. K. Lee in bibliography.

8 E. A. Ross, Victorian medicine in Penang, *Malaysia in History* 23 (1980): 84–9.

9 See H. L. Chee, Health status and the development of health services in a colonial state: The case of British Malaya, *IJHS* 12, 3 (1982): 397–417; Phua Kai Hong, Health and Development in Malaysia and Singapore, unpublished PhD dissertation (London: London School of Economics and Political Science, 1987); L. Manderson, Health services and the legitimation of the colonial state: British Malaya 1786–1941, *IJHS* 17, 1 (1987): 91–111.

10 C. Baker, The government medical service in Malawi: An administrative history, 1891–1974, *MH* 20 (1976): 296–311; A. Bayoumi, Medical administration in the Sudan, 1899–1970, *Clio Medica* 11, 2 (1976): 105–15; A. Beck, *A History of the British Medical Administration in East Africa, 1900–1950* (Cambridge, Mass.: Harvard University Press, 1970); A. Beck, The role of medicine in German East Africa, *BHM* 45 (1971): 170–178; E. K. Herrmann, Health care services in 19th century British Honduras, *SSM* 14A (1980): 353–356.

11 C. Baker, The government medical service in Malawi, p. 301.

12 A. Bopegamage, The military as a modernizing agent in India. *EDCC* 20, 1 (1971): 71–79.

13 See for example C. W. Hartwig, Church–state relations in Kenya: Health issues, *SSM* 13C (1979): 121–127.

14 See L. Manderson, Health services and the legitimation of the colonial state.

15 Edward W. Said, Secular criticism, in *The World, The Text and The Critic* (London: Vintage Books, 1991 [1st pub. 1984]), pp. 13–14; Eric Stokes, *The English Utilitarians and India* (Oxford: Clarendon Press, 1959); see also Edward W. Said, *Orientalism* (Harmondsworth: Penguin, 1991 [1st pub. 1978]).

16 L. Manderson, Social science research ...; Carol Vlassoff and Eva Rathgeber, Gender and tropical diseases: a new research focus, *SSM* 37, 4 (1993): 513–520; Carol Vlassoff and Elssy Bonilla, Gender-related differences in the impact of tropical diseases on women: what do we know? *JBS* 26 (1994): 37–53.

17 Australian Research Council, grant no. A 18085635.

1 Introduction: Imposing the empire

1 Colonial Malaya comprised the Straits Settlements (Singapore, Malacca and Penang), the Federated Malay States (FMS) (Selangor, Perak, Negri Sembilan and Pahang) and the Unfederated Malay States (UFMS) (Perlis, Kedah, Kelantan, Trengganu and Johore), with colonial rule least direct in the UFMS.

For a description of the history, politics and processes that characterised these arrangements, see R. Emerson, *Malaysia: A study of direct and indirect rule* (Kuala Lumpur: University of Malaya Press, 1964) (first pub. 1937); for more recent studies, see Hua Wu Yin, *Class and Communalism in Malaysia: politics in a dependent capitalist state* (London: Zed Books in conjunction with Marram Books, 1983), K. S. Jomo, *A Question of Class: Capital, the state and uneven development in Malaya* (New York: Monthly Review Press, 1988); and Edwin Lee, *The British as Rulers: Governing multiracial Singapore 1867–1914* (Singapore: Singapore University Press, 1991).

2 This is the proper task of the historian, of course, as it is for other social scientists engaged in individualistic projects of writing a reality from an always imperfect data set, stretching beyond empiricism to scholarly imaginations, see e.g. C. Wright Mills, *The Sociological Imagination* (New York: Oxford University Press, 1959) and Muriel Dimen-Schein, *The Anthropological Imagination* (New York: McGraw-Hill, 1977).

3 James Warren puts this data source to particularly good and imaginative use, see *Rickshaw Coolie: A people's history of Singapore*, (Singapore: Oxford University Press, 1986) and *Ah-Ku and Karayuki-san: Prostitution in Singapore, 1870–1940* (Singapore and New York: Oxford University Press, 1993).

4 The representation of a world order that has been directed by and was self-serving for colonialism has been addressed by Edward Said in *Orientalism* (Harmondsworth: Penguin, 1991). For further discussion of the authorial voice and representation from various disciplinary perspectives, see J. Clifford, and G. E. Marcus (eds), *Writing Culture* (Berkeley: University of California Press, 1986), H. L. Gates (ed.), *'Race', Writing and Difference* (Chicago and London: University of Chicago Press, 1986), R. Guha (ed.) *Subaltern Studies VI: Writings on South Asian History and Society* (Delhi: Oxford University Press, 1989), A. A. Malek, Orientalism in crisis, *Diogenes* 44 (1963): 107–108; Gayatri Chakravorty Spivak, Three women's texts and a critique of imperialism, *Critical Inquiry* 12, 1 (1985): 17–34, and *In Other Worlds: Essays in Cultural Politics* (New York and London: Methuen, 1987).

5 See Michael Stenson, *Class, Race and Colonialism in West Malaysia* (St. Lucia: University of Queensland Press, 1980), for discussions of conditions of labour and rebellion and resistance to this. It is noteworthy that many responded to colonialism formally, however, seeking to effect change to the structures and institutions of the regime from within.

6 See P. J. Rimmer, L. Manderson and C. Barlow, The underside of Malaysian history: A theoretical overview, in Rimmer and Allen (eds.), *The Underside of Malaysian History ...*, pp. 3–22.

7 Eric Hobsbawm, *Age of Empire: 1875–1914* (London: Weidenfeld and Nicholson, 1987).

8 Roy MacLeod, Introduction, in MacLeod and Lewis (eds), *Disease, Medicine, and Empire. Perspectives on Western medicine and the experience of European expansion* (London and New York: Routledge, 1988), p. 2.

9 *Ibid.*

10 Frantz Fanon, *Studies in a Dying Colonialism* (London: Earthscan Publications, 1989 [1st pub. 1961]), pp. 121, 131.

11 Jurgen Habermas, *Communication and the Evolution of Society* (London: Heinemann, 1979).

12 E. Said, Secular criticism. He refers particularly to the work of John Stuart Mill, who in his essay *Utilitarianism* (1861) argued for a hierarchy in terms of culture and morality which – whilst Mill himself did not carry this to its logical outcome – argued a moral basis for elite rule; this, Stokes argued, was the basis to British dominion over India, see Said, p. 12; see also Scott Gordon, *The History and Philosophy of Social Science* (London and New York: Routledge, 1991), p. 257.

13 David Arnold quotes a reference to Florence Nightingale, and her views of the 'civilising' aspects of sanitary reform in India, see Arnold, Introduction: Disease, medicine and empire, in Arnold (ed.), *Imperial Medicine and Indigenous Societies* (Manchester and New York: Manchester University Press, 1988), p. 3. Nightingale in 1863 had proposed unsuccessfully the establishment of a Sanitary Department and an enforceable sanitary code which would be 'the dawn of a new day for India', see Cecil Woodham-Smith, *Florence Nightingale, 1820–1910* (London: Fontana Books, 1968) (1st pub. 1951), p. 317.

14 Files of the Selangor Secretariat (hereafter Sel. Sec.) 223/1901, para. 17 (Treacher 1901).

15 C. A. Wiggins (1919), quoted in Beck, *A History of the British Medical Administration ...*, p. 67.

16 See Daniel R. Headrick, *The Tools of Empire. Technology and European imperialism in the nineteenth century* (New York and Oxford: Oxford University Press, 1981).

17 *Ibid.*, pp. 64–67.
18 On medical professionalisation, see E. Friedson, *Professional Powers. A study of the institutionalisation of formal knowledge* (Chicago and London: University of Chicago Press, 1986), N. Parry and J. Parry, *The Rise of the Medical Profession* (London: Croom Helm, 1976); I. Waddington, *The Medical Profession in the Industrial Revolution* (Dublin: Gill and Macmillan, 1984). On the demise of midwifery, see A. Oakley, Wisewoman and medicine man: Change in the management of childbirth, in Mitchell and Oakley (eds), *The Rights and Wrongs of Women* (Harmondsworth: Penguin, 1976), pp. 17–58.
19 Anne-Marie Moulin, Patriarchal science: The network of the overseas Pasteur Institutes, in P. Petitjean, C. Jami and A. M. Moulin (eds), *Science and Empires. Historical studies about scientific development and European expansion.* Boston Studies in the Philosophy of Science, vol. 136 (Dordrecht, Boston, London: Kluwer Academic Publishers, 1992), pp. 307–322. Moulin's work makes clear the extent to which science is a cultural product. With respect to bacteriology, and national styles of its pursuit, see O. Amsterdamska, Medical and biological constraints: Early research on variation in bacteriology, *SSS 17* (1987): 657–687; and as noted above, Worboys (in The emergence of tropical medicine) draws attention to nationalism in nineteenth and early twentieth-century medicine in his examination of 'styles' of intervention. See also Marcovich, French colonial medicine and colonial rule in MacLeod and Lewis (eds).
20 Anon., Neville Chamberlain opens Medical Research Bureau, *MMJ* I, III (1926), p. 77. The bureau was founded in 1913 to conduct research on diseases prevalent in both tropical and temperate climates, and reopened in December 1925.
21 Warwick Anderson, Immunities of empire: Race, disease and the new tropical medicine, 1900–1920, unpublished manuscript, History of Science Department, Harvard University, 1993; Mark Harrison, Tropical medicine in nineteenth-century India, *British Journal for the History of Science* 25 (1992): 299–318. Harrison draws attention to the historical depth of these views: both Lind (1768) and Johnson (from 1815) maintained (black) racial immunity and (white) susceptibility to tropical infection, and maintained that moral and physical degeneration would occur in the white man (*sic*) who stayed in the tropics too long.
22 E. A. Ross, Victorian medicine in Penang, p. 84. This fitted with contemporary British bathing practice, which was rather irregular. Until the decline in cost and increased availability of soap after 1853, and the installation of piped water to urban areas from the 1850s, few people bathed and health professionals saw little value in the practice. F. B. Smith, *The People's Health*, reports a male guardian of a workhouse in Dorchester who, objecting to the provision of baths for inmates, rolled back his sleeve saying 'white as a hare's tooth and hasn't been washed these forty years' (p. 399). Even with the introduction of antisepsis in the late nineteenth century, many doctors rejected the necessity of washing and sterilisation.
23 Philip D. Curtin, *Death by Migration. Europe's encounter with the tropical world in the nineteenth century* (Cambridge: Cambridge University Press, 1989), p. 157 ff; Anderson, Immunities of empire.
24 Again, see Anderson, Immunities of empire.
25 A-M. Moulin, Patriarchal science, p. 314; Headrick, *The Tools of Empire*, p. 65.
26 M. Worboys, Manson, Ross and colonial medical policy, p. 25.
27 J. L. Todd, Tropical medicine, 1898–1924, n.d. (25th Year Com-

memorative Talk for the United Fruit Company), cited by Maryinez
Lyons, Sleeping sickness, colonial medicine and imperialism: Some
connections in the Belgian Congo, in R. MacLeod and M. Lewis (eds),
p. 244, n. 16.

28 Lesley Doyal with Imogen Pennell, *The Political Economy of Health* (London:
Pluto Press, 1979), pp. 244–245.

29 B. G. Maegraith, History of the Liverpool School of Tropical Medicine, *MH*
16 (1972):354–368; John A. Shepherd, *A History of the Liverpool Medical
Institution*, (Chester: Liverpool Medical Institution, 1979), pp. 173–174;
M. Worboys, Manson, Ross and colonial medical policy: Tropical medicine
in London and Liverpool, 1899–1914, in R. MacLeod and M. Lewis (eds),
*Disease, Medicine, and Empire: Perspectives on Western Medicine and the Experience
of European Expansion*, pp. 21–37. See also M. Worboys, The emergence of
tropical medicine, and Moulin, Patriarchal science.

30 L. Doyal with Pennell, *The Political Economy of Health*, p. 245; A. Beck,
History of the British Medical Administration of East Africa, 1900–1950
(Cambridge, Mass.: Harvard University Press, 1970), pp. 32, 41, 107; J. A.
Shepherd, *A History of the Liverpool Medical Institution*, p. 173; Sir Malcolm
Watson, *Some Pages from the History of the Prevention of Malaria*, The Finlayson
Memorial Lecture, Glasgow, 29 November 1934 (Glasgow: Alex Macdougall,
1935), pp. 2–3; Worboys, Manson, Ross and colonial medical policy, p. 26.

31 R. Chatterton, The development of tropical medicine, p. 33.

32 For a discussion of this, in light of Patterson and Hartwig's claim that
1890–1930 was the 'unhealthiest time in all African history', see Arnold,
Introduction, pp. 5–6; K. D. Patterson and G. W. Hartwig, The disease
factor: An introductory overview, in G. W. Hartwig and K. D. Patterson
(eds), *Disease in African History: An introductory survey and case studies*
(Durham, NC: Duke University Press, 1978), pp. 3–24; cf. I. Klein, Death in
India, 1871–1921, *JAS* 32 (1973): 639–659.

33 A-M. Moulin, Patriarchal science, pp. 311–316.

34 G. M. van Heteren, A. de Knecht-van Eekelen and M. J. D. Poulissen (eds),
Dutch Medicine in the Malay Archipelago 1816–1942.

35 See for example works in N. Reingold and M. Rottenberg (eds), *Scientific
Colonialism: A cross-cultural comparison* (Washington: Smithsonian Institute
Press, 1987); Lewis Pyenson, *Cultural Imperialism and Exact Sciences. German
expansion overseas, 1900–1930* (New York: P. Lang, 1985); Lewis Pyenson,
Empire of Reason: Exact sciences in Indonesia, 1840–1940 (Leiden: E. J.
Brill, 1989); and V. V. Krishna, The colonial 'model' and the emergence
of national science in India, 1876–1920, in P. Petitjean, C. Jami and
A-M. Moulin (eds), *Science and Empires. Historical studies about scientific
development and European Expansion* (Dordrecht, Boston, London: Kluwer
Academic, 1992), pp. 57–72.

36 E.g. A-M. Moulin, Patriarchal science, p. 314.

37 H. C. Chai, *The Development of British Malaya*, p. 205. In his account, beri-beri
was 'decimating one of the most valuable sections of Malaya's population,
the Chinese miner', whilst 'tropical fevers were taking a heavy toll of labourers building the roads and railways'.

38 Sir Malcolm Watson, Malaria and mosquitos: Forty years on, *JRSA* LXXXVII,
No. 4505, (1939):489.

39 Sir Robert Chatterton, The development of tropical medicine, *Eastern
World* IV, II (1950): 33–34.

40 H. C. Chai, p. 202.

41 R. MacLeod, Introduction; MacLeod, Scientific advice for British India: Imperial perception and administrative goals, 1898–1923, *Modern Asian Studies* 9, 3 (1975):343–384; K. D. Patterson, *Health in Colonial Ghana: Disease, medicine and socio-economic change, 1900–1955* (Waltham, Mass.: Crossroads Press, 1981); Worboys, The emergence of tropical medicine; W. Anderson, Immunities of Empire.

42 Sir Andrew Balfour, The tropical field: The possibilities for medical women, *The Magazine of the London (Royal Free Hospital) School of Medicine for Women* XXIII, 101 (1928):84.

43 See Roy MacLeod and Milton Lewis, Preface, in MacLeod and Lewis (eds), *Disease, Medicine and Empire. Perspectives on Western medicine and the experience of European expansion*, pp. x–xii, and MacLeod, Introduction.

44 Denoon, Donald, with Kathleen Dugan and Leslie Marshall, *Public Health in Papua New Guinea. Medical possibility and social constraint, 1884–1984* (Cambridge: Cambridge University Press, 1989).

45 *Ibid.*, p. 52. Even so, government health services were extended to labour lines, and beyond the expatriate population, and to those people whose health had lesser impact on the colonial economy.

46 For examples of circumstances of colonialism elsewhere in the region, see A. L. Stoler, *Capitalism and Confrontation in Sumatra's Plantation Belt, 1870–1979* (New Haven and London: Yale University Press, 1985); Alfons van der Kraan, *Lombok: Conquest, colonization and underdevelopment, 1870–1940*, Southeast Asia Publication Series No. 5 (Singapore: Heinemann for the Asian Studies Association of Australia, 1980); R. E. Elson, *Javanese Peasants and the Colonial Sugar Industry*, Southeast Asia Publication Series No. 9 (Singapore: Oxford University Press for the Asian Studies Association of Australia, 1984); Norman G. Owen, *Prosperity without Progress: Manila hemp and material life in the colonial Philippines* (Berkeley: University of California Press, 1984); Cornelius Fasseur, *The Politics of Colonial Exploitation: Java, the Dutch and the cultivation system* (trans. R. E. Elson and A. Kraal, ed. R. E. Elson) (Ithaca: Southeast Asia Program, Cornell University, 1992).

47 Vicente Navarro, The political and economic origins of the underdevelopment of health in Latin America, in *Medicine under Capitalism* (London: Croom Helm, 1976); Vicente Navarro, *Imperialism, Health and Medicine* (London: Pluto Press, 1982); Meredith Turshen, The impact of colonialism on health and health services in Tanzania, *IJHS* 7, 1 (1977):7–35; Meredith Turshen, *The Political Ecology of Disease in Tanzania*, (New Brunswick, NJ: Rutgers University Press, 1984); Patrick A. Twumasi, Colonialism and international health: A study in social change in Ghana, *SSM* 15B (1981): 147–151; Kader A. Parahoo, Early colonial health developments in Mauritius, *IJHS* 16, 3 (1986): 409–423; L. Doyal with Pennell, *The Political Economy of Health*; and for Malaysia, H. L. Chee, Health status and the development of health services. See also MacLeod, Introduction, and Arnold, Introduction, for their overviews of the history of medicine and imperialism.

48 A. Beck, *A History of the British Medical Administration*; Beck, The role of medicine in German East Africa.

49 A. Beck, *A History of British Medical Administration*, p. 3.

50 *Ibid.*, p. 14.

51 *Ibid.*, p. 59, my emphasis, and p. 64, quoting C. J. Wilson on 'part of the cost of winning the war'.

52 See also C. W. Hartwig, Church–state relations in Kenya.

53 A. Beck, *A History of the British Medical Administration*, pp. 106, 114.
54 A. van Heteren, de Knecht-van Eekelen and Poulissen, *Dutch Medicine in the Malay Archipelago, 1816–1942.*
55 David Arnold, Smallpox and colonial medicine in nineteenth-century India, in Arnold (ed.), *Imperial Medicine and Indigenous Societies* (Manchester and New York: Manchester University Press, 1988), pp. 45–65.
56 A. M. Davis, What is climatic disease? *Transactions of the Epidemiological Society of London* XXII (New Series) (1902–1903):1–5, and discussion:6–10.
57 R. MacLeod, Introduction, p. 5, citing C. E. A. Winslow, *The Conquest of Epidemic Disease: A chapter in the history of ideas* (Princeton: Princeton University Press, 1967 [first pub. 1943]).
58 An example of this has been through biological adaptation and diversity, hence the failure to eradicate vector-borne diseases such as malaria due to mosquito vector resistance to pesticides, parasite resistance to drugs, human resistance to behavioural interventions (through non-compliance, failure to present for treatment, and so on), and by the inability of states to deliver the services that might best reduce the incidence of disease.
59 Although not necessarily, see chapters in E. E. Sabben-Clare, D. J. Bradley and K. Kirkwood (eds), *Health in Tropical Africa during the Colonial Period* (Oxford: Clarendon Press, 1980).
60 Frantz Fanon, *Studies in a Dying Colonialism*; see also Frantz Fanon, Medicine and colonialism, in J. Ehrenreich (ed.), *The Cultural Crisis of Modern Medicine* (New York: Monthly Review Press, 1978), pp. 229–251.
61 F. Fanon, *Studies in a Dying Colonialism*, pp. 121–145; R. MacLeod, Introduction, p. 1.
62 MacLeod, Introduction, p. 1; see also Dagmar Engels, Foundations of imperial hegemony: Western education, public health and policy in India and Africa, 1859 to independence. Conference Report, *Bulletin of the German Historical Institute*, London XI, 3 (1989):29–35; and L. Manderson, Health services and the legitimation of the colonial state.
63 See for example M. Vaughan, *Curing their Ills: Colonial power and African illness* (Cambridge: Polity Press, 1991).
64 D. R. Headrick, *The Tools of Empire*; and D. R. Headrick, The tools of imperialism: technology and the expansion of European colonial empires in the nineteenth century, *JMH* 57 (1979):231–263.
65 But see Denoon's book, *Public Health in Papua New Guinea*; Owen (ed.), *Death and Disease in Southeast Asia*; Cohen and Purcall (eds), *The Political Economy of Primary Health Care in Southeast Asia*, and papers in the edited collections of Arnold (*Imperial Medicine and Indigenous Societies*) and MacLeod and Lewis (*Disease, Medicine, and Empire*).
66 See L. Manderson, Wireless Wars in the Eastern Arena: Epidemiological surveillance, disease prevention and the work of Eastern Bureau of the League of Nations Health Organisation, 1925–1942, in P. Weindling (ed.), *International Health Organisations and Movements, 1918–1939* (Cambridge: Cambridge University Press, 1995), pp. 109–133.
67 Marcovich, French colonial medicine and colonial rule, p. 111.
68 See Y. K. Lee, Medical education in the Straits: 1786–1871, *JMBRAS* 46, 1 (1973):101–122.
69 See References for articles by Y. K. Lee on the General and Pauper Hospitals in early Singapore.
70 H. C. Chai, *The Development of British Malaya*, p. 198.
71 Doyal with Pennell, *The Political Economy of Health*, p. 239.

72 Institute of Medical Research (hereafter IMR), *Studies from the Institute of Medical Research, Federation of Malaya, Jubilee Volume*, No. 25 (Kuala Lumpur, Government Press, 1951), pp. 28, 34.

73 M. Turshen, *The Political Ecology of Disease*, p. 14.

74 *Ibid.*, Chapter 2.

75 M. Turshen (p. 54) continues her argument to identify three ways in which colonial capitalism affected rural women: it lowered their standard of living by exploiting rural areas; it imposed Victorian notions of women's inferiority and used them to deny women access to education and technical training; and it reduced the importance of women's work by substituting cash crops for food as the valued commodity. In arguing this, Turshen follows the arguments made by E. Boserup, *Women's Role in Economic Development* (London: Allen and Unwin, 1970), B. Rogers, *The Domestication of Women. Discrimination in developing societies* (London: Tavistock, 1980), and by contributors in Mona Etienne and Eleanor Leacock (eds), *Women and Colonization. Anthropological perspectives* (New York: Drager, 1980).

76 M. Turshen, *The Political Ecology of Disease*, pp. 63–64.

77 I. Fett, Land ownership in Negri Sembilan, 1900–1977, pp. 73–96, in L. Manderson (ed.), *Women's Work and Women's Roles. Economics and everyday life in Indonesia, Malaysia and Singapore*, Development Studies Centre Monograph No. 32 (Canberra: Australian National University, 1983).

78 See Chapter 7, this volume.

79 Donn V. Hart, *Bisayan Filipino and Malayan Humoral Pathologies: Folk medicine and ethnohistory in Southeast Asia.* Data Paper No. 76 (Ithaca, NY: Cornell University Department of Asian Studies Southeast Asia Program, 1969).

80 The nineteenth-century studies by Newbold and Maxwell, and the slightly later work of Skeat and Gimlette, in studying Malay religion, healing and magic, all make references to humoral pathology and interactions between different practitioners as a result of trade and cultural ties between the Malay states and Arabia. See T. J. Newbold, *Political and Statistical Account of the British Settlements in the Straits of Malacca, viz. Pinang, Malacca, and Singapore: with a history of the Malayan states on the peninsula* (London: John Murray, 1839); W. E. Maxwell, Shamanism in Perak, *Journal of the Straits Branch Royal Asiatic Society* 12 (1883):222–231; Walter W. Skeat, *Malay Magic: Being an introduction to the folklore and popular religion of the Malay Peninsula* (Singapore: Oxford University Press, 1984) (1st pub. 1900); and John D. Gimlette, *Malay Poisons and Charm Cures* (Kuala Lumpur: Oxford University Press, 1971 [1st pub. 1915]).

81 F. C. Colley, Traditional Indian medicine in Malaysia, *JMBRAS* LI, 1 (1978): 77–109; F. L. Dunn, Traditional beliefs and practices affecting medical care in Malaysian Chinese communities, *MJM* 29 (1974):7–10; Lenore Manderson, Traditional food classifications and humoral medical theory in Peninsular Malaysia, *Ecology, Food and Nutrition* 11 (1981): 81–93.

82 In particular, see W. Skeat, *Malay Magic,* J. D. Gimlette, *Malay Poisons and Charm Cures* and *A Dictionary of Malayan Medicine* (edited and completed by H. W. Thomson) (Oxford: Oxford University Press, 1939). Burkill's compendium of plants includes many of ethnopharmacological use and value, see I. H. Burkill, *A Dictionary of the Economic Products of the Malay Peninsula*, 2 vols. (London: Governments of the Straits Settlements and Federated Malay States, 1935).

83 Louis Golomb, *An Anthropology of Curing in Multiethnic Thailand* (Champaign/Urbana: University of Illinois Press, 1985), pp. 74–75.

84 C. Laderman, *Taming the Wind of Desire: Psychology, medicine and aesthetics in Malay Shamanic Performance* (Berkeley: University of California Press, 1991).
85 See Harrison, Tropical medicine in nineteenth-century India; T. J. S. Patterson, The transmission of Indian surgical techniques to Europe at the end of the eighteenth century, *Proceedings of the XXIII Congress of the History of Medicine* (London: Wellcome Institute for the History of Medicine, 1972), pp. 694–696; J. Masselos, The discourse from the other side: Perceptions of science and technology in Western India in the nineteenth century, Unpublished manuscript, University of Sydney, 1982.
86 M. Harrison, Tropical medicine in nineteenth-century India, p. 2; Arnold, Introduction, p. 11.
87 IMR, *Studies from the Institute of Medical Research*, p. 19; see I. M. Burkill and Mohammed Ariff, Malay village medicine, *Gardens Bulletin* 6, 2 (1930): 165–321, and 6, 3 (1930): 323–474.
88 See Charles S. Leslie (ed.), *Asian Medical Systems: A Comparative Study* (Berkeley: University of California Press, 1976).
89 Brenda Yeoh, Power and the People: Municipal control and plebeian agency in the control of disease and sanitary conditions in turn-of-the-century Singapore. Unpublished paper presented at the Regional Conference of the Asian Studies Association of Australia, Singapore, February 1989, p. 31.
90 *Ibid.*, pp. 32–33. Yeoh also provides a list of Chinese pharmacies established in Singapore between 1870 and 1928, which documents the location and year of establishment of 58 institutions.
91 Anon., Ayurvedic medicine. An ancient system, *MMJ* 6 July 1926:114–115. The departure point for a wider commentary on Ayurvedic medicine was the opening of the Lankan Ayurvedic Medical Hall. The author regarded the decision by the Ceylon Legislative Council, to ensure that people had a choice between biomedical and Ayurvedic care, as a 'black day for India' and that it was 'a little difficult to understand where the great merits of the Ayurvedic system come in, since its own advocates frankly confess to the need for grafting on so many of the branches of Western science' (p. 14).
92 B. Yeoh, Power and the people, p. 30.
93 IMR, *Studies from the Institute of Medical Research*, p. 23, and see D. Hooper, On Chinese medicine: drugs of Chinese pharmacists in Malaya, *Gardens Bulletin* 6,1 (1930):163–165.
94 *Ibid.*; *Malay Mail*, 6 July 1927.
95 G. I. H. Braine, *Trengganu. Annual Medical and Sanitary Report for the Year 1935* (Singapore: G. H. Kiat, 1936), p. 3.
96 FMS/P/KES/A11 (Perak), p. 5.
97 Sel. Sec. 3726/1918.
98 *ST* 30 July 1883, p. 3; 27 October 1883, p. 3.
99 *ST* 25 July 1883, p.3. Cf. advertisements for 'Wood's Great Peppermint Cure' in the 1920s, which promoted the pills to be taken at the first sign of a 'body chill' and which warned that '(i)n the moist heat of the tropical climate one can never feel safe from catching a chill', *ST* 6 January 1920, p. 10.

2 State statistics and corporeal reality

1 For an account of early measures, see Y. K. Lee, Smallpox and vaccination in early Singapore I. 1819–1829, *SMJ* 14 (1973): 525–531; II. 1830–1849.

252 NOTES (PAGES 28–34)

SMJ 17, 2 (1976): 202–206; III. 1850–1859. *SMJ* 18, 1 (1977): 16–20; and IV. 1860–1872. *SMJ* 18, 2 (1977): 126–135.

2 L. Manderson, Race, colonial mentality and public health in early twentieth century Malaya, in Rimmer and Allen (eds), *The Underside of Malaysian History*, pp. 193–213; on beri-beri, see Chai's chapter on the history of British medical administration in his *The Development of British Malaya, 1896–1909* (Kuala Lumpur: Oxford University Press, 1964).

3 See R. N. Jackson, *Immigrant Labour and the Development of Malaya, 1786–1920* (Kuala Lumpur: University of Malaya Press, 1961).

4 On rubber, see John H. Drabble, *Rubber in Malaya, 1876–1922: The genesis of the industry* (Kuala Lumpur: Oxford University Press, 1973); on agricultural enterprise, J. C. Jackson, *Planters and Speculators: Chinese and European agricultural enterprise in Malaya 1786–1921* (Kuala Lumpur: University of Malaya Press, 1968); on transport and communications, Amarjit Kaur, *Bridge and Barrier: Transport and Communications in colonial Malaya, 1870–1951* (Singapore: Oxford University Press, 1985); and various papers in Rimmer and Allen (eds), *The Underside of Malaysian History*.

5 To claim that beri-beri was caused solely by the consumption of highly-milled rice is to miss the point; tin miners and other workers ate from a narrow dietary selection and their nutritional status was equivocal, predisposing them to hypovitaminosis B_1 and B_2.

6 Tunku Shamsul Bahrin, The pattern of Indonesian migration and settlement in Malaya, *Asian Studies* 5, 2 (1967): 233–257.

7 Y. K. Lee, Singapore's Pauper and Tan Tock Seng Hospitals (1819–1873), Part I, *JMBRAS* 48, 2 (1975): 78–111; Y. K. Lee, The Pauper Hospital in early Singapore (Part I) (1819–1829) *SMJ* 14, 1 (1973): 49–54; Files of the British Adviser to Kelantan (hereafter BA Kel) 1887.

8 Straits Settlements, *Report of the Commissioners Appointed to Enquire into the State of Labour in the Straits Settlements and Protected Native States* (hereafter SS, *Labour Commission Report*) (Singapore: Government Printing Office, 1890), p. 8, citing an article in the *Journal of the Indian Archipelago* (1854).

9 D. Denoon, *Public Health in Papua New Guinea*, p. 31–32.

10 *Ibid.*

11 Robin J. Pryor, *Migration and Development in South-East Asia: A demographic perspective* (Kuala Lumpur: Oxford University Press, 1979), p. 79.

12 Ooi Jin Bee, *Land, People and Economy in Malaya* (London: Longman, 1963), p. 113; also V. W. W. S. Purcell, *The Chinese in Malaya* (London: Oxford University Press, 1948).

13 Simon Szreter, The GRO and the Public Health Movement in Britain, 1837–1914, *SHM* 4, 3 (1991): 443.

14 Simon Szreter, Introduction: The GRO and the Historians. *SHM* 4, 3 (1991): 401; also Szreter, The GRO and the Public Health Movement in Britain; on the development of social statistics/demography, see J. M. Eyler, Mortality statistics and Victorian public health policy: Program and criticisim. *BHM* 50 (1976): 355–365.

15 SS, *Labour Commission Report*, CO273/19 (1863).

16 IO/G134/5, Light to Cornwallis, 30 July 1792, f. 66.

17 Straits Settlements Records (hereafter SSR)/K5: f. 72, R. Caunter to R. Fullerton, 19 January 1827, enclosure of 30 July 1825.

18 SSR/N5, 1828: 75 (S. G. Bonham, Superintendent of Police).

19 SSR/N5, 1829: 150 (Bonham, 6 February 1829).

20 Malacca's population jumped from 26,024 in 1826 to 34,606 in April 1828 (SSR/O3, 1828: 215–216; SSR/O1, 1826–7: 352). The numbers for Malacca in 1826 were as follows: Malays 16,318, 'Christians' (a majority of Portuguese descent) 2,620, Chinese 4,478, 'Klings' (from southern India) 1,622, 'Hindoos' 986. The population included 1097 slaves from all ethnic groups, and 108 debtors (Malays and Christian).

21 39,721 in Penang Island; 60,036 in Province Wellesley; 57,421 in Singapore; and 52,713 in Malacca (SSR/R13, 1845–6: 679, 681).

22 SSR/T5, 1862–3: 26–27, 34–37 (these data are not extant); Files of the Colonial Office (hereafter CO) 273/30: 32.

23 SSR/S35, 1866: 104A (A. P. Howell to Governor, SS, 18 May 1866).

24 Viz., Europeans (not specified), Armenians, Jews, Eurasians, Abyssinians, Achinese, Africans, Andamanese, Arabs, Bengalees &c., Boyanese, Bugis, Burmese, Chinese, Cochinese, Dyaks, Hindoos, Japanese, Javanese, Jaweepakans (i.e. Jawi Peranakan), Klings, Malays, Manilamen, Mantras, Parsees, Persians, Siamese, and Singhalees.

25 W. A. Pickering, Journal of journey from Singapore to Sungei Ujong and of his story there from October 4 to November 29, 1874, Rhodes House Library, Colonial Records Project, Mss Indian Ocean S74, p. 12.

26 J. N. Lasker makes this same point in relation to the Ivory Coast. During the early colonial period to 1919, the delivery of medical care was associated with military posts. Health services were made available to the African population where such services might also promote pacification, and were designed and distributed to favour first French colonists and settlers, then the indigenous elite associated with colonial rule; services again were concentrated in areas of French settlement, in towns rather than rural areas, and in accordance with class and race, with individualised and expensive health care for the French and African elite and with rudimentary preventive care for the subject population. See J. N. Lasker, The role of health services in colonial rule: The case of the Ivory Coast, *CMP* 1 (1977): 277–297. The model is directly transported from the centre, and is therefore a feature of any hospital based medical system.

27 Colonial Office, *Papers Relating to Her Majesty's Possessions*, Part 1 (London: HMSO, 1878), p. 129.

28 *Ibid.*, pp. 326–331.

29 *Ibid.*, p. 329.

30 *Ibid.*, pp. 326, 328.

31 *Ibid.*, p. 329.

32 Files of the Selangor Secretariat (hereafter Sel. Sec.) 1330/1899; Sel. Sec. 5867/1895.

33 GB, Colonial Office, Accounts and Papers, ZHCI 6523, *Negri Sembilan Medical Report 1899*, pp. 255–256.

34 *Ibid.*, pp. 260, 265.

35 CO273/261/G1033, f. 571 (Report of Resident Surgeon, Negri Sembilan, 1897).

36 ZHCI 6411, no. 11, p. 255.

37 *Ibid.*, p. 256.

38 *Ibid.*, p. 222; for a social history of these workers see A. Kaur, *Bridge and Barrier* (Singapore: Oxford University Press, 1985), and his Working on the Railway: Indian workers in Malaya, 1880–1957, in Rimmer and Allen (eds), *The Underside of Malaysian History*, pp. 99–128. Ethnic variation was characteristic of this and later periods. The contrast is Perak where, at the same

time (1899), the Malay death rate was 23.61, Chinese 33.09, Indian 52.50 and European and Eurasian 6.65. During this year there were a total of 20,946 admissions at eleven hospitals, with a case mortality of 10.5 percent. Many of these were labourers working on railway and irrigation works.

39 Hospital deaths among infants were predominantly due to 'bowel complaints', convulsions and fever.

40 ZHCI 6523, *Negri Sembilan Medical Report 1899*, pp. 257–258.

41 *Ibid.*, p. 229.

42 *Ibid.*; *Pahang Medical Report 1899*, p. 282.

43 Files of the BA Kel, 339/1917: 2.

44 ZHCI 6523, *Report of the Medical Department, Pahang, 1900*.

45 For example, 26.25 percent of a total of 400 labourers working in the gold mines of Kelantan in 1905 had beri-beri and 16.2 percent died consequently, but this was due entirely to the labourers' poor quality diet; statewide beri-beri was not a major problem. BA Kel 153/1913: 3.

46 *ST* 21 May 1910.

47 Files of the Institute of Medical Research, Malaria Advisory Board (hereafter IMR/MAB) 5/1932: 13, Chief Health Officer.

48 See also L. Manderson, Blame, responsibility and remedial action: Death, disease and the infant in early twentieth century Malaya, in N. Owen (ed.), *Death and Disease in Southeast Asia*, pp. 257–282.

49 IMR, *Studies from the Institute of Medical Research*, p. 294.

50 CO273/33.

51 CO273/37, f. 420.

52 CO273/31, pp. 146–149. The Straits Settlements Association was formed on 21 January 1868 specifically to guard against any legislation that might be prejudicial to the interests of the Settlements and interfere with their role as free ports or with commercial prosperity, and to 'prevent unnecessary expenditure of the local Government'. The government in turn saw its role to be one of protecting the welfare of 'its people at large' (*ibid.*). Regulations remained unsystematic until the introduction of the International Sanitary Convention in 1912, in accordance with the Rome Convention (1906) and as administered by the Office International d'Hygiène publique. Even then, despite the obligations of signatories to collect and disseminate through the Office essential epidemiological information, it was to be argued that the convention was inappropriate for Asian conditions; this resulted in the establishment of the Eastern Bureau of the League of Nations Health Section in 1925 to collect and disseminate health statistics, quarantine procedures, and other information related to the control of disease, see Manderson, Wireless wars in the eastern arena.

53 League of Nations, Health Section, 12B/31959/23230, *Director's Report on the Singapore Bureau and its Work for the Year 1925* (Singapore: League of Nations, Health Section, Eastern Bureau, 1926), p. 1. White's report, dated 14 February 1914, refers to discussions between Gilbert Brooke, representing the Straits Settlements, and Dr de Vogel of the Netherlands East Indies in 1912 concerning the need for uniform quarantine procedures, in which context routine exchange of epidemiological information would have been required, p. 34. A full discussion of events leading up to the establishment of the Eastern Bureau is provided in L. Manderson, Wireless wars.

54 D. Arnold, Introduction, p. 13, comments that vaccination against smallpox and the segregation of lunatics and people with leprosy were the few 'medical services' that could be provided to the late nineteenth century.

55 See T. Horsfield, Report on the island of Banka, *Journal of the Indian Archipelago and Eastern Asia*, vol. II (1848): 323; see also Y. K. Lee, Smallpox and vaccination in early Singapore I–IV, *SMJ* (see References).

56 In 1825, the population had decreased by 335 persons, see SSR/H2, 1824–5, f. 112 (W. T. Cracroft, 28 January 1825), although the extent to which the smallpox epidemic directly contributed to the population decline remains open.

57 SSR/K14: 184 (Capt J. Low, 18 December 1829).

58 P. Aaby, Lessons from the past: Third World evidence and the reinterpretation of developed world mortality declines, *HTR* 2, Supp. (1992): 155–183.

59 CO273/38, pp. 226–227.

60 Sel. Sec. 824/1887, Collector and Magistrate of K. Selangor to Resident, 25 March 1887 and 8 April 1887.

61 BAKel 12/1913; BA Kel 263/1917.

62 Sel. Sec. 5168/1901, p. 16.

63 BAKel 12/1913.

64 E. W. Birch, *Papers of Sir Ernest W. Birch*, including correspondence 1889–1929, and diary of a voyage to the Malay Peninsula, 1920–1921, Mss Indian Ocean S242, ff. 42–43.

65 Sel. Sec.324/1886, p. 4.

66 BAKel 15B/1913.

67 BAKel 850/1914, f. 4; BA Kel 71/1918; Sel. Sec. 4968/1910.

68 Sel. Sec. 1287/1911; IMR 130/1921.

69 The expression is Gilbert Brooke's, reflecting on the inadequacy of control of shipping rather than of ports as a disease control measure, see G. E. Brooke, A system of intelligence as a handmaiden of hygiene, *MMJ* II (1927): 6–11.

70 *Penang Gazette* 21 May 1883.

71 R. C. Ileto, Cholera and the origins of the American sanitary order in the Philippines, in David Arnold (ed.) *Imperial Medicine and Indigenous Societies* (Manchester and New York: Manchester University Press, 1988), pp. 125–148.

72 John D.Gimlette, *Memorandum on Cholera: For the guidance of Europeans in the remote out-stations of British Malaya* (London: Waterlow, 1911).

73 IMR, *Studies from the Institute of Medical Research*, p. 241.

74 L. Manderson, Wireless wars.

75 IMR, *Studies from the Institute of Medical Research*, pp. 243–252.

76 *Ibid.*, p. 261.

77 For Indonesia, see Colin Brown, The influenza pandemic of 1918 in Indonesia, in N. Owen (ed.), *Death and Disease in Southeast Asia: Explorations in social, medical and demographic history* (Singapore: Oxford University Press for the Asian Studies Association of Australia), pp. 235–256; for colonial Ceylon, C. M. Langford and P. Story, Influenza in Sri Lanka, 1918–1919: The impact of a new disease in a pre-modern Third World setting, in *HTR* 2, Supp. (1992): 97–123. See also W. I. B. Beveridge, *Influenza: The last great plague* (London: Heinemann, 1977) and A.W. Crosby, *Epidemic and Peace, 1918* (Westport, Conn.: Greenwood Press, 1976).

78 Sel. Sec. 3832/1918; Sel.Sec. 3919/1918.

79 Sel. Sec. 4163/1918.

80 Sel. Sec. 613/1920.

81 Sel. Sec. 4017/1918.

82 Sel. Sec. 3910/1918; Sel. Sec. 4017/1918; Sel. Sec. 4061/1918; Sel. Sec. 4250/1918; Sel. Sec. 4298/1918, *Malay Mail* 11 June 1919.

83 Sel. Sec. 2627/1919.

84 Cited by J. E. Nathan, *The Census of British Malaya (The Straits Settlements, Federated Malay States and Protected States of Johore, Kedah, Perlis, Kelantan, Trengganu and Brunei, 1921* (London: Waterlow 1922), p. 19.

85 *Idem.* The Indian mortality rate was 372 for 1918, cf. 129.6 for Malays and 158.4 for Chinese.

86 C. A. Vlieland, *British Malaya. A Report on the 1931 Census and certain problems of vital statistics* (London: Crown Agents for the Colonies for the Colony of the Straits Settlements and the Malay States under British Protection, 1932), p. 105.

87 *Ibid.*

88 J. E. Nathan, *The Census of British Malaya*, p. 18.

89 For the years 1912, 1913 and 1914 respectively, the rate was 267.21, 271.34 and 250.23 according to departmental annual reports; however, the IMR continued to fall throughout this period.

90 A. Vlieland, p. 106.

91 *Ibid.*

92 Straits Settlements, *Annual Departmental Reports for the year 1934* (hereafter *SSAR 1934*) (Singapore: Government Printing Office, 1936), p. 721.

93 *SSAR 1936*, vol. 2, p. 1027.

94 C. A. Vlieland, *British Malaya*, p. 110.

95 *SSAR 1928*, p. 644.

96 *SSAR 1922*, p. 110.

97 *SSAR 1927*, p. 733, which notes for comparative purposes that the IMR in England and Wales for these periods were 138 (1901–5) and 80 (1921–5).

98 Federated Malay States, *Colonial Reports. Annual Reports on the Social and Economic Progress of the People of the Federated Malay States, 1931* (hereafter *FMSAR 1931*) (Kuala Lumpur, Government Printing Office, 1932), p. 12.

99 For example, the IMR declined in KL from 146 to 131 in the years 1933–1936, in Ipoh it was already 98 in 1933 and was 96 in 1936; in Seremban it dropped from 170 to 144 over these four years. See *FMSAR 1938*.

100 Files of the FMS, P/Kes/K.1, *Kedah and Perlis, Annual Report of the Medical and Health Department for the Year 1374 (1928–29)*, p. 2 and *Kedah and Perlis, Annual Report for the Medical and Health Department 1930*, p. 4.

101 Files of the BAT 481/1935, *Annual Medical and Sanitary Report for the Year 1934*, p. 4.

102 *SS/FMSAR 1937*, pp. 41, 82. Of course, it is not necessarily the case that the infant mortality rate would decline simply as an artefact of hospital delivery; rather the percentage has been used as an index of the proportion of women receiving medical care during pregnancy and parturition, including a small percentage who may have had complicated deliveries, stillbirths and/or post-partum haemorrhage without intervention. See Chapter 7 for a fuller discussion of antenatal and infant welfare work.

103 *SS/FMSAR 1937*, p. 12.

104 121 and 130.43 respectively, compared with a mean rate for the settlements of 180.65.

105 *SSAR 1931*, p. 694.

106 *SSAR 1905*, p. 189.

107 *FMSAR 1936*, p. 10.

108 BAKel 263/1917, *Annual Report of the Medical Department, 1916*, p. 3.

109 FMS/P/KES/K.1, *Kedah and Perlis Annual Report of the Medical and Health Departments*, p. 2.
110 *SSAR 1931*, p. 109.
111 *SSAR 1929*, p. 651.
112 BATr 481/1935: 4.
113 *SSAR 1925*, p. 566.
114 FMS, Commission of Inquiry, *Report of the Commission Appointed to Inquire into Certain Maters affecting the Health of Estates in the Federated Malay States together with a Memorandum by the Chief Secretary to Government* (Kuala Lumpur: Government Printer, 1924), p. B173.
115 Sel. Sec.1725/1921, Minutes of the Meeting of the Anti-Malaria Advisory Board, 23 April 1921, p. 4.
116 *SSAR 1936*, vol.II, pp. 911–2.
117 For malaria, this is a problem that pertains to the present. There is a substantial difference in endemic areas between the number of people sick with malaria (i.e. with clinical signs and symptoms) and those who are parasitaemic. With other parasitic infections, too, there may be no clinical indication of infection.
118 *SSAR 1937*, p. 1084.
119 L. Manderson, Health services and the legitimation of the colonial state; Manderson, Race, colonial mentality and public health.
120 J. Allgrove, Some recollections of rubber estate life in Malaya from 1920 to 1953, manuscript, British Association of Malaya Archives, BAM III/16, p. 9.
121 *FMSAR 1929*.

3 Biology, medical ideas and the social context of illness

1 H. Marriott, *Report of the Census of the Colony of the Straits Settlements taken on the 10th March, 1911* (Singapore: Government Printing Office, 1911), pp. 109–110. Forty of the doctors and all 132 midwives were women; a few women were employed in other categories except that of vaccinator (of whom there were only ten by this time).
2 *ST* 15 October 1882, p. 3.
3 For example, Japanese doctors ran a small hospital serving the Dungun and Kemaman mines in the 1920s, see A. J. Sturrock, *Trengganu. Annual Report for the Year AH 1348 (8 June 1929–27 May 1930)* (Singapore: Government Printing Office, 1930), and others provided medical care to Japanese prostitutes who worked in Singapore from the 1890s, see J. Warren, *Ah-Ku and Karayuki-san* (Singapore and New York: Oxford University Press, 1993).
4 FMS/P/KES/A.1, M. J. Wright, *State of Perak, Medical Report for the Year 1907*, p. 4.
5 FMS/P/KES/D.1, L.W.Evans, *Kelantan. The Annual Report on the Medical Department for the Year 1932* (Kota Bharu: Al-Asasiyah Press, 1933), p. 17; Birch, whilst Magistrate and Collector of Land Revenue in Malacca recalled much earlier – 1898 – complaints of hospitals that were reputed to be 'not fit for a bullock', although he disputed the claim and regarded the complaint from 'leading Chinese towkays' as 'an amusing incident', see E. W. Birch, *Papers of Sir Ernest W. Birch, including correspondence 1889–1929*, Mss Indian Ocean S242, Box 3/2, folio 42.
6 Sel. Sec.77/1876.
7 Sel. Sec.77/1876.
8 *Ibid.*; Sel. Sec.227/1892.

9˙ A press report from 1925, following the death of a woman from peritonitis after abdominal surgery in a private clinic, described the room and its walls as dirty; with an open drain down the middle that carried wet waste (a common feature of poor town housing, see chapter 4). The operating table was 'covered with rust', although the doctor said he covered this with a cloth before putting the patient on it. *ST* 11 September 1925, p. 8.

10 ZHCI 6523, *Report of the Medical Department, Pahang, 1900.*

11 Government reluctance to scrutinise too closely either the hospitals or conditions of labour frequently resulted in rather insipid accounts, occasioning one Selangor government official in 1901 to remark on the apparent anomaly of the high death rate of coolie immigrants if as claimed 'they are really cheerful, contented, well-fed and well-clothed and if the hospitals are really in excellent order', CO273/274/331, 25 November 1901.

12 J. W. W. Birch, *Diaries as British Resident in Perak, 1874–1875*, Entry for 13 February 1875, Larut, Mss Indian Ocean S242/1 (3).

13 *ST* 22 February 1883, p. 3.

14 Tan Chee Khoon, Memorandum on the Malayanization of the Medical Association of the Federation of Malaya by the Alumni Association of the King Edward VII College of Medicine and Faculty of Medicine, Univerity of Malaya, 5 December 1955, Mss Indian Ocean S39, p. 5.

15 FMS/P/KES/B.1, *State of Selangor. Annual Report on the Medical Department for the Year 1906*, p. 4.

16 Sel. Sec. 890/1900, Medical Report for the 4th Quarter, 1899.

17 Sel. Sec. 1030/1913, p. 9.

18 FMS/P/KES/B.1, *State of Selangor. Annual Report on the Medical Department for the Year 1905*, p. 6.

19 *Ibid.*

20 L. Manderson, Blame, responsibility and remedial action, in Owen (ed.) *Death and Disease in Southeast Asia*; FMS/P/KES/K.1, D. Bridges, *Kedah and Perlis. The Annual Report for the Medical and Health Departments for the Year 1347 AH (20th June 1928 to 8th June 1929 AD)* (Alor Star: Kedah Government Press, 1930), p. 5.

21 FMS/P/KES/D.1, L. W. Evans, *Kelantan. The Annual Report on the Medical Department for the Year 1932*, p. 4.

22 He cites the case of a 'Malay boy who was unable to walk owing to deformities and contractures of his limbs resulting from yaws, [who] submitted to amputation of both legs below the knees to enable him to walk on his stumps' and others who had part or the whole of their hands amputated following severe injuries. *Ibid.*, p. 13.

23 See for example G. S. Mowat, *Annual Report of Besut, 1947 and 1948*, Rhodes House Library, Colonial Records Project, Mss Indian Ocean S229, p. 7.

24 *SS/FMSAR 1937*, pp. 9–10.

25 Sel.Sec. 324/1886, f. 7.

26 Sel.Sec. 324/1886, f. 7.

27 Sel. Sec. 77/1876, ff. 11–12.

28 ZHCI 6411, Accounts and Papers 1901, XV, vi, No.13, *Perak Medical Report for 1899*, p. 301.

29 BAKel 153/1913, Annual Report, Medical Department, 1912.

30 Sel. Sec. 3920/1889.

31 Carlo Cipolla, *Miasmas and Disease, Public Health and the Environment in the Pre-Industrial Age* (New Haven: Yale University Press, 1991).

32 F. B. Smith's description of water, sanitation and housing in nineteenth-century England is apposite here, and he notes the difficulty now of recapturing the 'dirt, decay, disease and desolation' of the period (see *The People's Health* (London: Croom Helm: 1979), p. 195; also pp. 197–198, 218–226).

33 Victor R.Savage, *Western Impressions of Nature and Landscape in Southeast Asia* (Singapore: Singapore University Press, 1984), Chapter 4.

34 R. Little, On the medical topography of Singapore, pp. 458, 464.

35 CO 273/37, ff. 264–265 (Col. R. Woolley, Despatch from Singapore, 9 April 1870).

36 Colonial and Indian Exhibition, *Notes on the Straits Settlements and Malay States* (London: William Clowes and Sons Ltd, 1886), pp. 19–20.

37 ZHCI 6411/739, Negri Sembilan, *Annual Report of the Medical Department, 1899*, p. 306.

38 A. M. Davis, What is climatic disease? *Transactions of the Epidemiological Society* XXII (New Series) (1902–03). Davis included hepatitis as a possible third climatic disease.

39 D. Denoon *et al.*, *Public Health in Papua New Guinea*, p. 21; and see also Denoon Donald, Temperate medicine and settler capitalism: on the reception of Western medical ideas, in MacLeod and Lewis (eds), *Disease, Medicine, and Empire*, pp. 121–138.

40 M. Lyons, Sleeping sickness, colonial medicine and imperialism, in Macleod and Lewis (eds), *Disease, Mecicine and Empire*, p. 244. This included a wide variety of diseases including leprosy, plague, cholera and malaria, most occurring in parts of Europe and North America at the time of the publication of Manson's book.

41 See discussion following Davis' paper, What is climatic disease?, pp. 6–10.

42 *SSAR 1928*, p. 765.

43 Helen R. Woolcock, 'Our salubrious climate': attitudes to health in colonial Queensland, in MacLeod and Lewis (eds), *Disease, Medicine, and Empire*, pp. 182–183.

44 John G. Butcher, *The British in Malaya 1880–1941: The social history of a European community in colonial South-East Asia* (Kuala Lumpur: Oxford University Press, 1979); Philip Curtin, *Death by Migration. Europe's encounter with the tropical world in the nineteenth century* (Cambridge: Cambridge University Press, 1989), pp. 47–50; J. E. Spencer and W. L. Thomas, The hill stations and summer resorts of the Orient, *The Geographical Review* XXXVIII, 4 (1948): 637–651. Denoon, *Public Health in Papua New Guinea* (p. 25) argues that 'until the 1890s, it was commonly believed by Europeans that malaria was caused by 'miasma' in the air, best avoided by living at high altitudes, or at least in raised houses'. Indeed, the absence of breeding sites and vectors in high altitudes, and in some cases the flying patterns of vectors, meant that raised houses did offer some protection. The beliefs of early settlers, whilst consistent with their own understanding of the etiology and transmission of disease, were presumably reinforced empirically and by local knowledge and perceptions.

45 Col. R. Woolley, Despatch from Singapore, 9 April 1870, CO 273/37: ff. 264–265.

46 Woolcock, 'Our salubrious climate', pp. 183–184.

47 SS, *Labour Commission Report*, Appendix of Evidence, p. 36.

48 Butcher, *The British in Malaya, 1880–1941*.

49 ZHCI 411/739, Negri Sembilan, *Annual Report of the Medical Department, 1899*, p. 261.

50 *Ibid.*, p. 261.

51 *Ibid.*, pp. 260–1.

52 A. R. Wellington, *Hygiene and Sanitation in British Malaya.* Malayan Series No. XVI, British Empire Exhibition, London, 1924 (Singapore: Fraser and Neave, 1923), p. 4. See also Pahang, *Pahang Medical Report for 1900*, in Accounts and Papers ZHCI 6523 (London: Public Records Office), p. 260; S. C. G. Fox, *The Principles of Health in Malaya: Some suggestions to newcomers* (Taiping: Perak Government Printing Office, 1901), p. 1; Great Britain, Colonial and Indian Exhibition 1886, *Notes on the Straits Settlements and Malay States* (London: William Clowes, 1886), pp. 19–20; Great Britain Emigration Information Office, *Federated Malay States General Information for Intending Settlers* (London: HMSO, 1900), p. 5. For a summary of these views, see Butcher, *The British in Malaya*, pp. 68–72 and L. Manderson, Race, colonial mentality and public health in early twentieth century Malaya, pp. 193–194.

53 Anon., Acclimatisation of the white man in the tropics, *MMJES* 1 (May 1926), p. 31; *ST* 16 July 1926, p. 10.

54 K. Black, Health and climate – with special reference to British Malaya, Part I, *British Malaya* 3, 11 (1933), p. 253; also K. Black, Health and climate – with special reference to British Malaya, Part II, *British Malaya* 3, 12 (1933): 279–280.

55 P. D. Curtin, *Death by Migration*, p. 107.

56 Cuthbert Christy, *Notes on Prevention of Malaria* (London: Ross Institute of Tropical Hygiene, 1935), p. 51 ff. GB, Emigration Information Office, *Federated Malay States, General Information for Intending Settlers* (London: Her Majesty's Stationery Office, 1900), p. 12. The latter advice (wearing flannel), provided on a number of occasions, fits neatly with earlier advocacy of the use of the cummerbund to protect against chill, Harrison, Tropical medicine in nineteenth-century India, p. 16, citing J. Johnson, *The Influence of Tropical Climates* (1815). See also S. C. G. Fox, *The Principles of Health in Malaya: Some suggestions to newcomers* (Taiping: Perak Government Printing Office, 1901).

57 K. Black, Health and climate, Part II.

58 W. Anderson, Immunity of empire.

59 ZHCI 6523, *The Pahang Medical Report of 1900*, p. 260. See also Savage, *Western Impressions of Nature and Landscape*, pp. 109–126, for a discussion of the relationship between environment and character, here in the context of perceptions of the fecundity of the tropics and belief that the ready availability of abundant foodstuffs had contributed to native apathy and indolence. This view dated from the early eighteenth century and continued through to the mid-twentieth century. The negative aspect of this utopian image was that abundance caused mental as well as physical laziness; consequently people from cold climates had the intellectual edge, hence Black's idealisation of English 'slush and fog', Black, Health and climate – Part I, p. 253; see also L. Manderson, Race, colonial mentality and public health, pp. 195–198.

60 See S. Gordon, *The History and Philosophy of Social Science* (London and New York: Routledge, 1991), pp. 412–438, 499–510; Herbert Spencer, *Descriptive Sociology* (London: Williams and Norgate, 1873), and *Principles of Sociology* (London: Williams and Norgate, 1885–1896); Charles Darwin, *The Origin of the Species by Means of Natural Selection: or The preservation of favoured races in the struggle for life* (ed. J. W. Burrow) (London: John Murray, 1859); and see

Ernst Mayr, *The Growth of Biological Thought: Diversity, Evolution and Inheritance* (Cambridge, Mass.: Belknap Press, 1982) for an account of early theories of genetic transmission.

61 E. Said, *Orientalism*; Julie Marcus, *A World of Difference: Islam and gender hierarchy in Turkey*, Women in Asia Publications Series No. 3 (Sydney: Allen and Unwin, 1992); Donald Tuzin, Sex, culture and the anthropologist, *SSM* 33, 8 (1991): 867–874; Sara Suleri, *The Rhetoric of English India* (Chicago: University of Chicago Press, 1992) all address these issues.

62 See Mary Louise Pratt, *Imperial Eyes. Travel writings and transculturation* (London and New York: Routledge, 1992), pp. 151–153.

63 The 1890 Commission of inquiry into labour argued, in fact, that there was 'nothing to shew that the health of the coolies is materially injured by residence', see SS, *Labour Commission Report*, p. 15.

64 Dr A. W. Sinclair, in SS, *Labour Commission Report*, Appendix of Evidence, p. 166.

65 *Ibid.*, p. 12.

66 *Ibid.*, p. 24.

67 A. H. Cretch, *Malayan Mining Methods, with an Account of the Physique, Living Conditions and Food Requirements of the Asiatic Miner*, Mss Indian Ocean S96 (1933), pp. 44, 46, 49.

68 SS, *Labour Commission Report*, p. 15, citing the Journal of the Indian Archipelago.

69 CO273/275/332, 24 October 1901.

70 *Ibid.*, Report, p. 299; Appendix, Dr J. H. McClosky, Colonial Surgeon, Province Wellesley, p. 96.

71 *Ibid.*, Dr M. F. Simon, Acting Principal Civil Medical Officer, Straits Settlements, p. 37; Mr J. Turner, General Manager, Penang Sugar Estates Company, p. 85; and Mr W. F. B. Paul, British Resident, Sungei Ujong, p. 178.

72 C. W. C. Parr, *Report of the Commission appointed to inquire into the Conditions of Indentured Labor in the Federated Malay States, 1910*. Report No. 11 (Kuala Lumpur: Federated Malay States Labour Department, 1910), p. 15.

73 *ST* 21 August 1920, p.8.

74 A. H. Cretch, *Malayan Mining Methods, with an Account of the Physique, Living Conditions and Food Requirements of the Asiatic Miner*, pp. 37–48. Major G. St J. Orde-Browne, *Labour Conditions in Ceylon, Mauritius and Malaya*, Cmd 6423 (London: HMSO, 1943), pp. 101–102.

75 *SSAR 1904*, p. 706; GB, Economic Advisory Council, Committee on Nutrition in the Colonial Empire, *Nutrition in the Colonial Empire*. First Report, Part I, Cmd 6050 (London: HMSO, 1939), p. 27.

76 On the supposition that one vice would lead to another, see e.g. *SSAR 1904*, p. 706; *SSAR 1926*, p. 635. In the context of arguing against prohibition because opium use would be replaced by alcohol, the *Straits Times* argued that although the Chinese would be able to resist 'the spread of the drunken habit more successfully than the primitive tribes, yet the dangers to the family and to society are too serious to be lightly passed over', 7 January 1925, p. 11.

77 ZHCI 6411, Negri Sembilan, *Annual Report of the Medical Department, 1899*, p. 256.

78 *SSAR 1924*, p. 570.

79 In 1903 the death rate in Negri Sembilan was 35.75, 36.99 per 1,000 in Pahang, 35.03 in Selangor and 47.54 in Perak. Diarrhoea and dysentery

were the major causes of morbidity treated in hospital, Sel. Sec. 4025/1904. Dr E. A. O. Travers, then Registrar of Births and Deaths in Selangor, argued that 'the sickness and mortality from this class of disease has, during the last three years, increased out of all proportion to the increase of population of the state ... the discovery of a means of prevention and cure of dysentery and diarrhoea would be a far more important matter to this state and to the tropics generally, than any investigations, however successful, into the etiology of beri-beri or malarial fever', ZHCI 6737, Accounts and Papers, v.lix, 1904, no. 33, *Selangor, Medical Report for 1902*, p. 399.

80 Sel. Sec. 3678/1905.

81 A. R. Cretch, *Malayan Mining Methods*, p. 48–49.

82 Sel.Sec. 4853/1901.

83 Sel. Sec. 267/1910, no folio no.

84 Sel. Sec. 772/1885; Sel. Sec. 1800/1885.

85 Parr, *Report of the Commission*, pp. 29, 32.

86 Sel.Sec, P/KES/A.1, pp. 1–2, S. C. G. Fox, *Federated Malay States, State of Perak, The Medical Report for the Year 1906*.

87 Sel. Sec. 529/1908.

88 A. R. Cretch, *Malayan Mining Methods*, p. 42.

89 A. W. Sinclair, Notes on beri–beri, as observed in the Malay Peninsula from 1882 to 1888. *Transactions of the British Medical Association on Meeting held at Leeds, 1889* (London: British Medical Association, 1889), p. 2; Sel. Sec. 1958/1912; *FMSAR 1932*, p. 11; Files of the British Adviser of Trengganu (BATr) 1242/1937.

90 Sel. Sec. 165/1900.

91 Sel. Sec. 424/1915, Report of 10 April 1915.

92 See *inter alia* Sel. Sec. 2217/1905; 2366/1906; 864/1904; 6723/1904.

93 C. W. C. Parr, *Report of the Commission*, Report No. 11 (Kuala Lumpur: Federated Malay States Labour Department, 1910).

94 E. W. F. Gilman, *Labour in British Malaya*, Malayan Series No. XI, British Empire Exhibition, London, 1924 (Singapore: Fraser and Neave Ltd., 1923), p. 16.

95 BATr 481/1935, *Annual Medical and Sanitary Report for the Year 1934*.

96 BATr 1242/1937, Brown, Medical Officer, Trengganu to British Adviser, 2 November 1937.

97 *ST* 24 July 1925, p. 8.

98 BATr 1355/1938, f. 20A.

99 For details of estate conditions, see Chapter 5.

100 Sel. Sec. P/KES/A.1, S. C. G. Fox, *Federated Malay States, State of Perak, The Medical Report for the year 1906*, p. 2.

101 Sel.Sec. 2468/1910, D. K. McDowell, Principal Medical Officer to Federal Secretary, Federated Malay States, 19 March 1910.

102 See, for example, E. W. Birch, *A memorandum upon the subject of irrigation for the Resident-General (Sir F. A. Swettenham)* (Kuala Lumpur: Selangor Government Printing Office, 1898), p. 19.

103 Sel. Sec. 181/1883.

104 See e.g. *SSAR/FMSAR 1938*, p. 83.

105 Sel. Sec. 19/1894, District Officer, Kuala Selangor, 23 December 1893.

106 A. R. Cretch, *Malayan Mining Methods*, p. 52; cf. W. C. Caique, S. M. Knight, and W. Toodayan, Risk factors for the transmission of diarrhoeal disease in children in the Tumpat District, Kelantan, Malaysia: a case-control study, unpublished report, Master of Tropical Health (Brisbane: Tropical Health Program, University of Queensland, 1989).

107 BAKel 349/1918, *Annual Report of the District Officer, Ulu Kelantan, 1917*, p. 3.

108 BAKel 75/1918, p. 13.

109 L. W. Evans, *Kelantan. The Annual Report on the Medical Department for the Year 1932*, p. 7. The Institute of Medical Research in 1951 was to remark that 'Malays are not townsfolk and until recent years have been shy of the hospitals ... western methods are slowly diffusing into *kampung* life. Travelling dispensaries penetrate by road and river deep into the countryside bringing drugs and advice, and there are ambitious plans for future developments in rural health centres and clinics. Malaria control, developed at first for the towns, and then for the rubber plantations and mines, is now spreading to the Malay *kampungs*, and it is here that the main progress in future years is to be expected', see IMR, *Studies from the Institute of Medical Research*, p. 34.

110 See also Enid M. Wylie, Colonial administration and malaria in British Malaya 1900–1920, unpublished honours dissertation (Brisbane: Griffith University, 1989).

111 M. Worboys, The emergence of tropical medicine; Worboys, Manson, Ross and colonial medical policy.

112 Watson recalls that at a meeting of the Royal Society for the Arts on 28 November 1900, Ross both presented the life-cycle of malaria and argued for a comprehensive strategy of malaria control – avoiding bites by the use of bed nets and house screens, treating fever cases with quinine, and reducing larvae sites through clearing and drainage and the application of adulticides. He was many decades before his time. See Sir Malcolm Watson, Malaria and mosquitos: forty years on, *JRSA* LXXXVII, No. 4505 (1939), p. 483.

113 Sel. Sec. 6846/1901, Resident General, Kuala Lumpur 27 November 1901.

114 Sel. Sec. 6852/1901, General Manager FMS Railways to Resident General, 21 November 1901.

115 Sel. Sec. 6219/1901; Sel. Sec. 6847/1901.

116 FMS, *Report presented to Her Majesty's Secretary of State for the Colonies, 8 May 1904* (Kuala Lumpur: Federated Malay States Government Printing Office, 1905), p. 8.

117 L. D. Gammans, Anti-malaria work at Port Dickson, *MMJ* II, I (1927): 26.

118 ZHCI 6411, *Perak, Medical Department Report 1899*, p. 307.

119 *Ibid.*, p. 19.

120 *Ibid.*, p. 307. A paper published in the *Malayan Medical Journal*, reporting on the Mosquito Inspector's work since July 1924, lists 13 species of *Anopheles*, *A. maculatus* and *A. barbirostris* simply being the most common of these, see Anon., Anti-malarial work in Straits Settlements, *MMJES* I, IV (1926): 29.

121 Pahang, *Annual Medical Report, 1931* (Kuantan: Government Printing Office, 1932), pp. 7–8.

122 Sir Malcolm Watson, *Some Pages from the History of the Prevention of Malaria*, The Finlayson Memorial Lecture, Glasgow, 29 November 1934 (Glasgow: Alex Macdougall, 1935), p. 35.

123 E. P. Hodgkin and R. S. Johnston, Malaria at Batu Gajah, Perak: Transmitted by *Anopheles Barbirostrus* Van Der Welp, *BIMR* No. 1 (Kuala Lumpur: FMS Government Press, 1935), p. 7.

124 W. E. Holmes, The control of urban malaria (Kuala Lumpur), *BIMR* No. 2 (Kuala Lumpur: FMS Government Press, 1939).

125 A. R. Wellington, *Hygiene and Sanitation in British Malaya*. Malayan Series No. XVI, British Empire Exhibition, London, 1924 (Singapore: Fraser and

264 NOTES (PAGES 88–92)

Neave, 1923), p. 4; see also A. R. Wellington, *The ways and means adopted by government for the control of malaria in the Federated Malay States*, Paper presented to the Far Eastern Association of Tropical Medicine, Tokyo, October 1925 (Kuala Lumpur: Federated Malay States Government Press, 1925).

126 Sir Malcolm Watson, 1935. *Some Pages from the History of the Prevention of Malaria*, p. 19.

127 A form of malignant tertian malaria in which haemoglobin is present in the urine as a result of the massive destruction of red cells.

128 BAKel 263/1917, pp. 22, 25.

129 BAKel 339/1917, pp. 26–29; emphasis in the original.

130 BAKel 263/1917, p. 25.

131 BAKel 339/1917, pp. 39–47.

132 *ST* 17 February 1935, Estate Health, Memorandum on Report of Commission, Government Views, pp. 2–3, 12–23.

133 IMR/MAB 11/30, f. i.18.

134 IMR/MAB 38/1930, f. i.19.

135 IMR/MAB 32/1930, f. i.11.

136 IMR/MAB 5/1932, f. i.25.

137 Y. Chai, *The Development of British Malaya*, p. 207.

138 *Ibid.*, p. 205.

139 IMR, *Studies from the Institute of Medical Research*, Chapter II.

140 ZHCI 6411, *Perak, Medical Department Report, 1899*, p. 306.

141 Sinclair, Notes on Beri-beri, p. 4; Federated Malay States, *Report presented to His Majesty's Secretary of State for the Colonies, 8 May 1904*, p. 36.

142 Sel. Sec. 5083/1901. For an evaluation of Braddon's role in establishing the etiology of beri-beri, see E. M. Wylie, The search for the cause of Beriberi in the Malay Peninsula: The contribution of Dr W. L. Braddon. *JMBRAS* LXI, 2 (1988): 93–122.

143 Sel. Sec. 3374/1907.

144 BAKel 153/1913, pp. 1–3.

145 BATr481/1936, p. 7; L. Manderson, Traditional food beliefs and critical life events; L. Manderson, Traditional food classification and humoral medical theory; L. Manderson, Roasting, smoking and dieting in response to birth: Malay confinement in cross-cultural perspective, *SSM* 15B (1981): 509–520.

146 BATr481/1935.

147 Cecily D. Williams and J. W. Scharff, *Preventive Paediatrics. An experiment in Health Work in Trengganu in 1940–41, with an Appendix containing notes for Dressers and Nurses* (Kuala Lumpur: Department of Public Relations, Federation of Malaya, 1948), p. 12.

148 CO859/14/3550/18/1939, p. 4.

149 *FMSAR 1927*, p. 47.

150 Sel. Sec. 4814/1911.

151 The District Officer of Ulu Selangor insisted 'I know of no area sufficiently large to be worth gazetting', see Sel. Sec. 1413/1919, p. 1, cf. Sel. Sec. 1544/1919.

152 CO859/14/3550/18/1939, p. 4.

153 See Michael Worboys, The discovery of colonial malnutrition between the wars, in Arnold (ed.), *Imperial Medicine and Indigenous Societies*, pp. 208–225.

154 IMR, *Studies from the Institute of Medical Research*, pp. 119–120.

155 IMR 90/1925, f. 124.

156 Sel.Sec. 1513/1926, Secretary for Chinese Affairs to Under-Secretary of Federated Malay States, 17 February 1926.

157 IMR, *Studies from the Institute of Medical Research*, pp. 124–125; IMR 54/1923; IMR 73/1923; M. Barrowcliff, The vitamins, Paper presented to the Fifth Congress of the Far Eastern Association of Tropical Medicine, Singapore September 1923 (Kuala Lumpur: St John's Press, 1923); R. C. Burgess and Laidin bin Alang Musa, *A Report on the state of Health, the diet and the economic conditions of groups of people in the lower income levels of Malaya*, Institute of Medical Research Report No. 13 (Kuala Lumpur: Charles Grenier and Sons, 1950).

158 W. J. Vickers and J. H. Strahan, *A Health Survey of the State of Kedah with special referent to rice field malaria, nutrition, and the water supply, 1935–1936* (Kuala Lumpur: Ryle, Palmer, 1936), BATr 1379/1937.

159 F. G. Bourne, *Coroner's Annual Report*, p. 5.

160 W. J. Vickers and J. H. Strahan, *A Health Survey of the State of Kedah*, p. 3.

161 GB, Economic Advisory Council, *Nutrition in the Colonial Empire*, p. 47; see also GB, Economic Advisory Council, Committee on Nutrition in the Colonial Empire, *Summary of Information regarding Nutrition in the Colonial Empire. First Report, Part II* (Cmd 6051) (London: HMSO, 1939).

162 Sir W. Peel, Notes covering his colonial service from 1897–1935. Rhodes House Library, Colonial Records Project, Mss Indian Ocean S208, p. 659.

163 BAKel 627/1918, 829/1918.

164 BAKel 684/1912.

165 The rat plague hit coconut and paddy fields in Bernam District, Selangor, and it was estimated that 2,000 traps were needed for villages alone to keep down the population. A bounty of 1 cent per tail was paid, Sel. Sec. 1350/1917.

166 Sir W. Peel, Notes covering his colonial service from 1897–1935, Mss Indian Ocean S208, p. 659.

167 *Ibid.*, p. 66.

168 See L. Manderson, Introduction: The anthropology of food in Oceania and Southeast Asia, in L. Manderson (ed.), *Shared Wealth and Symbol. Food, culture and society in Oceania and Southeast Asia* (New York and Cambridge: Cambridge University Press, 1986), pp. 7–8. Burgess and Laidin (*A Report on the State of Health*, p. 26) maintain that Malays had 'an infinite faith in its health and strength giving properties: *Apa juga dimakan jika tiada nasi tidak ada bermaya rasa badan* (regardless of what is eaten, if there is no rice then there is no life)'. McArthur makes the same point, that Malay villagers (in Malacca) believe that life itself is dependent on eating rice, see M. McArthur, *Malaya-12. Assignment Report June 1958–November 1959*, WPR/449/62 (Geneva: World Health Organisation, 1962), p. 127.

169 Sel. Sec. G1441/1932, ff. 7–8; Sel. Sec. G2060/1932.

170 Sel. Sec. G121/1933, ff. 1A, 24A.

171 Sel. Sec. 84/1937, *ST* Editorial, 7 July 1937, p. 8.

4 Public health and the pathogenic city

1 John K. Noyes, *Colonial Space. Spatiality in the discourse of German South West Africa 1884–1915* (Chur, Switzerland: Harwood Academic Publishers, 1991), p. 82.

2 Noyes, *Colonial Space*, p. 163. In Smith's words, 'the production of space ... implies product of meaning, concepts and consciousness of space which are

266   NOTES (PAGES 96–101)

inseparably linked to its physical production', see Neil Smith, *Uneven Development, Nature, Capital and the Production of Space* (Oxford: Blackwell, 1984), p. 77; and see Noyes, *Colonial Space*, p. 98 ff.

3 David Harvey, *The Condition of Postmodernity. An essay into the origins of cultural change* (Oxford: Basil Blackwell, 1989), p. 264.

4 Noyes, *Colonial Space*, pp. 106–107.

5 *Vide* Mary Douglas, *Purity and Danger* (Harmondsworth: Penguin Books, 1966).

6 I have failed to find the right metaphor for this. Imagine discrete discs that spin on one large turning ring, the vibrations of one capable of but not necessarily setting off those of the next.

7 According to the Governor of the Straits Settlements, Sir Laurence Guillemard, speaking at the opening of the new General Hospital at Sepoy Lines in Singapore in 1926, there were two only: the other was the maintenance of law and order. *ST* 30 March 1926, p. 9.

8 Savage's useful term for the period 1870–1942, *Western Impressions of Nature and Landscape in Southeast Asia* (Singapore: Singapore University Press, 1984), p. 148.

9 John V. Pickstone, Death, dirt and fever epidemics: rewriting the history of British 'public health', 1780–1850, in T. Ranger and P. Slack (eds), *Epidemics and Ideas. Essays on the historical perception of pestilence* (Cambridge: Cambridge University Press, 1992), p. 126. See also Richard J. Evans, Epidemics and revolutions: cholera in nineteenth century Europe, *idem.*, pp. 149–173; Margaret Pelling, *Cholera, Fever and English Medicine, 1825–1865* (Oxford: Oxford University Press, 1978); Anthony S. Wohl, *Endangered Lives. Public Health in Victorian Britain* (London: J. M. Dent, 1983).

10 The choice of adjective is intentional.

11 T. G. McGee, *The Southeast Asian City: A social geography of the primate cities of Southeast Asia* (London: G. Bell, 1967); Butcher, *The British in Malaya*; Noyes, *Colonial Space*; Savage, *Western Impressions*; and see various papers in R. Ross and G. J. Telkamp (eds), *Colonial Cities: Essays in urbanism in a colonial context* (Dordrecht: Martinus Nijhoff, 1985).

12 See Sharon Siddique, *Singapore's Little India, Past, Present, Future* (Singapore: Institute of South East Asian Studies, 1982); Barrington Kaye, *Upper Nankin Street, Singapore: A sociological study of Chinese households living in a densely populated area* (Singapore: University of Malaya Press, 1960); J. M. Gullick, Kuala Lumpur 1880–1895, *JMBRAS* 28, 4 (1955): 7–139; Song Ong Siang, *One Hundred Years of the Chinese in Singapore* (London: John Murray, 1923).

13 SSR, *Census Reports and Returns (Straits Settlements, 2nd April 1871)*, no publication details, Colonial Reports 1871, Papers relating to Her Majesty's Possessions, Part 11 (1873), p. 3; J. R. Innes, *Report on the Census of the Straits Settlements taken on the 1st March 1901* (Singapore: Government Printing Office, 1901), pp. 18–19. Note that Nathan's figures for 1871 and 1921 do not accord with those provided in the original censuses (see Nathan, *The Census of British Malaya*, p. 18), but the trends are the same.

14 *ST* 8 May 1983, p. 2.

15 J. F. Warren, *Rickshaw Coolie*, and a number of related essays in James F. Warren, *At the Edge of Southeast Asian History: Essays* (Quezon City: New Day Publishers, 1987).

16 Peter J. Rimmer, Hackney carriage syces and rikisha pullers in Singapore: A colonial registrar's perspective on public transport, 1892–1923, in Rimmer and Allen (eds), *The Underside of Malaysian History* (Singapore: Singapore

University Press, 1990) pp. 129–160, and for an incomparable people's history that centres on the rickshaw puller, Warren, *Rickshaw Coolie* (Singapore: Oxford University Press, 1986).

17 Nineteenth-century press reports refer on a number of occasions to the 'careless driving' of rickshaw coolies competing with the gharries, and the hazards of the narrow roads, *ST* 7 September 1883, p. 2.

18 Michel Foucault, *Power/Knowledge. Selected interviews and other writings, 1927–1977* (Brighton: Harvester Press, 1980), p. 175.

19 Sel. Sec. 427/1882, f. 2.

20 *ST* 26 January 1883, 14 February 1883 for Singapore examples.

21 *ST* 1 February 1883, p. 2.

22 Sel. Sec. 3354/1903, President, Sanitary Board, Kuala Lumpur to Resident of Selangor, 7 July 1903.

23 Sel. Sec. 3345/1903.

24 CO273/158, C. F. Bozzolo, 8 October 1881.

25 *ST* 9 July 1883, p. 2, and see *ST* 21 February, 19 May and 4 July 1883.

26 *ST* 4 April 1883, p. 2.

27 *ST* 13 April 1883, p. 3; 4 April 1883, p. 2; 6 June 1883, p. 3.

28 For example, see Song, *One Hundred Years of the Chinese in Singapore* (London: John Murray, 1923), p. 538, pp. 544–545, reporting fires in Kampong Martin in 1916 and Trengganu Street in 1918.

29 Sel. Sec. 438/1885.

30 Sel. Sec. 6849/1902; *Malay Mail* 12 December 1902, p. 3.

31 Sel. Sec., P/KES/K.1, *Kedah and Perlis Annual Report, 1937*, p. 10.

32 M. Worboys, Manson, Ross and colonial medical policy, p. 28.

33 Sel. Sec. 733/1911.

34 Sel.Sec. 1046/1911; *Quarantine and Prevention of Disease Enactment (FMS) 913/1903*. Similar Enactments existed in all UFMS and settlements as well.

35 Sel. Sec. 1306/1908.

36 Sel. Sec. G1009/1930, p. 17.

37 Sel. Sec. 960/1911.

38 Brenda Yeoh, Power and the people, p. 17.

39 Sel. Sec. 933/1915, pp. 14–15.

40 Sel. Sec. 1476/1907.

41 Sel. Sec. 933/1915.

42 *Ibid.*

43 Sel. Sec. 1306/1908.

44 Sel. Sec. 466/1940, f. 13; for a discussion of the effectiveness of the slow filter in breaking down bacteria, see Curtin, *Death by Migration*, pp. 112–116.

45 For example, Sel. Sec. 1306/1908.

46 Sel. Sec. 305/1913. The Chairman of the Sanitary Board commented that part of the problem of sanitation was internal, and that detailed and explicit instructions were necessary: 'If any else than Dr Reid were Health Officer I would not bother about such matters, but by experience I find that he is incapable of working *with* an officer so he must be under orders'.

47 Sel. Sec. 933/1915, ff. 15–16.

48 Sel. Sec. 140/1924. This was not the only perspective; others insisted that the use of nightsoil was 'unscientific' and helped increase if not cause diarrhoea, dysentery and typhoid, Anon., Chinese gardeners and disease, *MMJES* 1, 2 (1926), p. 33.

49 Pahang, *Annual Department Reports 1931* (Kuantan: Government Printer, 1932); ZHCI 6523, *Pahang Medical Report for 1900*, pp. 261–262.

50 Evans, *Kelantan Annual Report*, p. 7.
51 Sel. Sec. 1754/1914, J. T. Clarke, Health Officer, Kinta, 10 July 1914.
52 Sel. Sec. 933/1915.
53 Sel. Sec. 3080/1889.
54 Subsequent research in Australia by Thompson, Tidswell and Elkington and by Liston in India provided corroboration of Simond's work. See I. J. Catanach, Plague and the tensions of empire: India, 1896–1918, in Arnold (ed.), *Imperial Medicine and Indigenous Societies* (Manchester and New York: Manchester University Press, 1988), pp. 158, 162–3.
55 Sel. Sec. 1306/1908; Sel. Sec. 733/1911. Megan Vaughan similarly describes the rather creative approaches to rat-catching in Uganda in Chapter 2 in *Curing their Ills* (Cambridge: Polity Press, 1991).
56 *ST* 29 May 1920, p. 9.
57 *ST* 16 September 1925, p. 10; 17 September 1925, p. 8.
58 George Town, Penang, Municipality of, *Health Officer's Annual Report for the Year 1938* (Penang: Criterion Press, 1939), p. 39.
59 IMR, *Studies from the Institute of Medical Research*, pp. 243–252.
60 Sel. Sec. 1508/1902, Treacher, Resident General of the Federated Malay States to British Resident, Selangor, 4 March 1902.
61 Sel. Sec. 1657/1904, Kuala Lumpur, *Annual Report of the Sanitary Board, 1903*.
62 FMS/P/KES/A.1, Federated Malay States, *Perak Medical Report of the Year 1908* (M. J. Wright, State Surgeon), p. 2.
63 Sel. Sec. 1307/1908; Sel. Sec. 1476/1907.
64 Sel. Sec. 4568/1911.
65 Sel. Sec. 4827/1910, p. 6. There is no definition here, or in other documentation cited, of how the sanitary inspectors were to determine 'filth, light, or airiness'.
66 At the time (1920) the IMR was 245.99, the crude death rate 41.63, Sel. Sec. 762/1921, p. 3. In Kuala Lumpur and Penang as well as Singapore, the sex ratio was skewed in favour of men, and while infants would certainly have been vulnerable to respiratory infections, particularly pneumonia, not that many lived in the most congested tenements: housing inspection in Singapore in 1917, for instance, documented 877 residents in 25 houses, but only six of these residents were under twelve months and 48 under five years. Sixty percent of occupants were male, virtually all Chinese (SSR, *Proceedings and Report of the Commission appointed to enquire into the cause of the presenting housing difficulties in Singapore, and the steps which should be taken to remedy such difficulties.* Vol I, Instrument of Appointment and Report; Vol II, Evidence and Memoranda (hereafter Housing Commission) (Singapore: Government Printing Office, 1918), pp. A 71, B 84.
67 Sel. Sec. 1306/1908.
68 Sel. Sec. 3575/1912, F. W. Douglas, 6 August 1912, cf. Singapore, as described powerfully by James Warren in *Rickshaw Coolie*.
69 Sel. Sec. 1087/1916; Sel. Sec. G1009/1930, p. 17.
70 H. M. Hobbs, *Welfare Clinics in Malaya* (1962), Mss Indian Ocean S38, pp. 18, 21–22.
71 T. F. Strang, *State of Kelantan. Annual Report of the Medical Department for the Year 1936* (Kota Bharu: Cheong Fatt Press, 1936), p. 9.
72 Sel. Sec. 1476/1907.
73 Sel. Sec. 994/1927, Kuala Lumpur, *Annual Report of the Health Officer, 1926*.
74 Research on measles and relationship of intensity of exposure, virus dose and severity of infection suggests that this would be one virus which would

have had considerable impact on infant mortality, see P. Aaby, J. Bukh, I. M. Lisse and A. J. Smits, Overcrowding and intensive exposure as determinants of measles mortality, *AJE* 120 (1984): 49–63; P. Aaby, Social and behavioural factors affecting transmission and severity of measles infection, in J. C. Caldwell, *et al.* (eds), *What We Know about Health Transition: The cultural, social and behavioural determinants of health* (Canberra: Health Transition Centre, Australian National University, 1990), pp. 826–842.

75 *ST* 22 April 1926, p. 10; Sel. Sec. 466/1940, ff. 22–23.
76 E. G. Broadrick to E. L. Brockman, 29 July 1905, in SSR, *Housing Commission,* p. A 61.
77 I. J. Catanach, Plague and the tensions of empire, 155–158.
78 W. J. Simpson, *Report on the Sanitary Conditions of Singapore* (London: HMSO, 1907).
79 *Ibid,* p. A 63; see also Yeoh, Power and the people.
80 *ST* 8 June 1907, p. 8.
81 SSR, *Housing Commission,* Middleton, 30 May 1908, p. C 52.
82 *Ibid.*
83 *Ibid.*
84 *ST* 9 June 1907, p. 8.
85 SSR, *Housing Commission,* D. J. Galloway, p. B 84.
86 *Ibid.,* pp. A 71, C 54.
87 *Ibid.,* p. C 81.
88 *Ibid.,* vol. II (Evidence and Memoranda), p. B 158.
89 *Ibid.,* pp. A 7–8.
90 *Ibid.,* p. C 11; see also Warren, *Rickshaw Coolie* and various essays in his *At the Edge of Southeast Asian History.*
91 *Ibid.* p. A 6. This continued to be the case, see e.g., *ST* 28 October 1925, p. 10.
92 Sel. Sec. 1476/1907.
93 SSR, *Housing Commission,* p. B 118.
94 *Ibid.,* Mr Braddell, p. B 119.
95 Sel. Sec. 4827/1910.
96 Calculated from Anon., Tuberculosis in Malaya, *MMJES* I, 3 (1926): 33–37.
97 Anon., Tuberculosis in Malaya, 33; Strang, *State of Kelantan. Annual Report,* p. 7.
98 J. Tertius Clarke, Tuberculosis in the tropics, II, I (1927): 19–23.
99 FMS, *Medical Report 1904,* p. 6.
100 Sel. Sec. 4827/1910, f. 6
101 Sel. Sec. 4827/1910, p. 6.
102 *ST* 8 September 1925, p. 10.
103 *ST* 3 May 1920, p. 8.
104 *ST* 26 January 1921, p. 10.
105 *ST* 10 February 1925, p. 8.
106 *ST* 6 February 1925, p. 8.
107 *Ibid.,* see also 2 May 1925, p. 10; 31 August 1925, p. 8.
108 *ST* 5 February 1927, p. 9; 8 February 1927, pp. 8–10.
109 *ST* 11 February 1925, p. 10.
110 *ST* 2 August 1926, p. 8.
111 *ST* 12 September 1925, pp. 9–10.
112 *ST* 26 September 1925, pp. 9–10, quoting Lornie's speech to the Commissioners, 25 September.

113 George Town, Penang, *Health Officer's Annual Report for the Year 1938*, p. 19.
114 *Ibid.*, p. 39.
115 *FMSAR 1934*, p. 12.
116 A. R. Wellington, *Hygiene and Sanitation in British Malaya*, p. 15.
117 For example, *ST* 19 March 1883, p. 3; 10 May 1883, p. 2, 15 June 1883, p. 3.
118 J. T. Clarke, Tuberculosis in the tropics, *MMJ* II, I (1927): 19–23.
119 *ST* 30 June 1907, p. 8.
120 *SSAR 1934*, p. 1002.
121 P/KES/A11, *Perak, Annual Medical Report 1907*, p. 7.
122 See e.g. *ST* 16 and 18 June 1883, 23 July 1883.
123 L. Manderson, Race, colonial mentality and public health, in Rimmer and Allen (eds), *The Underside of Malaysian History*.
124 Sel. Sec. 3270/1911.
125 BATr 481/1935.
126 BAKel 1020/1914.

5 Sickness and the world of work

1 E. W. F. Gilman, *Labour in British Malaya*, Malayan Series No. XI, British Empire Exhibition, London, 1924 (Singapore: Fraser and Neave, 1923), p. 17.
2 *Ibid.* One home supported by the fund was established in Kuala Lumpur in 1914, a second in Penang in 1922, to accommodate and support unemployed labourers until they found new work.
3 G. St. J. Orde-Browne, *Labour Conditions in Ceylon, Mauritius and Malaya* (London: HMSO, 1943), p. 95.
4 SSR, *Labour Commission Report*; C. W. C. Parr, *Report of the Commission* (Kuala Lumpur: FMS Labour Department, 1910) p. 41. If they were still indebted at the end of the year, they were kept on for $3 per month plus food; in 1910 it was more usual for Chinese coolies to be on three-year contracts, during which time advances for passage and supplies were to be repaid.
5 The first appears to have been an inquiry into ill-treatment on estates in Province Wellesley, conducted in 1881, and this was followed by fuller inquiries in 1890, 1910 and 1924 (see below). An inquiry was also held concerning the recruitment of Chinese labourers, triggered by riots in Singapore in 1872, SSR, *Labour Commission Report*, p. 3.
6 Sel. Sec. 1977/2886/1888, and see Chapter 3 above.
7 Cretch, *Malayan Mining Methods*, 1933, pp. 37, 46.
8 SS, *Labour Commission Report*, p. 47.
9 The death rate was 68 per 1,000, although it was considerably higher on select estates. Whilst the Tamil population represented only 2.5 percent of the population, it contributed 25 percent of hospital admissions, compared with Chinese, European, and Malay hospital admission rates of 11.6, 1.2 and .01 percent respectively. See ZHCI 6411/1899, Negri Sembilan, *Annual Departmental Report for 1899*, p. 256.
10 *Ibid.*, p. 17, Acting Colonial Secretary A. P. Talbot, quoting the Acting Resident of Perak, 7 December 1889.
11 *Ibid.*, Appendix Insp. 5 (Report of visit to Gula Sugar Estate, Perak, 11 December 1890).
12 CO273/274, f. 332.
13 Some contract labour continued to the late 1940s, however; see CO859/148/12254.R/1948.

14 *SSAR 1928*, p. 777. The decline in hookworm infection among incoming coolies from an estimated 90 percent in 1916 to 44 percent by 1928 was attributed to the mass administration of antihelminths.
15 Sel. Sec. 5867/1895.
16 CO273/274/331.
17 Sel. Sec. 2541/1908; Sel. Sec. 1578/1911.
18 SSR, *Labour Commission Report*, p. 48.
19 *Ibid.*, p. 7.
20 Sel. Sec. 256, 1904.
21 Sel. Sec. 1593/1911, f. 2.
22 SSR, *Labour Commission Report*, Inspections Nos. 11 and 13.
23 Parr, *Report of the Commission*, p. 3.
24 *Ibid.*, p. 8.
25 *SSAR 1928*, p. 779.
26 Sel. Sec. 1844/1912.
27 There were peaks in malaria, for example, in 1907, 1911, 1920, 1928 and 1929; see IMR, *Studies from the Institute of Medical Research*; P/PERU 4.
28 Sel. Sec. 269/1906.
29 BAKel 170/1913, Report by J. Gimlette, Residency Surgeon, Kelantan.
30 FMS, *Report of the Commission Appointed to Inquire into Certain Matters Affecting the Health of Estates in the Federated Malay States together with a Memorandum by the Chief Secretary to Government* (Kuala Lumpur: Government Printer, 1925), p. A 29.
31 *Ibid.*, p. A 28. For a description of the commission and its findings, see Norman J. Parmer, Estate workers' health in the Federated Malay States in the 1920s, in Rimmer and Allen (eds), *The Underside of Malaysian History. Pullers, prostitutes, plantation workers*, pp. 179–192.
32 J. W. Scharff, *A Note on Public Health Administration in the Northern Settlement* (Penang: Criterion Press, n.d., c.1932), p. 31; *SSAR 1926*, p. 478. The ideal was one latrine per family, never realised, and most managers worked towards one per ten people, see Gordon Cameron, Estate medical and health practice in Malaya, *East African Medical Journal* 29, 4 (1952): 155–156.
33 Sel. Sec. 1584/1911.
34 BAKel 339/1917, ff. 39–47. In Selangor in 1920, of 3,000 labourers examined, around 90 percent were infected; in Perlis the estimate, for 1927–8, was virtually 100 percent infection; for Penang in 1928, over 73 percent, see *SSAR 1928*, p. 777.
35 FMS, *Report of the Commission*, p. A 13.
36 Curtin, *Death by Migration* (Cambridge: Cambridge University Press, 1989), pp. 134–139 and especially Table 6.3.
37 Hodgkin and Johnston, Malaria at Batu Gajah, Perak, p. 6.
38 Watson, *Some Pages from the History of the Prevention of Malaria*, BIMR, No.1 (Kuala Lumpur: FMS Government Presss, 1935), p. 17.
39 *Ibid.*, p. 18.
40 *FMSAR 1932*; P/KES 1: 52–62. For the FMS combined, there were 16,981 cases of malaria of a total of 78,195. This was followed by venereal disease (4,048), chronic ulcer (3,479), and flu (3,271).
41 P/KES/D, *Kelantan, Annual Medical Department Report*.
42 Sel. Sec. 35/1936; L. D. Gammans, Anti-malaria work at Port Dickson, *MMJES* II, I (1927): 24–28.
43 '(I)n the interests of the labour force and of the owners and of the estate

managers themselves, the last mentioned should be warned where estates
have been closed down that a labour force should not be recruited and
brought on to the estate again until anti-malarial work has been effectively
carried out by a skeleton gang for three weeks or more previous to the date
of the intended reopening of the lines', IMR/MAB 38/1930, P. S. Selwyn-
Clark to Senior Health Officers, 26 September 1933.

44 Sel. Sec. 1593/1911, f. 7.
45 Sel. Sec. 218, Acting British Resident of Negri Sembilan, D. H. Wise, 1900.
46 SSR, *Labour Commission Report*, pp. 63–67.
47 Sel. Sec. 223/1901.
48 BAKel 170/1913.
49 M. Watson, *Some Pages from the History of the Prevention of Malaria* (Glasgow:
   Alex Macdougall, 1935), p. 18; see also BAKel 302/1918, f. 31, and
   Kelantan, *Annual Report of the Medical Department 1937*, p. 14.
50 IMR 54/1931, Annual Report 1930 of Pathological Division.
51 FMS, *Report of the Commission*, p. B 124, see also B 125; CO859/53/12257/5
   (1941).
52 *Ibid.*
53 FMS, *Report of the Commission*, p. B 125; CO859/53/12257/5 (1941) citing
   the *JMBMA*, Sept 1940: 157.
54 BAKel 75/1913.
55 Sel. Sec. 1581/1911.
56 Parr, *Report of the Commission*, p. 9.
57 SSR, *Labour Commission Report*, p. 23.
58 Parr, *Report of the Commission*, p. 5.
59 *Ibid.*, p. 32.
60 Parr, *Report of the Commission*, Suppl. p. 44.
61 *Ibid.*, p. 13.
62 *Ibid.*, p. 33, J. R. Delmege, Medical Officer, Krian; pp. 22, 25–6. On the role
   of sexual abuse as a mechanism of terror to control a wider population, see
   Anne-Marie Cass, Gender and Violence in the Philippines, unpublished
   PhD dissertation, (Brisbane: University of Queensland, 1992).
63 The Acting Protector of the Chinese for Selangor, Pahang and Negri
   Sembilan States in 1910, William Cowan, in Parr, *Report of the Commission*,
   p. 29; Orde-Browne, *Labour Conditions in Ceylon, Mauritius and Malaya*
   (London: HMSO, 1943), p. 95.
64 CO273/353/1907, ff. 183–199.
65 Sel. Sec. 1427/1918, p. 10.
66 Cameron, Estate medical and health practice, p. 155.
67 Parr, *Report of the Commission*, pp. 36–37.
68 Sel. Sec. 1313/1915, f. 19.
69 Sel. Sec. 5047/1916.
70 Sel. Sec. 4816/1916, f.7.
71 Sel. Sec. 3034/1917.
72 BATr 1355/1938, p. 20A.
73 Government Notification No. 170, 15 April 1886.
74 SSR, *Labour Commission Report*, p. 7.
75 *Ibid.*, p. 49.
76 Sel. Sec. 264/1906.
77 Sel. Sec. 129/1907. Estates not taking part in the scheme were charged a
   daily charge by government for the cost of hospitalisation of sick labourers,
   but this arrangement ceased in the 1930s with the depression.

78 FMS, *Report of the Commission*, p. A4; Sel. Sec. 2542/1908; Sel. Sec. 2541/1908.

79 Sel. Sec. 1605/1911, see 'Highlands (New Division) Estate Hospital. Superintendent Indian Immigrants Inspector's Reports for 1911'. It had 4 wards and 2 dressers to 50 patients and was regarded by the inspector, Haynes, as 'the most favorable estate hospital that I have yet seen in Selangor'.

80 BAKel 263/1917, *Annual Report Medical Department, 1916*; BAKel 339/1917, ff. 39–47.

81 Sel. Sec. 271/1911, f. 1.

82 Sel. Sec. 271/1911; Sel. Sec. 286/1911.

83 Sel. Sec. 807/1911.

84 Sel.Sec. 289/1911, f. 7.

85 *Ibid.* Similarly, the Kent Estate hospital was clean, but the estate did not provide clothing nor a bathing place for patients. Both were common omissions, Sel. Sec. 1607/1911.

86 Parr, *Report of the Commission*, p. 33; Sel. Sec. 142/1911.

87 Sel. Sec. 2542/1908, f. 1; Sel. Sec. 1582/1911.

88 Sel. Sec. 1585/1911.

89 Sel. Sec. 1313/1915.

90 Society of Estate Medical Officers, *An open letter to the unofficial members of the Legislative Federal Councils (SS and FMS)* (Kuala Lumpur: M. J. Rattray for the Society of Estate Medical Officers, 1918), p. 2.

91 *Ibid.*, p. 5.

92 *Ibid.*, p. 7.

93 Recommendations made during the Second World War in expectation of reinstatement of British rule were that all health services and medical care be a government responsibility. However, many continued to argue the preferability of hospitals remaining with the private sector, see Files of the British Military Administration, BMA PH/2.

94 FMS, *Report of the Commission*, p. A 15.

95 *Ibid.*, p. B 16.

96 G. St. J. Orde-Browne, *Labour Conditions in Ceylon, Mauritius and Malaya*, p. 99.

97 FMS, *Report of the Commission*, pp. A 5, A 6.

98 G. St. J. Orde-Browne, *Labour Conditions in Ceylon, Mauritius and Malaya*, p. 99.

99 Sel. Sec. 1582/1911; *SS/FMSAR 1937*, p. 10.

100 FMS, *Report of the Commission*, p. A 75.

101 W. Stark, in R. W. Heussler, Papers of Professor Robert W. Heussler, Rhodes House Library, MSS Brit.Emp. s.480. Box 17, History of the Malayan Civil Service 1853–1984. File 3. Letters, memoirs and notes on the M. C. S. and Heussler's research into its history. Correspondence from W. J. K. Stark (1910–1933), p. 7.

102 Sel. Sec. 2046/1920.

103 BAKel 263/197, f. 25.

104 Sel. Sec. 1610/1911.

105 The Colonial Office Committee on Emigration from India to the Crown Colonies and Protectorates, 1910, cited in Malcolm Watson, *Some Pages from the History of the Prevention of Malaria*, p. 16.

106 Jelf, president of the commission, was Acting Controller of Labour for the Straits Settlements and the Federated Malay States. Other members included Dr R. Dowden, Principal Medical Officer, FMS; J. Bruce, J. W. Campbell and Choo Kia Peng, planters; Dr D. C. Macaskill, Member of

Parliament; and Pattinarapat Kelunni Nambyar, Member of the Straits Settlements Legislative Council. The commission met 17 times, heard evidence from 57 individuals, and conducted interviews with 51 labourers chosen randomly from various estates.

107 C. W. C. Parr, *Report of the Commission*, pp. 9–10.
108 Under Section 70 and Section 82 (1) of the Labour Code, CO 859/1752/7, 1939, ff. 47–48.
109 IMR 59/1923, f. B 126.
110 FMS, *Report of the Commission*, p. B 173.
111 D. W. G. Faris, File of medical papers, 1931–1946, *Selangor Coast District Annual Report 1931*, Mss Indian Ocean S135, p. 12.
112 Cameron, Estate medical and health practice, p. 154.
113 W. J. Vickers and J. H. Strahan, *A Health Survey* (Kuala Lumpur: Ryle, Palmer, 1936), p. 38.
114 P/KES/K.1, *Annual Report of Kedah and Perlis 1937*.
115 R. W. Heussler, Interview with W. J. A. Stark, OBE, MSS Brit.Emp. s.480.
116 J. A. Kempe, *Perak, Annual Report of Medical Department*, 1932.
117 *SSAR 1923*, p. 629; see Manderson, Race, colonial mentality and public health.
118 W. G. Maxwell, Some problems of education and public health in Malaya. United Empire. *The Royal Colonial Institute Journal* XVIII, 1 (1927): 215; IMR, *Studies from the Institute of Medical Research*; P/PERU 4.
119 W. G. Maxwell, Some problems of education and public health, p. 219.
120 *FMSAR 1932*, pp. 3–4.
121 W. J. Vickers and J. H. Strahan, *A Health Survey*, p. 47.
122 *SSAR 1934*, p. 1003.
123 Scharff, *A Note on Public Health Administration*, p. 32.
124 CO859/39/12827, f. 12.
125 See e.g. J. W. Hoflin, *Malaria* (Kuala Lumpur: Federated Malay States, Malaria Advisory Board, 1934), a bilingual pamphlet (English and Chinese) which was built around the message 'No mosquitos, no malaria'.
126 J. Curtin, *Death by Migration*, p. 132, notes that among British troops malaria began to decline as a killing disease with the introduction of quinine, and he argues that the decline of morbidity from malaria was one of the most dramatic changes in the nineteenth century. Headrick, *The Tools of Empire*, shares this view.
127 There was some disagreement between the Health Officer and the Chairman of the Sanitary Board over the success of this approach, given the continuing increase of malaria. The Health Officer's concern related to compliance if the drug were free; the Board maintained that request for the drug was an indication of intended compliance. Sel. Sec. 284; also SU274.
128 Curtin, *Death by Migration*, p. 134; Ronald Ross, *Malaria Fever: Its Cause, Prevention, and Treatment* (Liverpool: Liverpool School of Tropical Medicine, 1902), pp. 46–47.
129 Cuthbert Christy, *Notes on the Prevention of Malaria* (London: Ross Institute of Tropical Hygiene, 1935).
130 Vickers and Strahan, *A Health Survey*, p. 48.
131 S. C. Howard, The practical application of anti-malarial measures on Malayan estates, *BIMR* 2 (1939), p. 4.
132 Sel. Sec. 1341/1911.
133 Watson, *Some Pages from the History of the Prevention of Malaria*, p. 17.
134 Sir Robert Chatterton, The development of tropical medicine, *Eastern World* IV, 11 (1950), p. 34.

135 *SSAR 1936*, vol.II, pp. 911–912.

136 B. Anantaswami Rao, *Malaria Control in Malaya, Java, Ceylon and South India*, Mysore State Department of Public Health, Bulletin No. 15 (Bangalore: Government Press, 1939), p. 4. He was also to suggest that, 'One cannot escape the feeling that the permanent anti-malarial measures involving heavy capital outlay, most in evidence in Singapore, are gradually replaced by the recurrent measures like oiling, as one moves north towards Kedah', p. 14. See also Lt. Col. J. A. Sinton and Professor Raja Ram, *Man-made Malaria in India*, Health Bulletin No. 22, Malaria Bureau No. 10, 2nd ed. (Simla: Government of India Press, 1938).

137 SSR, *Labour Commission Report*, Evidence, p. 113.

138 Sel. Sec. 223/1901, para. 17.

139 IMR, *Studies from the Institute of Medical Research*, p. 119.

140 Sel. Sec. 254/1904.

141 Sel. Sec. 4369/1901.

142 Dr Freer, in Sel. Sec. 237/1901, pp. 4–5.

143 Sel. Sec. 133/1935.

144 Sel. Sec. 3973/1917.

145 Sel. Sec. 1248/1918, p. 1. There was pressure from some estates for an increased allocation of subsidised rice, although officers argued that if estate managers wanted to increase subsidised rice to labourers, they could do so by reducing their own family's allocation, see E. S. Hose, District Officer, Teluk Anson, in Sel. Sec. 755/1919, p. 6.

146 FMS, High Commission Despatch to Colonial Advisory Medical Committee, No. 102, 25 Nov 1941.

147 Cretch, *Malayan Mining Methods*, pp. 46–47.

148 R. C. Burgess, *The Nutrition of the Kampong Malays in the Coast District of Selangor.* Interim Report of the Standing Committee on Nutrition in Malaya (Kuala Lumpur: FMS Government Press, 1937); C. D. Williams, The life of a Malay child, *JMBMA* 2, 2 (1938): 73–81; C. D. Williams, Common diseases of children as seen in the General Hospital, Singapore, *JMBMA* 2, 3 (1938): 113–123; A. L. Hoops, Causes of death amongst southern Indian labour populations of Malacca rubber estates, *JMBMA* 3, 3 (1939): 213–227; R. A. Pallister, Some observations on deficiency diseases in Malaya, *JMBMA* 4, 2 (1940): 191–197.

149 Audrey I. Richards, *Hunger and Work in a Savage Tribe* (London: Routledge, 1932) and *Labour, Land and Diet in Northern Rhodesia. An economic study of the Bemboi tribe* (Oxford: Oxford University Press, 1939). For a comprehensive discussion of the interest in nutrition in the 1930s, see Michael Worboys, The discovery of colonial malnutrition between the wars, in Arnold (ed.), *Imperial Medicine and Indigenous Societies* (Manchester and New York: Manchester University Press, 1988), pp. 208–225.

150 GB, Economic Advisory Council, *Summary of Information regarding Nutrition*, p. 61.

151 *Ibid.*

152 *Ibid.*, pp. 60–61.

153 *Ibid.*

154 Sel. Sec. 135/1937. An inquiry by the Government of India, which sent a deputation to Malaya from 6 December 1936 to 1 January 1937, concluded that wages were no higher than they had been on some estates at the turn of the century, although they fluctuated.

155 Sel. Sec. 269/1906.

156 CO273/265/1900, p. 20.
157 Sel. Sec. 397/1932.
158 FMS, *Report of the Commission*, p. A 62.
159 Faris, Selangor Coast District Annual Report 1931, p. 15; Scharff, *A Note on Public Health Administration*.
160 IMR/MAB 38/1930, Selwyn Clarke, Chief Health Officer, Prevention of Malaria on Estates, 15 September 1930.
161 *SSAR 1923*, p. 93.
162 *FMSAR 1930*, p. 55.
163 *SSAR 1935*, vol. II, p. 162. Other commentators were less generous, although workers rather than employers were usually at fault. Cretch, *Malayan Mining Methods*, pp. 36–37, observed that '(o)n rubber estates the Tamil enjoys comparatively better housing than the Chinese on tin mines, there is no overcrowding and the sanitation is under European Supervision. Away from rubber estates the housing and sanitation of the Tamil is very bad. They appear to be naturally dirty both in regard to their person and habits. They spend as little as possible on food and they are therefore badly nourished and of very poor physique'.

6 Brothel politics and the bodies of women

1 Sections of this paper appear in L. Manderson, Migration, prostitution and medical surveillance in early twentieth-century Malaya, in L. Marks and M. Worboys (eds), *Migrants, Minorities and Medicine* (London: Routledge, in press). The focus of this chapter should not be taken to imply that women did not work in other capacities; as already indicated, the history of their roles as rubber tappers and labourers, as well as in the tertiary sector, has still to be written.
2 ZHCI 6737, Accounts and Papers v.lix, no. 29, 1904, Pahang, *Medical Report for the State of Pahang, 1901*, p. 350.
3 GB, *Contagious Diseases Regulations (Perak and Malay States), Copy of Correspondence relative to proposed introduction of Contagious Diseases Regulations in Perak or other Protected Malay States*, H.C.146 (London: HMSO, 1894), p. 10, F. A. Swettenham to Colonial Secretary, Straits Settlements, 16 September 1891.
4 GB, *Correspondence regarding the measures to be adopted for checking the spread of venereal disease, Ceylon, Hong Kong and Straits Settlements*, H.C.147, June 1894, C.9523 (London: HMSO, 1899), p. 75, Third day of Committee Proceedings, 12 May 1898.
5 CO273/261/1900, f. 328, A. H. Capper, Acting Protector of Chinese, Memorandum on Registration of Chinese prostitutes in the Federated Malay States, 6 April 1900, p. 9.
6 GB, *Correspondence*, p. 90, E. A. O. Travers, Memorandum by the State Surgeon, Selangor, May 1897.
7 CO273/261/1900, f. 324.
8 GB, *Contagious Diseases Regulations*, p. 10.
9 GB, *Correspondence*, p. 71.
10 S. E. Nicoll–Jones, *Report on the Problem of Prostitution in Singapore, 1940*, Mss Indian Ocean S27, p. 17.
11 CO273/2258/30403/1900, f. 41.
12 FMS, *Memorandum on the Protection of Chinese and other Asiatic Women and Girls* (Selangor: Government Press, 1900), p. 1; Great Britain, *Correspondence*, p. 79, Jane McBreen.

13 GB, *Correspondence*, p. 84, G. T. Hare, Secretary, Chinese Affairs, 12 June 1898.
14 GB, *Contagious Diseases Regulations*, p. 6, F. A. Swettenham to the Colonial
    Secretary, 16 September 1891.
15 GB, *Correspondence*, p. 79.
16 CO273/265/22834/1900, f. 838.
17 Sel. Sec. 1461/1885.
18 S. E. Nicoll-Jones, *Report on the Problem of Prostitution*, p. 28.
19 FMS, *Memorandum*, pp. 3–4.
20 CO273/261/1900, A. H. Capper, Memorandum. Registration of Chinese
    Prostitutes in the Federated Malay States, 6 April 1900.
21 GB, *Contagious Diseases Regulations*, p. 6; Great Britain, *Correspondence*, p. 68.
22 Sel. Sec. 4434/1893.
23 Sel. Sec. 375/1886, f. 4.
24 J. Warren, *Ah-Ku and Karayuki-san* (Singapore and New York: Oxford Uni-
    versity Press, 1993).
25 CO273/261, p. 17, f. 346.
26 *Ibid.*
27 *Ibid.*, p. 8, f. 337.
28 Sel. Sec. 1030/1913.
29 Sel. Sec. G1171/1928.
30 Residency Surgeon's Report, Sel. Sec. 5068/1890, f. 3.
31 Sel. Sec. 1018/1893, p. 2; Sel. Sec. 1985/1894.
32 GB, *Correspondence*, p. 89, E. A. O. Travers, Memorandum, May 1897.
33 Sel. Sec. 691/1885, f. 2.
34 Sel. Sec. 3080/1889, p. 1.
35 *Ibid.*, Sel. Sec. 5068/1890, f. 7–8; Sel. Sec. 5062/1894.
36 *Ibid.*, Sel. Sec. 2962/1894; Sel. Sec. 5068/1890.
37 Sel. Sec. 4459/1907, f. 1, list of brothels and number of cubicles, 13 August
    1907; Memorandum (no folio number), S. Hose to Protector of Chinese,
    19 August 1909. According to A. M. Pountney, Acting Protector of Chinese
    in Selangor and Negri Sembilan, around 60 percent of prostitutes (in 1907)
    paid rent for these cubicles, Sel. Sec. 2735/1907, Memorandum, A. M.
    Pountney, 15 May 1907.
38 GB, *Correspondence*, p. 65, Dr Mugliston Colonial Surgeon, is only one ex-
    ample, although the more common metaphor was 'slave' or 'chattel'.
39 Sel. Sec. 657/1884.
40 Sel. Sec. 1018/1893; Sel. Sec. 4434/1893.
41 Sel. Sec. 6054/1894; Sel. Sec. 1695/1895.
42 Sel. Sec. 1985/1894.
43 GB, *Correspondence*, p. 81, F. A. Swettenham to the High Commissioner, 23
    August 1898.
44 *Ibid.*, p. 85, G. T. Hare, Memorandum, 12 June 1898.
45 Sel. Sec. 4903/1902.
46 GB, *Contagious Diseases Regulations*, p. 7.
47 *Ibid.*
48 Sel. Sec. 2435/1925, Minutes sheet, 13 July 1925.
49 Sel. Sec. 3080/1889; CO273/278/884/1900, ff. 157–162.
50 Sel. Sec. 167/1886.
51 CO273/277/37833/1901, ff. 278–279.
52 CO273/278/884/1902, ff. 156–157.
53 For a meticulous ethnohistory of women sex workers in Singapore, see J. F.
    Warren, *Ah-Ku and Karayuki-san*; also his Prostitution in Singapore society

278 NOTES (PAGES 176–182)

and the *Karayuki-san*, in P. J. Rimmer and L. M. Allen (eds), *The Underside of Malaysian History: Pullers, Prostitutes, Plantation Workers* (Singapore: Singapore University Press, 1990), pp. 161–176.
54 GB, *Correspondence*, p. 86.
55 CO273/265, No. 22834/1900, f. 838.
56 D. Galloway, On inguinal lymphadenitis, *MMJ* 1, 1 (1926): 1–6. See Edward Shorter, *The History of Women's Bodies* (New York: Basic Books, 1982) for an account of the gynaecological gaze at this time.
57 Sel. Sec. 2735/1907; also CO273/258/30403/1900.
58 GB, *Correspondence*, p. 87, Memorandum by Dr J. Welch, District Surgeon, Selangor, 21 April 1897.
59 *Ibid.*, pp. 52–53, 87.
60 Straits Settlements Association, Minute Book 11 August 1887–21 February 1899, Adamson, Chairman of the SSA, to Chamberlain, Secretary of State for the Colonies, 8 November 1897, Table A.
61 This estimate of 50 percent infection among prisoners was one sustained into the twentieth century, see e.g. CO273/270/34212/1901, f. 245.
62 GB, *Correspondence*, p. 87.
63 D. Galloway, On inguinal lymphadenitis 1.
64 CO273/262/25598/1900, f. 100, *Medical Report for Selangor, 1900*.
65 For example, a man with bubo (swollen lymph nodes) would be described as suffering from adenitis, CO273/263/3482/1900, f. 281, S. C. G. Fox to Acting State Surgeon, Perak, 17 September 1900.
66 Straits Settlements Association, Minute Book 11 August 1887–21 February 1899, pp. 4, 7.
67 GB, *Correspondence*, p. 87.
68 CO273/1018/1893, f. 3.
69 GB, *Correspondence*, p. 56, Report of the Committee.
70 *Ibid.*, pp. 55–56; also CO273/261, f. 358, A. H. Capper, Acting Protector of Chinese, Memorandum 6 April 1900.
71 GB, *Correspondence*, p. 46.
72 GB, *Correspondence*, p. 47.
73 Sel. Sec. 1731/1903, E. A. O. Travers, State Surgeon, Selangor, Memorandum on private medical examination of inmates of brothels and establishment of private hospitals, 14 April 1903, p. 1.
74 *Ibid.*, p. 73.
75 *Ibid.*, pp. 49, 62.
76 *Ibid.*, p. 113, Gan Eng Seng, Memorandum, 20 February 1899; see also other enclosures, pp. 111–114.
77 CO273/256/4829/1900.
78 CO273/258/30403/1900, f. 39.
79 CO273/256/4829/1900, ff. 56–57.
80 CO273/258/30403/1900, f. 40.
81 GB, *Correspondence*, p. 115.
82 CO273/256/4829/1900, f. 56, Report by the Acting Colonial Surgeon (E. W. von Tunzelmann) on the working in Singapore of Ordinance XIII of 1899, 15 January 1900.
83 *Ibid.*, pp. 7–9, Report, T. C. Mugliston, 3 April 1895; Report, G. T. Hare, 12 September 1894.
84 CO273/256/4829/1900, ff. 57–58.
85 *Ibid.*, f. 59, Table 2.
86 Sel. Sec. 4902/1902, British Resident, 29 September 1902.

87 Sel. Sec. 4902/1902, GB, *Correspondence*, p. 86.
88 Sel. Sec. 4902/1902.
89 *Ibid.*, f. 3.
90 *Ibid.*
91 CO273/339/G1121, FMS 9181/1908, f. 230A, Evans, Chinese Protector in Singapore.
92 Sel. Sec. 1731/1903.
93 Sel.Sec. 1731/1903, f. 3.
94 *Ibid.*, f. 4.
95 CO273/339/FMS 4535/1908, f. 74–77.
96 CO2732/339/FMS 4535/1908, f. 73.
97 CO273/339/G1121/FMS4535/198, Dr Travers' Private Hospital, f. 56.
98 CO273/339/FMS 4535/1908, f. 79.
99 *Ibid.*
100 CO273/339/G1121/FMS 11053/1908, f. 65, Brockman to High Commissioner, FMS, 6 January 1908, p. 4.
101 CO273/340/G1122/FMS 16686/1908, ff. 108–125, Conduct of Mr Birch.
102 CO273/339/FMS 11053/1908, f. 317; CO273/340/FMS 16686/1908, f. 86.
103 CO273/339/FMA 11053/1908, f. 442, f. 465.
104 Sel. Sec. 2078/1906. Signatories included Travers, the State Surgeon of Selangor; G. F. Leicester, Acting Director of the IMR, A. J. McClosky, W. Fletcher, M. Watson, J. R. Delmege, and H. M. Harrison, District Surgeons respectively of Selangor, Kuala Lumpur, Klang, Ulu Selangor and Pekan; and W. L. Braddon, W. S. Milne, P. N. Gerrard, J. E. M. Brown, M. P. Meldrum, R. Dowden, J. G. D. Cooper, S. C. G. Fox, W. H. Fry, and A. A. Woods.
105 Sel. Sec. 2152/1906, Federal Secretary, FMS to British Resident, Selangor, 3 July 1906.
106 L. M. Woodward, *Commission of Inquiry into the Conduct of Government Medical Officers, Report* (Kuala Lumpur: Government Printing Office, 1908).
107 CO273/339/FMS 9181/1908, ff. 207–209.
108 CO273/339/FMS 9181/1908, f. 220.
109 *Ibid.*, f. 197. Fox himself wrote to Connolly: 'Regarding the Chinese Prostitutes of Papan or of anywhere else, you know as well as I do that, if unsolicited these women are not in the habit of writing to anyone new to come and visit them regularly. You cannot get over the fact that these Papan prostitutes have been and are all my patients for the last 3½ years', CO273/339/FMS 11053/1908, f. 386, Fox to Connolly, 21 July 1906.
110 CO273/339/FMS 9181/1908.
111 *Ibid.*, f. 221.
112 CO273/339/FMS 9181/1908, ff. 228–229, Exhibit to Commission of Inquiry, Brothel Keepers of Kampar, 14 October 1906, emphasis in the original; Testimony from Brothel Keepers of Papan, 17 October 1906.
113 CO273/339/FMS 11053/1908, f. 422.
114 *Ibid.*, f. 406.
115 *Ibid.*, ff. 386–392, 428.
116 *Ibid.*, ff. 270–271.
117 CO273/339/FMS 11053/1908, f. 423.
118 *Ibid.*, ff. 384, 436.
119 *Ibid.*, ff. 361–370; CO273/340/FMS 16686/1908, f. 72.
120 CO273/339/FMS 11053/1908, f. 418.
121 CO273/340/FMS 16686/1908, f. 120.

122 Sel. Sec. 5405/1907, Circular 20/1907 (Private Practice of Government Medical Officers), 27 September 1907.
123 Sel. Sec. 5404/1907.
124 See for example Sel. Sec. Misc. 6334/1893; Sel. Sec. 4466/1891.
125 Sel. Sec. 769/1918, f. 2; also Sel. Sec. 1030/1913; Sel. Sec. 0672/1915; Sel. Sec. 1006/1916, f. 4.
126 Sel. Sec. 1030/1913, f. 4.
127 CO273/258/30403/1900, ff. 38–41.
128 Sel. Sec. 769/1918, Chinese Secretariat, Annual Report, 1917, p. 2.
129 S.E.Nicoll-Jones, *Report*.
130 Sel. Sec. 861/1940, f. 8.
131 Sel. Sec. 6860/1893; Sel. Sec. 2100/1902.
132 Sel. Sec. 838/1932, f. 3.
133 Sel. Sec. 2111/1907, f. 2.
134 Sel. Sec. 2374/1911; Sel. Sec. 2950/1911.
135 Sel. Sec. 1879/1911; Sel. Sec. 5419/1911.
136 Sel. Sec. 838/1932.
137 Sel. Sec. 1852/1912.
138 Sel. Sec. 902/1911.
139 Sel. Sec. 5419/1911.
140 Sel. Sec. 2374/1911.
141 Sel. Sec. 1879/1911.
142 Sel. Sec. 3532/1914; Sel. Sec. 2374/1911.
143 Sel. Sec. 1027/1914.
144 Sel. Sec. 1879/1911, f. 4.
145 Sel. Sec. 2950/1911.
146 BA Kel 263/1917, f.3.
147 G. Hutchinson, *Rubber planting in Malaya, 1928–1932*, BAM III/15, pp. 41–42.
148 For background to the international context, see Paul Weindling, The politics of international co-ordination to combat sexually transmitted diseases, 1900–1980s, in V. Berridge and P. Strong (eds), *AIDS in Contemporary History* (Cambridge: Cambridge University Press, forthcoming); Bridget A. Towers, Health education policy 1916–1926: Venereal disease and the prophylaxis dilemma, *Medical History* 24, 1 (1980), pp. 70–87. International and regional meetings, including the International Congresses for the Suppression of Traffic in Women and Children and Imperial Social Hygiene Congresses, maintained pressure on the Colonial Office and its responsible governments.
149 Files of the League of Nations, Health Committee 12B/12345/5923 (1921), VD in Seaports, f. 14–15.
150 *ST* 13 January 1921, p. 8; 19 January 1921, p. 8; 24 January 1921, p. 8
151 Straits Settlements, *First Report of the Advisory Committee on Social Hygiene*, No. 48 of 1925, in Sel. Sec. 3830/1925; Sel. Sec. 4825/1925.
152 Anon., Social hygiene and the Federated Malay States, *Health and Empire* II, 4 (1927): 259; *ST* 25 August 1925, p. 11. For example, asymptomatic infections, constant reinfection of 'cured' women, and an illusion of security that medical checks would give to clients, Sel. Sec. 3830/1925.
153 E. B. Turner, British Social Hygiene Council notes, *Health and Empire* I, 4 (1926), p. 328.
154 Malinowski was a member, and both Raymond Firth and Audrey Richards represented him on occasions when he was unavailable.

155 Anon., Editorial comments, *Health and Empire* I, 1 (1926), p. 3; Sel. Sec. 4147/1926.
156 Anon., Social hygiene and the Federated Malay States, p. 261; R. W. C. Kelly, Social hygiene work in Singapore, *Health and Empire* IV, 1 (1929), p. 47.
157 Anon., British Social Hygiene Council, Imperial Conference, September 27th, 1928 (Report of proceedings), *Health and Empire* III, 4 (1928): 267; *SSAR 1927*; Kelly, Social hygiene work, pp. 50–51.
158 Sel. Sec. 546/1923.
159 Anon., Social hygiene and the Federated Malay States, pp. 257–258.
160 *Ibid.*, pp. 258–259.
161 *FMSAR 1925*; *FMSAR 1927*.
162 *FMSAR 1925*.
163 E. O. Grant, Fifth Imperial Social Hygiene Congress. Summary of Proceedings, *Health and Empire* VI, 3 (1931), p. 218.
164 Sel. Sec. G1203/1931, f. 64.
165 Douglas White, The Straits Settlements Ordinance, October 1930, *Health and Empire* VI, 1 (1931): 18–21. White recognised that this did not deal with the problem of 'sly' prostitution, which some people, such as Chen Su Lan, a Singapore medical practitioner, estimated to exceed the number of known prostitutes fourfold. Chen however maintained that the two were correlated, that is that the legal toleration of brothels encouraged sly prostitution and that concomitantly, the end of registered brothels would lead to a decrease in sly brothels also; see Anon., Points for speakers, *Health and Empire* VI, 1 (1931), p. 79.
166 Sel. Sec. G2411/1931, f. 1.
167 G. Hutchinson, *Rubber Planting*, p. 42.
168 Sel. Sec. G485/1930, f. 1.
169 *Ibid.*, f. 3, P. T. Allen, Secretary of Chinese Affairs, 10 March 1930.
170 Sel. Sec. G477/1929; Sel. Sec. G2103/1931, f. 64.
171 Sel. Sec. G477/1929, Tan Hock Choon, Ipoh, to Chief Secretary, Kuala Lumpur, 22 December 1928.

7 Domestic lives

1 See Y. K. Lee's history of smallpox and vaccination in early Singapore (entries in References). There is some evidence of parental resistance to vaccination, see BA Kel 263/1917.
2 Margaret Pelling makes this point especially with respect to older children, since government attention focused on the health of infants and paid little attention to the illnesses of older children or to their care, see M. Pelling, Child health as a social value in early modern England, *SHM* 1, 2 (1988): 135–164.
3 Anna Davin, Imperialism and motherhood, *History Workshop* 5 (1978): 11.
4 *Ibid.*, pp. 10–11; Jane Lewis, *The Politics of Motherhood: Child and maternal welfare in England, 1900–1939*, (London: Croom Helm, 1980); Jane Lewis, The social history of social policy: infant welfare in Edwardian England, *Journal of Social Policy* 9 (1980): 403–486; Milton Lewis, The 'health of the race' and infant health in New South Wales: perspectives on medicine and empire, in MacLeod and Lewis (eds), *Disease, Medicine, and Empire. Perspectives on Western medicine and the experience of European expansion* (London and New York: Routledge, 1988), p. 307. See also S. Szreter, The GRO and the Public Health Movement, *SHM* 4, 3 (1991): 459.

5 In Fiji, concern with the infant mortality rate and the dramatic depopulation of the islands led to an inquiry that predates these developments, and a committee appointed to inquire into these matters reported in 1896. See Nicholas Thomas, Sanitation and seeing: The creation of state power in early colonial Fiji, *Comparative Studies in Social History* 32 (1990):153–158.

6 Sel. Sec. 3006/1915, J. T. Clarke, Report on Conference of the National Association for the Prevention of Infant Mortality and for the Welfare of Infancy, London, 4–5 August 1913, p. 4.

7 See also L. Manderson, Blame, responsibility and remedial action: death, disease and the infant in early twentieth century Malaya, pp. 257–282; Political economy and the politics of gender: Primary health care in colonial Malaya, in Paul Cohen and John Purcal (eds), *The Political Economy of Primary Health Care in Southeast Asia* (Bangkok: Australian Development Studies Network and the ASEAN Training Centre for Primary Health Care Development, 1989), pp. 76–94; Women and the state: maternal and child health in colonial Malaya, in V. Fildes, L. Marks and H. Marland (eds), *Women and Children First: International maternal and infant welfare 1870–1950* (London: Routledge, 1992), pp. 154–177; and Colonising Reproduction: Motherhood and maternity in early twentieth-century Malaya, in M. Jolly and K. Ram (eds), *Maternity in Colonial and Post-Colonial Asia and the Pacific*, (forthcoming).

8 Sel. Sec. 1754/1915, Sansom, Memorandum, 14 December 1914, p. 2; Ian D. Gebbie, Some aspects of the venereal disease problem in the Federated Malay States, with a serological survey of Indian labourers, *BMJ* 1 (4 March 1939): 438–441.

9 *SSAR 1909*, p. 469; around 20 percent were from neonatal tetanus.

10 S. Szreter, The GRO and the Public Health Movement, pp. 459–60.

11 Sel. Sec. 1476/1907, Acting Chairman of the Sanitary Board, Kuala Lumpur, 12 March 1907.

12 Sel. Sec. 3006/1915, Memorandum, Sheet no. 4.

13 *ST* 22 May 1907, p. 8.

14 For example, *SSAR 1904*, p. 731, the Maternity Hospital was closed from 23 March–23 May following a case of septicaemia; *SSAR 1908*, p. 538, the maternity ward of the General Hospital was closed for renovation.

15 Singapore Malay rituals c.1949–1950 are described in Judith Djamour, *Malay Kinship and Marriage in Singapore* (London: Athlone Press, 1965 [1st pub. 1959]), pp. 89–92. See also K. B. Kuah, Malay customs in relation to childbirth, *MJM* 15.2220 27, 2 (1972): 81–84; Paul C. Y. Chen, An analysis of customs related to childbirth in rural Malay culture, *Tropical Geography and Medicine* 25 (1973): 197–204, and for Trengganu practices in the 1970s, Carol Laderman, *Wives and Midwives: Childbirth and nutrition in rural Malaysia* (Berkeley: University of California Press, 1983). For an overview and summary of various confinement practices, see L. Manderson, Roasting, smoking and dieting in response to birth: Malay confinement in cross-cultural perspective, *SSM* 15B (1981): 509–520.

16 J. A. Kempe, *Perak Administration Report for the year 1932* (Kuala Lumpur: Government Printing Office, 1933), p. 6.

17 J. Lewis, *The Politics of Motherhood*; Ann Oakley, Wisewoman and medicine man; for the US see B. Ehrenreich and D. English, *Witches, midwives and nurses: A history of women healers* (Old Westbury, NY: Feminist Press, 1973).

18 W. Williams, Puerperal mortality, *Transactions of the Epidemiological Society of London* XV (New Series, 1895–1896): 100–133.
19 *SSAR 1905*, pp. 232, 715.
20 W. Williams, Puerperal mortality, p. 103, provides figures for the period 1847–1894 for England and Wales to illustrate the steady decline in the maternal death rate from accidents of childbirth such as haemorrhage and placenta praevia (as well as a few unclear causes such as 'puerperal mania') (3.01 per 1,000 live births in 1847–1854 to 2.41 in 1885–1894). Over the same period, however, deaths from puerperal fever rose (1.72 to 2.53 women dying per 1,000 births), a clear indicator of risks of infection in hospitals.
21 *SSAR 1904*, p. 482.
22 Sel. Sec. 3006/1915, Clarke, 10 July 1914, p. 13. See also L. Manderson, Blame, responsibility and remedial action, pp. 264 ff. and L. Manderson, Women and the state, p. 158.
23 CO859/154/12402/11, 1947–8.
24 Sel. Sec. 3006/1915, Memorandum, Sheet no. 4.
25 Sel. Sec. 1754/1915, ff. 3, 5.
26 *Ibid.*, f. 35.
27 Files of the Institute of Medical Research, IMR 59/1923, 2.
28 L. Manderson, Women and the state, p. 160; H. G. R. Leonard, *Annual Report on the Social and Economic Progress of the People of Pahang for the year 1931* (Kuala Lumpur: Government Printing Office, 1932), p. 4.
29 Carson, *Kedah and Perlis. Annual Report of the Medical Department for 1938* (Alor Star: Kedah Government Press, 1940), p. 6.
30 *SSAR/FMSAR 1937*, p. 44.
31 R. M. MacGregor, *Annual Reports of the Medical Departments, Straits Settlements and Federated Malay States for the year 1937* (Singapore: Government Printing Office, 1938), p. 44.
32 Sel. Sec. G2142/1931.
33 E. W. Darville, *Maternity and child welfare work in Penang, 1927–35, 1935–41.* Lectures given at the London School of Hygiene and Tropical Medicine, Mss Indian Ocean S134, p. 19.
34 A. J. Sturrock, *Annual Report of the British Adviser, Trengganu, for the years A.H.1346 and 1347 (30 June 1927–18 June 1928; 19 June 1928–7 June 1929)* (Singapore: Government Printing Office, 1929), p. 10.
35 CO859/1/1201/19, 1939, p. 7.
36 L. W. Evans, *Kelantan. Annual Report of the Medical Department for 1930* (Penang: Criterion Press, 1931), p. 16.
37 J. Portelly, *Kedah and Perlis. Annual Report for the Medical Department, 1936* (Alor Star: Kedah Government Press, 1937), p. 2.
38 CO859/46/12101/3D, p. 7, Medical Education, Committee on Training of Nurses for Colonial Territories, Minutes of the 4th meeting, 9 March 1944, Dr Mabel Brodie.
39 J. Portelly, *Kedah and Perlis. Annual Report of the Medical Department for 1937* (Alor Star: Kedah Government Press, 1938), p. ii.
40 CO859/46/12101/3D, p. 7, Dr Brodie.
41 J. C. Carson, p. 6
42 From 1927 Asian women began to work as nurses in general hospitals in the FMS, and the gradual increase of women presenting to outpatients departments was attributed to this, *FMSAR 1927*, p. 55.
43 Sel. Sec. G118/1937.

44 Sel. Sec. 3006/1915, Memorandum, 6 June 1915.
45 Celia Davies, The Health Visitor as mother's friend: A woman's place in public health, 1900–1914, *SHM* 1, 1 (1988): 39–59; Simon Szreter, The importance of social intervention in Britain's mortality decline c. 1850–1914: A re-interpretation of the role of public health. *SHM* 1, 1 (1988): 1–37.
46 Davies, The Health Visitor as mother's friend, p. 44.
47 *SSAR 1936*, vol. II, p. 952.
48 Sel. Sec. 3006/1915, ff. 11–12.
49 CO859/46/12101/3D, p. 6.
50 Sel. Sec. 3006/1915, f. 13.
51 SSR, *Proceedings and Report*, p. B 84.
52 FMS, *Report of the Commission*, p. B 24, J. H. Ponnampalam.
53 Sel. Sec. 3156/1915, p. 20.
54 CO859/46/12101/4A, 1943, f. 6.
55 See Davin, Imperialism and motherhood, pp. 47–48; for details of Truby King's ideas see Philippa Mein Smith, 'That welfare warfare': sectarianism in infant welfare in Australia, 1918–1939, in V. Fildes, L. Marks and H. Marland (eds), *Women and Children First: International maternal and infant welfare 1870–1950* (London: Routledge, 1992), pp. 230–256.
56 *SSAR 1933*, vol. II, p. 945.
57 L. Manderson, Infant feeding practice, market expansion, and the patterning of choice, Southeast Asia, 1880–1980, *New Doctor* 26 (1982):27–32; L. Manderson, Bottle feeding and ideology in colonial Malaya: the production of change, *IJHS* 12 (1982): 597–616.
58 Sel. Sec. 1307/1908, f. 4.
59 *ST* 2 May 1907, p. 7; *SSAR 1910*, p. 581; Sel. Sec. 3006/1915, f. 9.
60 Sel. Sec. 3006/1915, p. 9; Carson, *Kedah and Perlis*, p. 6.
61 See L. Manderson, Roasting, smoking and dieting; P/KES/K/1, *Kedah and Perlis Annual Report 1938*, p. 43.
62 *SSAR 1910*, p. 581.
63 T. F. Strang, *State of Kelantan. Annual Report of the Medical Department for the Year 1936* (Kota Bharu: Cheong Fatt Press, 1936), p. 15.
64 The Singapore Children's Welfare Society was a voluntary organisation of expatriate and local elite women, which ran the clinics and conducted home visiting from 1923–33; it suspended all services in 1935 due to lack of funds, see *SSAR 1935*, p. 844.
65 *ST* 27 April 1926, p. 10.
66 L. Manderson, Women and the state, pp. 164–168; and Carson, *Kedah and Perlis*, p. 7.
67 *Ibid.*, *ST* 6 February 1925, p. 8.
68 *SSAR 1926*, pp. 423–434; L. Manderson, Blame, responsibility and remedial action, pp. 274–275.
69 *FMSAR 1926*, p. 38.
70 D. Bridges, *Kedah and Perlis*, p. 7; CO859/46/12101/32, p. 2.
71 In 1939, a total of 35 lady doctors were employed in the Colonial Medical Services, fifteen of whom were in the settlements and states of Malaya. Malaya also had the most nurses (178 of a total of 800, followed by Hong Kong with 66), and after Hong Kong had the most female teachers, including two senior education officers and 19 school mistresses of a total 94 women posted from Britain. See CO859/1/1201/19, 1939, ACEC (Advisory Committee on Education in the Colonies) 5/1939, 'Teaching of

Domestic Science in England and its application to work in the colonies', 21 April 1937.

72 *FMSAR 1904*, p. 7.
73 *FMSAR 1932*, p. 13, for example.
74 J. Lewis, *The Politics of Motherhood*, p. 33. In England and Wales, the rate was around five from 1910 through to the mid-1930s, excepting only 1918–19 when it jumped as a result of the influenza epidemic and an outbreak of sepsis ('puerperal fever'). While far more women died of tuberculosis, maternal mortality was the second cause of death of women aged 15–44, pp. 36–37.
75 D. Bridges, *Kedah and Perlis*, p. 12.
76 *SSAR 1936*, pp. 949–951.
77 *SSAR 1936*, vol. I, p. 920.
78 This compares with an estimated rate of less than four in the UK at this time; *FMSAR 1936*, p. 10.
79 FMS/P/KES/K.1, *Kedah and Perlis Annual Report (1928–29)*, p. 12.
80 See, for example, *FMSAR 1926*, p. 35, which comments on the poor health of Tamil women and their children's poor physique; IMR 54/1931, pp. 22–23; *FMSAR 1937*, p. 10.
81 CO859/53/12257/5, 1941
82 Loretta Brabin and Bernard J. Brabin, Parasitic infections in women and their consequences, *Advances in Parasitology* 31 (1992): 1–81. See also N. J. White and D. A. Warrell, The management of severe malaria, in W. H. Wernsdorfer and I. A. McGregor (eds), *Malaria. Principles and Practice of Malariology*, vol. I (Edinburgh: Churchill Livingstone, 1988), p. 865.
83 *SSAR 1910*, p. 581.
84 In general, the curriculum was not dissimilar to that given to working-class girls in the UK at around the same time, see A. Davin, Imperialism and motherhood, p. 26, and her account of the School for Mothers, pp. 38–43. See also Great Britain, Ministry of Agriculture and Fisheries, *The Practical Education of Women for Rural Life*. Report of the Sub-Committee of the Interdepartmental Committee of the Ministry of Agriculture and Board of Education (Chaired by Lady Denham) (London: HMSO, 1928).
85 Sel. Sec. 1307/1908, p. 4.
86 L. Manderson, The development and direction of female education in Peninsular Malaysia, *JMBRAS* LI (1978): 100–122; *SSAR 1928*, p. 770.
87 *SSAR 1927*, p. 730. At the time Brooke was concurrently Health Officer in Singapore and Director of the Eastern Bureau of the League of Nations Health Committee.
88 Sel. Sec. 2056/1914; CO859/1/1201/19, 1939.
89 H. G. R. Leonard, *Annual Report on the Social and Economic Progress of the People of Pahang for the Year 1931* (Kuala Lumpur: FMS Government Printing Office, 1932), pp. 28–29.
90 *SSAR 1928*, p. 770.
91 Sel. Sec. G544/1937, f. 17.
92 CO859/4/1241/A, 1939, p. 3.
93 Mary Blacklock, Certain aspects of the welfare of women and children in the colonies, *ATMP* 30 (1936): 221–264.
94 *Ibid.*, p. 261.
95 CO859/89/12065/1, 1944, f. 1.
96 Fabian Colonial Bureau, *Hunger and Health in the Colonies* (London: Fabian Colonial Bureau and Gollancz, 1944), p. 22. Not all agreed. Drummond Shiels, former Undersecretary of State for the Colonies, argued that the

employment of women within the colonial administration might be valuable with respect to other wider issues affecting women and children (for instance, conditions of employment, the traffic in women and children, and so on), but that women would 'complicate' the general administrative work of the colonies; he described the colonial administration, which did not recruit women, as 'one of the last citadels to withstand the assaults of the conquering sex' and observed that the 'economic situation' (i.e. the Depression) had 'saved the position for the exclusionists', p. 327. See Drummond Shiels, Social hygiene and human welfare. The task of colonial administration, *Health and Empire* VII, 4 (1933): 319–331.

97 CO859/1/1201/19, SCWE 9/1939, p. 3.
98 *Ibid.*, p. 6.
99 CO859/1/SCWE6/39, p. 1.
100 *Ibid.*
101 *Ibid.*, Education. Advisory Committee. Sub-committee on education and welfare of women and girls, p. 2.
102 CO859/20/12001/10, p. 3.
103 See also L. Manderson, Political economy and the politics of gender.
104 Davies, The Health Visitor, p. 57.
105 CO859/46/12101/4A, 1943, ff. 7–8.
106 Blacklock, Certain aspects of the welfare of women, p. 224.
107 Davin, Imperialism and motherhood, p. 26.
108 CO953/2/51032, 1948, p. 7, 19 December 1947.
109 Paul C. Y. Chen, Providing maternal and child health care in rural Malaysia, *Tropical Geography and Medicine* 29 (1977): 441–448; Malaysian Medical Association, *The Future of Health Services in Malaysia* (Kuala Lumpur: Malaysian Medical Association, 1980), pp. 23–25.

8 Conclusion: The moral logic of colonial medicine

1 Following J. Habermas, *Communication and the Evolution of Society* (London: Heinemann, 1979), p. 195.
2 Gauri Viswanathan, *Masks of Conquest. Literary Study and British Rule in India* (London: Faber and Faber, 1990), p. 165, my emphasis. Her book is a compelling discussion of the paradoxes of education under colonialism.
3 Roy MacLeod, Introduction, in MacLeod and Lewis (eds), *Disease, Medicine, and Empire. Perspectives on Western Medicine and the Experience of European Expansion* (London and New York: Routledge, 1988), p. 1.
4 Certainly for those trained during the first half of the twentieth century, see Y. K. Lee, Medical education in the Straits: *1786–1871, JMBRAS* 46, 1 (1973): 103–122.
5 CO859/46/12101/4A, 1943, f. 16.
6 M. Vaughan, *Curing their Ills*, p. 39.
7 P. N. Gerrard, *On the Hygienic Management of Labour in the Tropics* (Singapore: Methodist Publishing House, 1913), p. 1.
8 Major G. St J. Orde-Browne, Some problems of recruited labour, *Health and Empire* XII, 3 (1937): 208–218.
9 CO859/42/12001/11, 1941; CO859/46/12101/4A, 1943.
10 Carol Smart, Disruptive bodies and unruly sex: the regulation of reproduction and sexuality in the nineteenth century, in Carol Smart (ed.), *Regulating Womanhood. Historical essays on marriage, motherhood and sexuality* (London and New York: Routledge, 1992), p. 12. Colonial officers were not

unreflexive in this regard. In 1935, J. W. Scharff, then Registrar of Births and Deaths in the Straits Settlements, pointed out that '(t)he value of health activities, particularly in the direction of child welfare work, can never be expressed completely in terms of mathematics', *SSAR 1935*, pp. 523–524.

11 *SSAR 1928*, p. 785 (Paul F. Russell and Clark H. Yeager, Extracts from the Straits Settlements Rural Sanitation Survey and Campaign Final Report and Tables, 1925–1928). For a detailed discussion of the campaign, see L. Manderson, Race, colonial mentality and public health, pp. 206–210.

12 See L. Manderson, Health services, in which I explore the application of Habermas' notion of legitimation. This is also what members of the Colonial Advisory Committee thought when they met during the war years, and a statement on medical policy notes that '(t)he medical services should be conceived as part of a co-operative effort for improving the well-being of the community ... It follows that progress of medical activities should form an integral part of a general plan for social welfare', CO859/46/12101/4A, 1943, f. 1, 10 December 1943.

13 The medical and pharmacological taxonomic work of the Botanic Gardens in Singapore, in addition to its more conventional botanic research, is of interest here, see I. H. Burkhill and M. Haniff, Malay village medicine, *Garden Bulletin* 6, 2 (1930); Ismail Munshi, *The Medical Book of Malayan Medicine*, ed. with notes by J. D. Gimlette and determinations of drugs by I. H. Burkhill (Singapore: Botanic Gardens, 1930); D. Hooper, *On Chinese medicine* (Singapore: Botanic Gardens, 1929).

14 *FMSAR 1905*, pp. 36–37, Abstract of a report presented to H.M. Secretary of State for the Colonies, 8 May 1904.

15 M. Vaughan, *Curing their Ills*, p. 6.

16 This is a point that Nicholas Thomas, in Sanitation and seeing, p. 157, makes, when he notes also the association of vice, disease and disorder, and the importance of description and regulation in the creation of order in the sanitising projects of the late nineteenth century.

17 See N. Thomas, Sanitation and seeing, p. 160, on the operationalisation of 'crowding' in colonial Fiji.

18 *SSAR 1928*, pp. 778–779.

19 See Robert Winzeler's account of the cultural construction of madness in colonial Malaya in his Malayan *amok* and *latah* as 'history bound' syndromes, in P. J. Rimmer and L. M. Allen (eds), *The Underside of Malaysian History*, pp. 214–229.

20 CO273/267, p. 144.

21 *SSAR 1906*, p. 354. For papers on the institutional history of leprosy and developments, in terms of treatment and control, to the present, see A. Joshua-Raghavar, *Leprosy in Malaysia. Past, present and future* (edited by K. Rajagopalan), (Sungai Buluh, Selangor: A. Joshua-Raghavar, 1983).

22 F. G. Bourne, *Coroner's Annual Report*, p. 5.

23 League of Nations, Health Organisation, *Report of the Intergovernmental Conference of Far-Eastern Countries on Rural Hygiene*, A19.1937.III (III.Health. 1937.III.17) (Geneva: League of Nations, 1937); League of Nations, Health Organisation, *Report of the Malayan Delegation. Preparatory Paper for Intergovernmental Conference of Far Eastern Countries on Rural Hygiene*, CH.1235 (c) (Geneva: League of Nations, 1937). For a description of the interest in the nutritional status of colonial subjects in this period, see Worboys, The

discovery of colonial malnutrition, in D. Arnold (ed.), *Imperial Medicine and Indigenous Societies* (Manchester and New York: Manchester University Press, 1988).

24 A. H. Cretch, *Malayan Mining Methods*, p. 93.
25 B. A. Rao, *Malaria Control in Malaya, Java, Ceylon and South India*, pp. 12–13.
26 K. C. Blackwell, *Malay Curry*, p. 60; GB, Economic Advisory Council, *Nutrition in the Colonial Empire*, (London: HMSO, 1939).
27 D. Shiels, Social hygiene and human welfare, *Health and Empire* VII, 4 (1933): 319–331.
28 R. C. Burgess, *The Nutrition of the Kampong Malays in the Coast District of Selangor.* Interim Report of the Standing Committee on Nutrition in Malaya (Kuala Lumpur: FMS Government Press, 1937); Vickers and Strahan, *A Health Survey of the State of Kedah*, p. 60.
29 *Ibid.*, p. 60.
30 G. A. de C. de Moubray, *Letter 17 January 1967, Jersey, to I. Lloyd Philips, describing achievement as administrative officer in Malaya, 1920–1946*, Mss Indian Ocean S159.
31 CO859/31/12415/1, 1940, Malaria Advisory Board, Malay States, f. 1.
32 GB, Economic Advisory Council, *Nutrition in the Colonial Empire*, pp. 40–45.
33 CO859/46/12101/3D, no folio no., Memorandum by Dr Mary Blacklock, Nursing problems in the colonies and methods adopted to deal with them.
34 CO859/19/7595/1939, notes on file, ff. 4, 12.
35 *Ibid.*, note on file, no folio no., A. J. Dawe, 12 January 1940.
36 *Ibid.*, note on file, no folio no., Sir George Macdonald, 14 January 1940.

References

Note: See also Archival sources p. 308; Abbreviations p. x.

Aaby, Peter, Lessons from the past: Third World evidence and the reinterpretation of developed world mortality declines, *HTR* 2, Supp. (1992): 155–183.

Aaby, Peter, Social and behavioural factors affecting transmission and severity of measles infection, in J. C. Caldwell, S. Findley, P. Caldwell, G. Santow *et al.* (eds), *What We Know about Health Transition: the cultural, social and behavioural determinants of health* (Canberra: Health Transition Centre, Australian National University, 1990), pp. 826–842.

Aaby, P., J. Bukh, I. M. Lisse and A. J. Smits, Overcrowding and intensive exposure as determinants of measles mortality, *AJE.* 120 (1984): 49–63.

Allgrove, Joe, Some recollections of rubber estate life in Malaya from 1920 to 1953, Ms., files of the British Association of Malaya, BAM III/16.

Amsterdamska, O., Medical and biological constraints: early research on variation in bacteriology, *SSS* 17 (1987): 657–687.

Anderson, Warwick, Immunities of Empire: Race, disease and the new tropical medicine, 1900–1920, unpublished manuscript, History of Science Department, Harvard University, 1993.

Anon., Editorial comments, *Health and Empire* I, 1 (1926): 1–12.

Anon., Acclimatisation of the white man in the tropics, *MJES* I (May 1926): 31–33.

Anon., Ayurvedic medicine: An ancient system. *MMJ* I (July 1926): 114–115.

Anon., Chinese gardeners and disease, *MMJES* I, 2 (1926): 33.

Anon., Tuberculosis in Malaya, *MMJES* I, 3 (1926): 33–37.

Anon., Neville Chamberlain opens Medical Research Bureau, *MMJ* I, 3 (1926): 71–78.

Anon., Anti-malarial work in Straits Settlements, *MMJES* I, 4 (1926): 27–31.

Anon., Social hygiene and the Federated Malay States, *Health and Empire* II, 4 (1927): 256–262.

Anon., British Social Hygiene Council, Imperial Conference, September 27th, 1928 (Report of proceedings), *Health and Empire* III, 4 (1928): 267–282.

Anon., Points for speakers, *Health and Empire* VI, 1 (1931): 79.

Arnold, David, Introduction: Disease, medicine and empire, in David Arnold (ed.), *Imperial Medicine and Indigenous Societies* (Manchester and New York: Manchester University Press, 1988), pp. 1–26.

289

Arnold, David, Smallpox and colonial medicine in nineteenth-century India, in David Arnold (ed.), *Imperial Medicine and Indigenous Societies* (Manchester and New York: Manchester University Press, 1988), pp. 45–65.

Bahrin, Tunku Shamsul, The pattern of Indonesian migration and settlement in Malaya, *Asian Studies* 5, 2 (1967): 233–257.

Baker, C., The government medical service in Malawi: An administrative history, 1891–1974, *MH* 20 (1976): 296–311.

Balfour, Sir Andrew, The tropical field: The possibilities for medical women, *The Magazine of the London (Royal Free Hospital) School of Medicine for Women* XXIII, 101 (1928): 80–101.

Balfour, Sir Andrew, Health in the tropics, *The Medical Officer*, 15 March (Offprint, LSHTM Library).

Barrowcliff, M., *The vitamins*, Paper presented to the Fifth Congress of the Far Eastern Association of Tropical Medicine, Singapore September 1923 (Kuala Lumpur: St John's Press, 1923).

Bayoumi, A., Medical administration in the Sudan, 1899–1970, *Clio Medica* 11, 2 (1976): 105–115.

Beck, Ann, *A History of the British Medical Administration of East Africa, 1900–1950*, (Cambridge, Mass.: Harvard University Press, 1970).

Beck, Ann, The role of medicine in German East Africa, *BHM* 45 (1971): 170–178.

Beck, Ann, Medical administration and medical research in developing countries: Remarks on their history in colonial East Africa, *BHM* 46 (1972): 349–358.

Beveridge, W. I. B., *Influenza: The last great plague* (London: Heinemann, 1977).

Bilson, Geoffrey, Public health and the medical profession in nineteenth-century Canada, in Roy MacLeod and Milton Lewis (eds), *Disease, Medicine, and Empire. Perspectives on Western Medicine and the Experience of European Expansion* (London and New York: Routledge, 1988), pp. 156–175.

Birch, E. W., *A Memorandum upon the Subject of Irrigation for the Resident-General (Sir F. A. Swettenham)* (Kuala Lumpur: Selangor Government Printing Office, 1898).

Birch, E. W., *Papers of Sir Ernest W. Birch*, including correspondence 1889–1929, Rhodes House Library, Colonial Records Project, Mss Indian Ocean S242.

Birch, J. W. W., *Diaries as British Resident in Perak, 1874–1875*, Entry for 13 February 1875, Larut, Rhodes House Library, Colonial Records Project, Mss Indian Ocean S242/1 (3).

Black, K., Health and climate – with special reference to British Malaya, Part I, *British Malaya* 3, 11 (1933): 253–256.

Black, K., Health and climate – with special reference to British Malaya, Part II, *British Malaya* 3, 12 (1933): 279–280.

Blacklock, Mary, Certain aspects of the welfare of women and children in the colonies, *ATMP* 30 (1936): 221–264.

Blackwell, K. C., *Malay Curry* (Autobiography 1921–1944), Rhodes House Library, Colonial Records Project, Mss Indian Ocean S90.

Bopegamage, A., The military as a modernizing agent in India, *EDCC* 20, 1 (1971): 71–79.

Boserup, Esther, *Women's Role in Economic Development* (London: Allen and Unwin, 1970).

Bourne, F. G., *Coroner's Annual Report, Singapore 1933*, Rhodes House Library, Colonial Records Project, Mss Indian Ocean S203.

Brabin, Loretta, and Bernard J. Brabin, Parasitic infections in women and their consequences, *Advances in Parasitology* 31 (1992): 1–81.

Braine, G. I. H., *Trengganu, Annual Medical and Sanitary Report for the Year 1935* (Singapore: G. H. Kiat, 1936).

Bridges, D., *Kedah and Perlis. The Annual Report for the Medical and Health Departments for the Year 1347 AH. (20th June 1928 to 8th June 1929 A.D.)* (Alor Star: Kedah Government Press, 1930).

Brooke, G. E., A system of intelligence as a handmaiden of hygiene, *MMJ* II (1927): 6–11.

Brown, Colin, The influenza pandemic of 1918 in Indonesia, in Norman Owen (ed.), *Death and Disease in Southeast Asia: Explorations in social, medical and demographic history* (Singapore: Oxford University Press for the Asian Studies Association of Australia, 1987), pp. 235–256.

Burgess, R. C., *The Nutrition of the Kampong Malays in the Coast District of Selangor.* Interim Report of the Standing Committee on Nutrition in Malaya (Kuala Lumpur: FMS Government Press, 1937).

Burgess, R. C. and Laidin bin Alang Musa, *A Report on the State of Health, the Diet and the Economic Conditions of Groups of People in the Lower Income Levels of Malaya.* Institute of Medical Research Report No. 13 (Kuala Lumpur: Charles Grenier and Sons, 1950).

Burkill, I. H., *A Dictionary of the Economic Products of the Malay Peninsula,* 2 vols. (London: Governments of the Straits Settlements and Federated Malay States, 1935).

Burkill, I. M., and Mohammed Ariff, Malay village medicine, *Garden Bulletin* 6, 2 (1930): 165–321; 6, 3 (1930): 323–474.

Butcher, John G., *The British in Malaya 1880–1941: The social history of a European community in colonial South-East Asia* (Kuala Lumpur: Oxford University Press, 1979).

Caique, W. C., S. M. Knight and W. Toodayan. Risk factors for the transmission of diarrhoeal disease in children in the Tumpat district, Kelantan, Malaysia: A case-control study. Unpublished report, Master of Tropical Health (Brisbane: Tropical Health Program, University of Queensland, 1989).

Cameron, Gordon, Estate medical and health practice in Malaya, *East African Medical Journal* 29, 4 (1952): 153–158.

Cameron, Thomas W. M., On the centenary of the birth of Patrick Manson, the father of modern tropical medicine, *McGill Medical Journal* XIII, 3 (1944) (Offprint, LSHTM library, no page nos.).

Carson, J. C., *Kedah and Perlis. Annual Report of the Medical Department for 1938* (Alor Star: Kedah Government Press, 1940).

Cass, Anne-Marie, Gender and Violence in the Philippines. Unpublished PhD dissertation (Brisbane: University of Queensland, 1991).

Catanach, I. J., Plague and the tensions of empire: India, 1896–1918, in David Arnold (ed.), *Imperial Medicine and Indigenous Societies* (Manchester and New York: Manchester University Press, 1988), pp. 149–171.

Chai, H. C., *The Development of British Malaya, 1896–1909* (Kuala Lumpur: Oxford University Press, 1964).

Chatterton, Sir Robert, The development of tropical medicine, *Eastern World* IV, 11 (1950): 33–34.

Chee Heng Leng, Health status and the development of health services in a colonial state: The case of British Malaya, *IJHS* 12, 3 (1982): 397–417.

Chen, Paul C. Y., An analysis of customs related to childbirth in rural Malay culture, *Tropical and Geographical Medicine* 25 (1973): 197–204.

Chen, Paul C. Y., Providing maternal and child health care in rural Malaysia, *Tropical and Geographical Medicine* 29 (1977): 441–448.

Christy, Cuthbert, *Notes on Prevention of Malaria* (London: Ross Institute of Tropical Hygiene, 1935).

Cipolla, Carlo, *Miasmas and Disease, Public Health and the Environment in the Pre-Industrial Age* (New Haven: Yale University Press, 1991).

Clarke, J. Tertius, Tuberculosis in the tropics, *MMJ* II, I (1927): 19–23.

Clifford, J. and G. E. Marcus (eds), *Writing Culture* (Berkeley: University of California Press, 1986).

Clifford, Sir Hugh, *Address of His Excellency the High Commissioner Sir High Clifford, M.C.S., G.C.M.E., G.B.E., at the meeting of the Federal Council, 16th November, 1927* (Kuala Lumpur: Federated Malay States Government Printing Office, 1927).

Cohen, Paul and Purcal, John (eds), *The Political Economy of Primary Health Care in Southeast Asia* (Bangkok: Australian Development Studies Network and the ASEAN Training Centre for Primary Health Care Development, 1989).

Colley, F. C., Traditional Indian medicine in Malaysia, *JMBRAS* LI, 1 (1978): 77–109.

Cretch, A. H., *Malayan Mining Methods, with an Account of the Physique, Living Conditions and Food Requirements of the Asiatic Miner, 1933*, Rhodes House Library, Colonial Records Project, Mss Indian Ocean S96.

Crosby, A. W., *Epidemic and Peace, 1918* (Westport, Conn.: Greenwood Press, 1976).

Curtin, Philip D., *Death by Migration. Europe's encounter with the tropical world in the nineteenth century* (Cambridge: Cambridge University Press, 1989).

Darwin, Charles. *The Origin of the Species by Means of Natural Selection: or The preservation of favoured races in the struggle for life*, ed. J. W. Burrow (Harmondsworth: Penguin, 1968) (1st pub. London: John Murray, 1859).

Darville, E. W., *Maternity and Child Welfare Work in Penang, 1927–35, 1935–41.* Lectures given at the London School of Hygiene and Tropical Medicine. Rhodes House Library, Colonial Records Project, Mss Indian Ocean S134.

Davies, Celia, The Health Visitor as mother's friend: a woman's place in public health, 1900–1914, *SHM* 1, 1 (1988): 39–59.

Davin, Anna, Imperialism and motherhood, *History Workshop* 5 (1978): 9–66.

Davis, A. M., What is climatic disease? *Transactions of the Epidemiological Society of London* XXII (New Series) (1902–1903): 1–5, and discussion: 6–10.

de Moubray, G. A. de C., *Letter 17 January 1967, Jersey, to I. Lloyd Philips, describing achievement as administrative officer in Malaya, 1920–1946*, Rhodes House Library, Colonial Records Project, Mss Indian Ocean S159.

Denoon, Donald, Temperate medicine and settler capitalism: on the reception of western medical ideas, in R. MacLeod and M. Lewis (eds), *Disease, Medicine, and Empire. Perspectives on Western medicine and the experience of European expansion* (London and New York: Routledge, 1988), pp. 121–138.

Denoon, Donald, with Kathleen Dugan and Leslie Marshall, *Public Health in Papua New Guinea. Medical possibility and social constraint, 1884–1984* (Cambridge: Cambridge University Press, 1989).

Dimen-Schein, Muriel, *The Anthropological Imagination* (New York: McGraw-Hill, 1977).

Djamour, Judith, *Malay Kinship and Marriage in Singapore* (London: Athlone Press, 1965) (1st pub. 1959).

Doyal, Lesley with Imogen Pennell, *The Political Economy of Health* (London: Pluto Press, 1979).

Drabble, John H., *Rubber in Malaya, 1876–1922: The genesis of the industry* (Kuala Lumpur: Oxford University Press, 1973).

Dunn, F. L., Traditional beliefs and practices affecting medical care in Malaysian Chinese communities, *MJM* 29 (1974): 7–10.

Ehrenreich, B. and D. English, *Witches, Midwives and Nurses: A history of women healers* (Old Westbury, NY: Feminist Press, 1973).

Ehrenreich, J. (ed.), *The Cultural Crisis of Modern Medicine* (New York: Monthly Review Press, 1978).

Elson, R. E., *Javanese Peasants and the Colonial Sugar Industry: Impact and change in an East Java residency, 1830–1940*, Southeast Asia Publication Series/Asian Studies Association of Australia No. 9 (Singapore: Oxford University Press, 1984).

Emerson, Rupert, *Malaysia: A study of direct and indirect rule* (Kuala Lumpur: University of Malaya Press, 1964) (1st pub. 1937).

Engels, Dagmar, Foundations of imperial hegemony: Western education, public health and policy in India and Africa, 1859 to independence. Conference Report, *Bulletin of the German Historical Institute, London* XI, 3 (1989): 29–35.

Etienne, Mona, and Eleanor Leacock (eds), *Women and Colonization. Anthropological perspectives* (New York: Drager, 1980).

Evans, L. W., *Kelantan. The Annual Report on the Medical Department for the Year 1930* (Penang: Criterion Press, 1931).

Evans, L. W., *Kelantan. The Annual Report on the Medical Department for the Year 1932* (Kota Bharu: Al-Asasiyah Press, 1933).

Evans, Richard J., Epidemics and revolutions: Cholera in nineteenth century Europe, in T. Ranger and P. Slack (eds), *Epidemics and Ideas. Essays on the historical perception of pestilence* (Cambridge: Cambridge University Press, 1992), pp. 149–173.

Eyler, J. M. Mortality statistics and Victorian public health policy: program and criticism. *BHM* 50 (1976): 355–365.

Fabian Colonial Bureau, *Hunger and Health in the Colonies* (London: Fabian Colonial Bureau and Victor Gollancz, 1944).

Fanon, Frantz, Medicine and colonialism, in J. Ehrenreich (ed.), *The Cultural Crisis of Modern Medicine* (New York: Monthly Review Press, 1978).

Fanon, Frantz, *Studies in a Dying Colonialism* (London: Earthscan Publications, 1989) (1st pub. 1961).

Faris, D. W. G., *File of Medical Papers, 1931–1946*, including Selangor Coast District Annual Report 1931, when Health Officer; reports on the working of the government Health department, Singapore, 1941–45; reports on the hospital and nutrition at the civilian internment camp, Rhodes House Library, Colonial Records Project, Mss Indian Ocean S135.

Federated Malay States, *Colonial Reports. Annual Reports on the Social and Economic Progress of the People of the Federated Malay States* (Kuala Lumpur: Government Printing Office and London: HMSO, various years).

Fasseur, Cornelius, *The Politics of Colonial Exploitation: Java, the Dutch and the cultivation system* (trans. R. E. Elson and A. Kraal, ed. R. E. Elson) (Ithaca: Southeast Asia Program, Cornell University, 1992).

Faure, Olivier, The social history of health in France: a survey of recent developments (trans. Roger Griffin), *SHM* 3, 3 (1990): 437–451.

Federated Malay States, *Memorandum on the Protection of Chinese and other Asiatic Women and Girls* (Selangor: Government Press, 1900).

Federated Malay States, *Report presented to Her Majesty's Secretary of State for the Colonies, 8 May 1904* (Kuala Lumpur: Federated Malay States Government Printing Office, 1905).

Federated Malay States, *Report of the Commission Appointed to Enquire into Certain Matters Affecting the Health of Estates in the Federated Malay States together with a Memorandum by the Chief Secretary to Government* (Kuala Lumpur: Government Printer, 1925).

Fett, I., Land ownership in Negri Sembilan, 1900–1977, in Lenore Manderson (ed.), *Women's Work and Women's Roles. Economics and Everyday Life in Indonesia, Malaysia and Singapore*, Development Studies Centre Monograph No. 32 (Canberra: Australian National University, 1983), pp. 73–96.

Fletcher, William, *Incubation and Contact Carriers of Enteric Fever* (Kuala Lumpur: Federated Malay States Government Printing Office, 1921).

Foucault, Michel, *Power/Knowledge. Selected interviews and other writings, 1927–1977* (Brighton: Harvester Press, 1980).

Fox, S. C. G., *The Principles of Health in Malaya: Some suggestions to newcomers* (Taiping: Perak Government Printing Office, 1901).

Friedson, E., *Professional Powers. A study of the institutionalisation of formal knowledge* (Chicago and London: University of Chicago Press, 1986).

Galloway, D., On inguinal lymphadenitis, *MMJ* 1, 1 (1926): 1–6.

Gammans, L.D., Anti-malaria work at Port Dickson, *MMJES* II, I (1927): 24–28.

Gates H. L. (ed.), *'Race', Writing and Difference* (Chicago and London: University of Chicago Press, 1986).

Gebbie, Ian D., Some aspects of the venereal disease problem in the Federated Malay States, with a serological survey of Indian labourers, *BMJ* 1 (4 March 1939): 438–441.

George Town, Penang, Municipality of, *Health Officer's Annual Report for the Year 1938* (Penang: Criterion Press, 1939).

Gerrard, P. N., *On the Hygienic Management of Labour in the Tropics* (Singapore: Methodist Publishing House, 1913).

Gilman, E. W. F., *Labour in British Malaya*, Malayan Series No XI, British Empire Exhibition, London, 1924 (Singapore: Fraser and Neave, 1923).

Gimlette, John D., *Memorandum on Cholera: For the guidance of Europeans in remote out-stations of British Malaya* (London: Waterlow, 1911).

Gimlette, J. D., *Malay Poisons and Charm Cures* (Kuala Lumpur: Oxford University Press, 1971) (1st pub. 1915).

Gimlette, J. D., *A Dictionary of Malayan Medicine* (ed. and completed by H. W. Thomson) (Oxford: Oxford University Press, 1939).

Golomb, Louis, *An Anthropology of Curing in Multiethnic Thailand* (Champaign/Urbana: University of Illinois Press, 1985).

Gordon, Scott, *The History and Philosophy of Social Science* (London and New York: Routledge, 1991).

Grant, E. O., Fifth Imperial Social Hygiene Congress. Summary of Proceedings, *Health and Empire* VI, 3 (1931): 211–236.

Great Britain, Colonial Office, *Papers Relating to Her Majesty's Possessions, Part 1* (London: HMSO, 1876).

Great Britain, *Contagious Diseases Regulations (Perak and Malay States), Copy of Correspondence relative to proposed introduction of Contagious Diseases Regulations in Perak or other Protected Malay States*, H.C.146 (London: HMSO, 1894).

Great Britain, *Correspondence regarding the Measures to be adopted for checking the spread of venereal disease, Ceylon, Hong Kong and Straits Settlements*, H.C.147, June 1894, C.9523 (London: HMSO, 1899).

Great Britain, Colonial Office, *Colonial Office Conference Proceedings*, London 10–31 May 1927. Cmd 2883 and 2884. (London: HMSO, 1927).

Great Britain, Colonial Office, *Information for the Use of Candidates for Appointments in the Malayan Medicine Service* (London: Colonial Office, 1929).

Great Britain, Colonial Office, *Memorandum showing the progress and development in the Colonial Empire and in the machinery for dealing with colonial questions from November, 1924, to November, 1928.* Presented by the Secretary of State for the Colonies to Parliament by Command of His Majesty, January 1929. Cmd. 3268 (London: HMSO, 1929).

Great Britain, Colonial Office, *Report of the Colonial Development Public Health Committee.* Miscellaneous No. 413(London: Colonial Office, 1930).

Great Britain, Colonial Office, *Nutrition Policy in the Colonial Empire.* No. 121 (London: Colonial Office, 1936).

Great Britain, Colonial and Indian Exhibition, *Notes on the Straits Settlements and Malay States* (London: William Clowes, 1886).

Great Britain, Economic Advisory Council, Committee on Nutrition in the Colonial Empire, *Nutrition in the Colonial Empire.* First Report, Part I, Cmd 6050. (London: HMSO, 1939).

Great Britain, Economic Advisory Council, Committee on Nutrition in the Colonial Empire, *Summary of Information regarding Nutrition in the Colonial Empire.* First Report, Part II, Cmd 6051. (London: HMSO, 1939).

Great Britain, Emigration Information Office, *Federated Malay States, General Information for Intending Settlers* (London: HMSO, 1900).

Great Britain, Ministry of Agriculture and Fisheries, *The Practical Education of Women for Rural Life.* Report of the Sub-Committee of the Interdepartmental Committee of the Ministry of Agriculture and Board of Education (Chaired by Lady Denham) (London: HMSO, 1928).

Guha, R., (ed.), *Subaltern Studies VI: Writings on South Asian History and Society* (Delhi: Oxford University Press, 1989).

Gullick, J. M., Kuala Lumpur 1880–1895, *JMBRAS* 28, 4 (1955): 7–139.

Habermas, Jurgen, *Communication and the Evolution of Society* (London: Heinemann, 1979).

Harrison, Mark, Tropical medicine in nineteenth-century India, *BJHS* 25 (1992): 299–318.

Harrison, Mark, *Public Health in British India: Anglo-Indian preventive medicine 1859–1914* (Cambridge: Cambridge University Press, 1994).

Hart, Donn V., *Bisayan Filipino and Malayan Humoral Pathologies: Folk medicine and ethnohistory in Southeast Asia,* Data Paper No. 76 (Ithaca, N.Y: Cornell University, Department of Asian Studies Southeast Asia Program, 1969).

Harvey, David, *The Condition of Postmodernity. An essay into the origins of cultural change* (Oxford: Basil Blackwell, 1989).

Hartwig, C. W., Church-state relations in Kenya: Health issues, *SSM* 13C (1979): 121–127.

Headrick, Daniel R., The tools of imperialism: technology and the expansion of European colonial empires in the nineteenth century, *JMH* 57 (1979): 231–263.

Headrick, Daniel R., *The Tools of Empire. Technology and European imperialism in the nineteenth century* (New York and Oxford: Oxford University Press, 1981).

Herrmann, E. K., Health care services in 19th century British Honduras, *SSM* 14A (1980): 353–6.

van Heteren, G.M., A. de Knecht-van Eekelen and M. J. D. Poulissen, (eds), *Dutch Medicine in the Malay Archipelago, 1816–1942.* Articles presented at a symposium held in honour of Prof. Dr D. de Moulin. Nieuwe Nederlandse Bijdragen tot de Gescgiendenis der Geneeskunde en der

Natuurwtenschappen No. 35 (Chief editor A. M. Luyendijk–Elshout) (Amsterdam and Atlanta, GA.: Rodopi, 1989).

Heussler, Robert W., Papers of Professor Robert W. Heussler, Rhodes House Library, Mss Brit. Emp. s.480. Box 17, History of the Malayan Civil Service 1853–1984. File 3. Letters, memoirs and notes on the M.C.S. and Heussler's research into its history. Correspondence from W. J. K. Stark (1910–1933).

Hobbs, H. M., *Welfare Clinics in Malaya* (1962), Rhodes House Library, Colonial Records Project, Mss Indian Ocean S38.

Hobsbawm, Eric, *Age of Empire: 1875–1914* (London: Weidenfeld and Nicholson, 1987).

Hodgkin, E. P., Naturalistic methods of malaria control. *JMBMA* 2, 1 (1938): 24–29.

Hodgkin, E. P. and R. S. Johnston, Malaria at Batu Gajah, Perak: Transmitted by *Anopheles barbirostrus* Van Der Wulp, *BIMR,* No. 1 (Kuala Lumpur: FMS Government Press, 1935).

Hoflin, J. W., *Malaria* (Kuala Lumpur: Federated Malay States, Malaria Advisory Board, 1934).

Holmes, W. E., The control of urban malaria (Kuala Lumpur), *BIMR* No. 2 (Kuala Lumpur: FMS Government Press, 1939).

Hooper, D., *On Chinese medicine: drugs of Chinese pharmacies in Malaya* (Singapore: Botanic Gardens, 1929).

Hooper, D., On Chinese Medicine: Drugs of Chinese pharmacists in Malaya, *Gardens Bulletin* 6, 1 (1930): 163–165.

Hoops, A. L., Causes of death amongst southern Indian labour populations of Malacca rubber estates, *JMBMA* 3, 3 (1939): 213–227.

Horsfield, T. Report on the island of Banka, *Journal of the Indian Archipelago and Eastern Asia,* vol.II (1848): 299–336, 373–397, 398–427, 705–824.

Howard, S. C., The practical application of anti-malarial measures on Malayan estates. *BIMR* No. 2 (Kuala Lumpur: FMS Government Press, 1939).

Hua Wu Yin, *Class and Communalism in Malaysia: Politics in a dependent capitalist state* (London: Zed Books in conjunction with Marram Books, 1983).

Hutchinson, G., *Rubber Planting in Malaya, 1928–1932,* Files of the British Association of Malaya, BAM III/15.

Ileto, Reynaldo C., Cholera and the origins of the American sanitary order in the Philippines, in David Arnold (ed.), *Imperial Medicine and Indigenous Societies* (Manchester and New York: Manchester University Press, 1988), pp. 125–148.

Imperial Bureau of Animal Nutrition, *Nutrition Research in the British Colonial Empire.* Technical Communications No 8. (Aberdeen: Imperial Bureau of Animal Nutrition, 1937).

Innes, J. R., *Report on the Census of the Straits Settlements taken on the 1st March 1901* (Singapore: Government Printing Office, 1901).

Institute of Medical Research, *Studies from the Institute of Medical Research, Federation of Malaya, Jubilee Volume,* No. 25 (Kuala Lumpur, Government Press, 1951).

Ismail Munshi, *The Medical Book of Malayan Medicine,* ed. with notes by J. D. Gimlette and determinations of drugs by I. H. Burkhill (Singapore: Botanic Gardens, 1930).

Jackson, J. C., *Planters and Speculators: Chinese and European agricultural enterprise in Malaya 1786–1921* (Kuala Lumpur: University of Malaysia Press, 1968).

Jackson, R. N., *Immigrant Labour and the Development of Malaya, 1786–1920* (Kuala Lumpur: University of Malaya Press, 1961).

Jomo, Kwame Sundaram, *A Question of Class: Capital, the state and uneven development in Malaya* (New York: Monthly Review Press, 1988).

Joshua-Raghavar, A., *Leprosy in Malaysia. Past, present and future* (ed. by K. Rajagopalan) (Sungai Buluh, Selangor: A. Joshua-Raghavar, 1983).

Kaur, Amarjit, *Bridge and Barrier: Transport and communications in colonial Malaya, 1870–1951* (Singapore: Oxford University Press, 1985).

Kaur, Amarjit, Working on the railway: Indian workers in Malaya, 1880–1957, in P. J. Rimmer and L. M. Allen (eds), *The Underside of Malaysian History: Pullers, prostitutes, plantation workers* (Singapore: Singapore University Press, 1990), pp. 99–128.

Kaye, Barrington, *Upper Nankin Street, Singapore: A sociological study of Chinese households living in a densely populated area* (Singapore: University of Malaya Press, 1960).

Kelly, R. W. C., Social hygiene work in Singapore, *Health and Empire* IV, 1 (1929): 47–52.

Kempe, J. A., *Perak Administration Report for the year 1932* (Kuala Lumpur: Government Printing Office, 1933).

Klein, I., Death in India, 1871–1921, *Journal of Asian Studies* 32 (1973): 639–659.

Knight, A., Tan Tock Seng's Hospital, Singapore, *JMBRAS* 42, 1 (1969): 252–255 (1st pub. 1913).

van der Kraan, Alfons, *Lombok: Conquest, Colonization and Underdevelopment, 1870–1940*, Southeast Asia Publication Series No. 5 (Singapore: Heinemann for the Asian Studies Association of Australia, 1980).

Krishna, V. V., The colonial 'model' and the emergence of national science in India, 1876–1920, in P. Petitjean, C. Jami and A. M. Moulin (eds), *Science and Empires. Historical studies about scientific development and European expansion.* Boston Studies in the Philosophy of Science, vol.136 (Dordrecht, Boston, London: Kluwer Academic, 1992), pp. 57–72.

Kuah, K. B., Malay customs in relation to childbirth, *MJM* 27, 2 (1972): 81–84.

Laderman, C., *Wives and Midwives: Childbirth and nutrition in rural Malaysia* (Berkeley: University of California Press, 1983).

Laderman, C., *Taming the Wind of Desire: Psychology, medicine and aesthetics in Malay shamanic performance* (Berkeley: University of California Press, 1991).

Langford C. M. and P. Story, Influenza in Sri Lanka, 1918–1919: The impact of a new disease in a pre–modern Third World setting, *HTR* 2, Supp. (1992): 97–123.

Lasker, J. N., The role of health services in colonial rule: the case of the Ivory Coast, *CMP* 1 (1977): 277–297.

League of Nations, Health Organisation, *Report of the Malayan Delegation.* Preparatory Paper for Inter-Governmental Conference of Far Eastern Countries on Rural Hygiene, CH.1235 (c) (Geneva: League of Nations, 1937).

League of Nations, Health Organisation, *Report of the Intergovernmental Conference of Far-Eastern Countries on Rural Hygiene*, A19.1937.III (III.Health.1937. III.17) (Geneva: League of Nations, 1937).

League of Nations, Health Organisation, *Intergovernmental Conference of Far-Eastern Countries on Rural Hygiene (Bandoeng, August 3rd to 13th, 1937), Country Reports*, CH12.53, No.1 (Geneva: League of Nations, 1937).

Lee, Edwin, *The British as Rulers: Governing multiracial Singapore 1867–1914* (Singapore: Singapore University Press, 1991).

Lee, Y. K., The first anaesthetic in the Straits Settlements (Singapore, Penang and Malacca) – 1847, *BJA* 44 (1972): 408–411.

Lee, Y. K., Dental practice in early Singapore 1819–1869, *BJD* 133 (1972): 155–160.

Lee, Y. K., The general hospital in early Singapore (Part I) (1819–1829), *SMJ* 14 (1973): 37–41.

Lee, Y. K., The general hospital in early Singapore (Part II) (1830–1839), *SMJ* 14 (1973): 519–524.

Lee, Y. K., Cholera in early Singapore I. 1819–1849, *SMJ* 14 (1973): 42–48.

Lee, Y. K., Smallpox and vaccination in early Singapore 1. 1819–1829, *SMJ* 14 (1973): 525–531.

Lee, Y. K., Medical education in the Straits: 1786–1871, *JMBRAS* 46, 1 (1973): 101–122.

Lee, Y. K., Lunatics and lunatic asylums in early Singapore (1819–1869), *MH* 17 (1973): 11–36.

Lee, Y. K., The Pauper Hospital in early Singapore (Part I) (1819–1829), *SMJ* 14, 1 (1973): 49–54.

Lee, Y. K., The Pauper Hospital in early Singapore (Part II) (1830–1839), *SMJ* 15, 1 (1974): 72–83.

Lee, Y. K., The Pauper Hospital in early Singapore (Part III) (1840–1849) – Section I, *SMJ* 16, 1 (1975): 106–121.

Lee, Y. K., The Pauper Hospital in early Singapore (Part III) (1840–1849) – Section II, *SMJ* 16, 3 (1975): 208–223.

Lee, Y. K., The Pauper Hospital in early Singapore (Part IV) (1850–1859) – Section I, *SMJ* 16, 3 (1975): 269–289.

Lee, Y. K., The Pauper Hospital in early Singapore (Part IV) (1850–1859) – Section II, *SMJ* 17, 1 (1976): 16–31.

Lee, Y. K., The Pauper Hospital in early Singapore (Part V) (1860–1873) – Section I, *SMJ* 17, 2 (1976): 74–83.

Lee, Y. K., The Pauper Hospital in early Singapore (Part V) (1860–1873) – Section II, *SMJ* 17, 3 (1976): 138–149.

Lee, Y. K., Forensic medicine in early Singapore I. 1819–1839, *SMJ* 15 (1974): 84–90.

Lee, Y. K., Singapore's pauper and Tan Tock Seng hospitals (1819–1873). Part 1, *JMBRAS* 48, 2 (1975): 78–111.

Lee, Y. K., Singapore's pauper and Tan Tock Seng hospitals (1819–1873). Part 2, *JMBRAS* 49, 1 (1976): 113–133.

Lee, Y. K., Singapore's pauper and Tan Tock Seng hospitals. Part 3: The new hospital 1860, *JMBRAS* 49, 2 (1976): 164–183.

Lee, Y. K., Singapore's pauper and Tan Tock Seng hospitals. Part 4: The government takes over, *JMBRAS* 50, 2 (1977): 111–135.

Lee, Y. K., Smallpox in early Singapore II. 1830–1849, *SMJ* 17, 2 (1976): 202–206.

Lee, Y. K., Smallpox in early Singapore III. 1850–1859, *SMJ* 18, 1 (1977): 16–20.

Lee, Y. K., Smallpox in early Singapore IV. 1860–1872, *SMJ* 18, 2 1977): 126–135.

Lee, Y. K., The origins of the municipal health department, Singapore, *SMJ* 18, 3 (1977): 189–191.

Leonard, H. G. R., *Annual Report on the Social and Economic Progress of the People of Pahang for the Year 1931* (Kuala Lumpur: FMS Government Printing Office, 1932), pp. 28–29.

Leslie, Charles S. (ed.), *Asian Medical Systems: A comparative study* (Berkeley: University of California Press, 1976).

Lewis, Jane, *The Politics of Motherhood: Child and maternal welfare in England, 1900–1939* (London: Croom Helm, 1980).

Lewis, Jane, The social history of social policy: Infant welfare in Edwardian England, *JSP* 9 (1980): 463–486.

Lewis, Milton, The 'health of the race' and infant health in New South Wales: Perspectives on medicine and empire, in Roy MacLeod and Milton Lewis (eds), *Disease, Medicine, and Empire. Perspectives on Western medicine and the experience of European expansion* (London and New York: Routledge, 1988), pp. 301–315.

Little, R. An essay on coral reefs as the cause of Blakan Mati fever and of the fevers in various ports of the East. Part I. On the medical topography of Singapore particularly in its marshes and malaria. *Journal of the Indian Archipelago and Eastern Asia* I, 2 (1848): 450–492.

Little, R. An essay on coral reefs as the cause of Blakan Mati fever and of the fevers in various ports of the East. Part II. On coral reefs as a cause of the fever of the islands near Singapore. *Journal of the Indian Archipelago and Eastern Asia* I, 2 (1848): 572–599.

Loudon, Irvine, Maternal mortality: 1880–1950. Some regional and international comparisons. *SHM* 1, 2 (1988): 183–228.

Lyons, Maryinez, Sleeping sickness, colonial medicine and imperialism: Some connections in the Belgian Congo, in Roy MacLeod and Milton Lewis (eds), *Disease, Medicine, and Empire. Perspectives on Western medicine and the experience of European expansion* (London and New York: Routledge, 1988), pp. 242–256.

McArthur, M., *Malaya–12. Assignment Report June 1958–November 1959*, WPR/449/62 (Geneva: World Health Organisation, 1962).

McFarlane, Neil, Hospitals, housing and tuberculosis in Glasgow, 1911–1951. *SHM* 2, 1 (1989): 59–85.

McGee, T. G., *The Southeast Asian City: A social geography of the primate cities of Southeast Asia* (London: G. Bell, 1967).

MacGregor, R. M., *Annual Reports of the Medical Departments, Straits Settlements and Federated Malay States for the year 1937* (Singapore: Government Printing Office, 1938).

MacLeod, Roy and Lewis, Milton (eds), *Disease, Medicine and Empire. Perspectives on Western medicine and the experience of European expansion* (London and New York: Routledge, 1988).

MacLeod, Roy and Milton Lewis, Preface, in MacLeod and Lewis (eds), *Disease, Medicine and Empire. Perspectives on Western medicine and the experience of European expansion* (London and New York: Routledge, 1988), pp. x–xii.

MacLeod, Roy, Introduction, in MacLeod and Lewis (eds), *Disease, Medicine, and Empire. Perspectives on Western medicine and the experience of European expansion* (London and New York, Routledge, 1988), pp. 1–18.

MacLeod, Roy, Scientific advice for British India: Imperial perception and administrative goals, 1898–1923, *Modern Asian Studies* 9, 3 (1975): 343–384.

Maegraith, B. G., History of the Liverpool School of Tropical Medicine, *MH* 16 (1972): 354–368.

Malaysian Medical Association, *The Future of Health Services in Malaysia* (Kuala Lumpur: Malaysian Medical Association, 1980).

Malek, A. A., Orientalism in crisis, *Diogenes* 44 (1963): 107–108.

Manderson, Lenore, The development and direction of female education in Peninsular Malaysia, *JMBRAS* LI, 2 (1978): 100–22.

Manderson, Lenore, Traditional food classifications and humoral medical theory in Peninsular Malaysia, *Ecology, Food and Nutrition* 11 (1981): 81–93.

Manderson, Lenore, Traditional food beliefs and critical life events in Peninsular Malaysia, *SSI* 20, 6 (1981): 947–975.

Manderson, Lenore, Roasting, smoking and dieting in response to birth: Malay confinement in cross-cultural perspective, *SSM* 15B (1981): 509–520.

Manderson, Lenore, Infant feeding practice, market expansion, and the patterning of choice, Southeast Asia, 1880–1980, *New Doctor* 26 (1982a): 27–32.

Manderson, Lenore, Bottle feeding and ideology in colonial Malaya: The production of change, *IJHS* 12, 4 (1982b): 597–616.

Manderson, Lenore (ed.), *Women's Work and Women's Roles: Economics and everyday life in Indonesia, Malaysia and Singapore*, Development Studies Centre Monograph No. 32 (Canberra: Australian National University, 1983).

Manderson, Lenore, Introduction: The anthropology of food in Oceania and Southeast Asia, in Lenore Manderson (ed.), *Shared Wealth and Symbol. Food, culture and society in Oceania and Southeast Asia* (New York and Cambridge: Cambridge University Press, 1986), pp. 1–25.

Manderson, Lenore, Health services and the legitimation of the colonial state: British Malaya 1786–1941, *IJHS* 17, 1 (1987): 91–111.

Manderson, Lenore, Blame, responsibility and remedial action: Death, disease and the infant in early twentieth century Malaya, in Norman Owen (ed.), *Death and Disease in Southeast Asia: Explorations in social, medical and demographic history* (Singapore: Oxford University Press for the Asian Studies Association of Australia, 1987), pp. 257–282.

Manderson, Lenore, Political economy and the politics of gender: Primary health care in colonial Malaya, in Paul Cohen and John Purcal (eds), *The Political Economy of Primary Health Care in Southeast Asia* (Bangkok: Australian Development Studies Network and the ASEAN Training Centre for Primary Health Care Development, 1989), pp. 76–94.

Manderson, Lenore, Race, colonial mentality and public health in early twentieth-century Malaya, in Peter J. Rimmer and Lisa M. Allen (eds), *The Underside of Malaysian History. Pullers, prostitutes, plantation workers* (Singapore: Singapore University Press, 1990), pp. 193–213.

Manderson, Lenore, Women and the state: maternal and child health in colonial Malaya, in Valerie Fildes, Lara Marks and Hilary Marland (eds), *Women and Children First: International Maternal and Infant Welfare 1870–1950* (London: Routledge, 1992), pp. 154–177.

Manderson, Lenore, Social science research and tropical disease, *MJA*, 160 (1994): 289–292.

Manderson, Lenore, Wireless wars in the eastern arena: Epidemiological surveillance, disease prevention and the work of Eastern Bureau of the League of Nations Health Organisation, 1925–1942, in Paul Weindling (ed.), *International Health Organisations and Movements, 1918–1939* (Cambridge: Cambridge University Press, 1995), pp. 109–133.

Manderson, Lenore, Migration, prostitution and medical surveillance in early 20th century Malaya, in L. Marks and M. Worboys (eds), *Migrants, Minorities and Medicine* (London: Routledge, in press).

Manderson, Lenore, Colonising reproduction: Motherhood and maternity in early twentieth-century Malaya, in Margaret Jolly and Kalpana Ram (eds), *Maternity in Colonial and Post-Colonial Asia and the Pacific* (forthcoming).

Marcovich, Anne, French colonial medicine and colonial rule: Algeria and Indochina, in Roy MacLeod and Milton Lewis (eds), *Disease, Medicine, and Empire. Perspectives on Western medicine and the experience of European expansion* (London and New York: Routledge, 1988), pp. 103–117.

Marcus, J., *A World of Difference: Islam and gender hierarchy in Turkey*, Women in Asia Series No. 3 (Sydney: Allen and Unwin, 1992).

Marriott, H., *Report of the Census of the Colony of the Straits Settlements taken on the 10th March, 1911* (Singapore: Government Printing Office, 1911).

Masselos, J., The discourse from the other side: Perceptions of science and technology in western India in the nineteenth century, unpublished manuscript, University of Sydney, 1982.

Maxwell, W. E., Shamanism in Perak, *Journal of Straits Branch Royal Asiatic Society*, 12 (1883): 222–231.

Maxwell, W. G., Some problems of education and public health in Malaya. United Empire, *Royal Colonial Institute Journal*, XVIII, 1 (1927): 206–219.

Mayr, Ernst, *The Growth of Biological Thought: Diversity, evolution and inheritance* (Cambridge, Mass.: Belknap Press, 1982).

Merewether, E. M., *Report on the Census of the Straits Settlements, taken on the 5th April 1891* (Singapore: Government Printer's Officer, 1892).

Mills, C. Wright, *The Sociological Imagination* (New York: Oxford University Press, 1959).

Mitchell, Allan, An inexact science: the statistics of tuberculosis in late nineteenth-century France, *SHM* 3, 3 (1990): 387–404.

Moulin, Anne-Marie, Patriarchal science: The network of the overseas Pasteur Institutes, in P. Petitjean, C. Jami and A. M. Moulin (eds), *Science and Empires. Historical Studies about Scientific Development and European Expansion.* Boston Studies in the Philosophy of Science, vol.136 (Dordrecht, Boston, London: Kluwer Academic, 1992), pp. 307–322.

Mowat, G. S., *Annual Report of Besut, 1947 and 1948*, Rhodes House Library, Colonial Records Project, Mss Indian Ocean S229.

Nathan, J. E., *The Census of British Malaya (The Straits Settlements, Federated Malay States and Protected States of Johore, Kedah, Perlis, Kelantan, Trengganu and Brunei, 1921* (London: Waterlow, 1922).

Navarro, Vicente, The political and economic origins of the underdevelopment of health in Latin America, in Vicente Navarro, *Medicine under Capitalism* (London: Croom Helm, 1976).

Navarro, Vicente, *Imperialism, Health and Medicine* (London: Pluto Press, 1982).

Newbold, T. J., *Political and Statistical Account of the British Settlements in the Straits of Malacca, viz. Pinang, Malacca, and Singapore: with a history of the Malayan states on the peninsula* (London: John Murray, 1839).

Nicoll-Jones, S. E., *Report on the Problem of Prostitution in Singapore, 1940*, Rhodes House Library, Colonial Records Project, Mss Indian Ocean S27.

Noyes, John K., *Colonial Space. Spatiality in the discourse of German South-West Africa 1884–1915* (Chur, Switzerland: Harwood Academic, 1991).

Oakley, Ann, Wisewoman and medicine man: Change in the management of childbirth, in Juliet Mitchell and Ann Oakley (eds), *The Rights and Wrongs of Women* (Harmondsworth: Penguin, 1976), pp. 17–58.

O'Connor, Francis W., The teaching of tropical medicine in Europe. *Rockefeller Foundation Quarterly Bulletin* (1929), (Offprint, LSHTM Library, no page nos.).

Ooi Jin Bee, *Land, People and Economy in Malaya* (London: Longman, 1963).

Orde-Browne, Major G. St J., Some problems of recruited labour, *Health and Empire* XII, 3 (1937): 208–218.

Orde-Browne, Major G. St J., *Labour Conditions in Ceylon, Mauritius and Malaya*, Cmd 6423 (London: HMSO, 1943).

Owen, Norman G., *Prosperity without Progress: Manila Hemp and Material Life in the Colonial Philippines* (Berkeley: University of California Press, 1984).

Pahang, *Annual Department Reports 1931* (Kuantan: Government Printer, 1932).

Pallister, R. A., Some observations on deficiency diseases in Malaya, *JMBMA* 4, 2 (1940): 191–197.

Parahoo, Kader A., Early colonial health developments in Mauritius, *IJHS* 16, 3 (1986): 409–423.

Parr, C. W. C., *Report of the Commission appointed to enquire into the Conditions of Indentured Labor in the Federated Malay States, 1910*. Report No 11. (Kuala Lumpur: Federated Malay States Labour Department, 1910).

Parry, N. and J. Parry, *The Rise of the Medical Profession* (London: Croom Helm, 1976).

Patterson, K. D. and G. W. Hartwig, The disease factor: An introductory overview, in G. W. Hartwig and K. D. Patterson (eds), *Disease in African History: An introductory survey and case studies* (Durham, NC: Duke University Press, 1978), pp. 3–24.

Patterson, K. D., *Health in Colonial Ghana: Disease, Medicine and socio-economic change, 1900–1955* (Waltham, Mass.: Crossroads Press, 1981).

Patterson, T. S. J., The transmission of Indian surgical techniques to Europe at the end of the eighteenth century, *Proceedings of the XXIII Congress of the History of Medicine* (London: Wellcome Institute for the History of Medicine, 1972), pp. 694–696.

Peel, Sir W., *Notes covering his colonial service from 1897–1935*. Rhodes House Library, Colonial Records Project, Mss Indian Ocean S208.

Penang, Municipality of George Town, *Health Officers' Annual Report for the Year 1938* (Penang: Criterion Press, 1939).

Pelling, Margaret, *Cholera, Fever and English Medicine, 1825–1865* (Oxford: Oxford University Press, 1978).

Pelling, Margaret, Child health as a social value in early modern England, *SHM* 1, 2 (1988): 135–164.

Petitjean, P., C. Jami and A-M. Moulin (eds), *Science and Empires. Historical studies about scientific development and European expansion*. Boston Studies in the Philosophy of Science, vol.136 (Dordrecht, Boston, London: Kluwer Academic, 1992).

Phua Kai Hong, Health and Development in Malaysia and Singapore, unpublished PhD dissertation (London: London School of Economics and Political Science, 1987).

Pickstone, John V., Death, dirt and fever epidemics: Rewriting the history of British 'public health', 1780–1850, in Terence Ranger and Paul Slack (eds), *Epidemics and Ideas. Essays on the historical perception of pestilence* (Cambridge: Cambridge University Press, 1992), pp. 125–148.

Portelly, J., *Kedah and Perlis. Annual Report for the Medical Department, 1936* (Alor Star: Kedah Government Press, 1937).

Portelly, J., *Kedah and Perlis. Annual Report of the Medical Department for 1937* (Alor Star: Kedah Government Press, 1938).

Poynton, Sir Hilton, The View from the Colonial Office, in E. E. Sabben-Clare, D. J. Bradley and K. Kirkwood (eds), *Health in Tropical Africa during the Colonial Period*, (Oxford: Clarendon Press, 1980), pp. 195–204.

Pratt, Mary Louise, *Imperial Eyes. Travel writings and transculturation* (London and New York: Routledge, 1992).

Pryor, Robyn J., *Migration and Development in South-East Asia: A demographic perspective* (Kuala Lumpur: Oxford University Press, 1979).

Purcell, V. W. W. S., *The Chinese in Malaya* (London: Oxford University Press, 1948).

Pyenson, Lewis, *Cultural Imperialism and Exact Sciences. German expansion overseas, 1900–1930* (New York: P. Lang, 1985).

Pyenson, Lewis, *Empire of Reason: Exact sciences in Indonesia, 1840–1940* (Leiden: E. J. Brill, 1989).

Ramasubban, Radhika, Imperial health in British India, 1857–1900, in Roy MacLeod and Milton Lewis (eds), *Disease, Medicine, and Empire. Perspectives on Western medicine and the experience of European expansion* (London and New York: Routledge, 1988), pp. 38–60.

Rao, B. Anantaswami, *Malaria Control in Malaya, Java, Ceylon and South India*, Mysore State Department of Public Health, Bulletin No. 15 (Bangalore: Government Press, 1939).

Reingold, N. and M. Rottenberg (eds), *Scientific Colonialism: A cross-cultural comparison* (Washington: Smithsonian Institute Press, 1987).

Richards, Audrey I., *Hunger and Work in a Savage Tribe* (London: Routledge, 1932).

Richards, Audrey I., *Labour, Land and Diet in Northern Rhodesia. An economic study of the Bemboi tribe* (Oxford: Oxford University Press, 1939).

Ridley, Hugh, *Images of Imperial Rule* (London and Canberra: Croom Helm, 1983).

Rimmer, Peter J., Hackney carriage syces and rikisha pullers in Singapore: A colonial registrar's perspective on public transport, 1892–1923, in Peter J. Rimmer and Lisa M. Allen (eds), *The Underside of Malaysian History. Pullers, prostitutes, plantation workers* (Singapore: Singapore University Press, 1990), pp. 129–160.

Rimmer, Peter J. and Lisa M. Allen (eds), *The Underside of Malaysian History. Pullers, prostitutes, plantation workers* (Singapore: Singapore University Press, 1990).

Rimmer, Peter J., Lenore Manderson and Colin Barlow, The underside of Malaysian history: A theoretical overview, in Peter J. Rimmer and Lisa M. Allen (eds), *The Underside of Malaysian History. Pullers, prostitutes, plantation workers* (Singapore: Singapore University Press, 1990), pp. 3–22.

Rogers, Barbara, *The Domestication of Women. Discrimination in developing societies* (London: Tavistock, 1980).

Rosenfield, P. L., The potential of transdisciplinary research for sustaining and extending linkages between the health and social sciences, *SSM* 35 (1992): 1343–1358.

Ross, E. A., Victorian medicine in Penang, *Malaysia in History* 23 (1980): 84–89.

Ross, R. and G. J. Telkamp (eds), *Colonial Cities: Essays in urbanism in a colonial context* (Dordrecht: Martinus Nijhoff, 1985).

Ross, Ronald, *Malaria Fever: Its cause, prevention, and treatment* (Liverpool: Liverpool School of Tropical Medicine, 1902).

Sabben-Clare, E. E., D. J. Bradley and K. Kirkwood (eds), *Health in Tropical Africa during the Colonial Period* (Oxford: Clarendon Press, 1980).

Said, Edward W., *Orientalism* (Harmondsworth: Penguin, 1991) (1st pub. 1978).

Said, Edward W., *The World, The Text and The Critic* (London: Vintage Books, 1991) (1st pub. 1984).

Savage, Victor R., *Western Impressions of Nature and Landscape in Southeast Asia* (Singapore: Singapore University Press, 1984).

Scharff, J. W., *A Note on Public Health Administration in the Northern Settlement* (Penang: Criterion Press, n.d. c. 1932).

Shepherd, John A., *A History of the Liverpool Medical Institution* (Chester: Liverpool Medical Institution, 1979).

Shiels, Drummond, Social hygiene and human welfare. The task of colonial administration, *Health and Empire* VII, 4 (1933): 319–331.

Shorter, Edward, *The History of Women's Bodies* (New York: Basic Books, 1982).

Siddique, Sharon, *Singapore's Little India, Past, Present, Future* (Singapore: Institute of South East Asian Studies, 1982).

Simpson, W. J., *Report on the Sanitary Conditions of Singapore* (London: HMSO, 1907).

Sinclair A. W., Notes on beri-beri, as observed in the Malay Peninsula from 1882 to 1888. *Transactions of the British Medical Association, Meeting held at Leeds, 1889* (London: British Medical Association, 1889).

Sinton, Lt. Col. J. A. and Professor Raja Ram, *Man-made Malaria in India.* Health Bulletin No. 22, Malaria Bureau No. 10, 2nd ed. (Simla: Government of India Press, 1938).

Skeat, W. W., *Malay Magic: Being an introduction to the folklore and popular religion of the Malay Peninsula* (New York: Dover Publications, 1967) (1st pub. 1900).

Smart, Carol, Disruptive bodies and unruly sex: the regulation of reproduction and sexuality in the nineteenth century, in Carol Smart (ed.), *Regulating Womanhood. Historical essays on marriage, motherhood and sexuality* (London and New York: Routledge, 1992), pp. 7–32.

Smith, F. B., *The People's Health, 1830–1910* (London: Croom Helm, 1979).

Smith, Neil, *Uneven Development, Nature, Capital and the Production of Space* (Oxford: Blackwell, 1984).

Society of Estate Medical Officers, *An open letter to the unofficial members of the Legislative Federal Councils (S.S. and F.M.S.)* (Kuala Lumpur: M. J. Rattray for the Society of Estate Medical Officers, 1918).

Song Ong Siang, *One Hundred Years of the Chinese in Singapore* (London: John Murray, 1923).

Spencer, Herbert, *Descriptive Sociology* (London: Williams and Norgate, 1873).

Spencer, Herbert, *Principles of Sociology* (London: Williams and Norgate, 1885–1896).

Spencer, J. E. and W. L. Thomas, The hill stations and summer resorts of the Orient, *The Geographical Review* XXXVIII, 4 (1948): 637–651.

Spivak, Gayatri Chakravorty, Three women's texts and a critique of imperialism, *Critical Inquiry* 12, 1 (1985): 17–34.

Spivak, Gayatri Chakravorty, *In Other Worlds: Essays in cultural politics* (New York and London: Methuen, 1987).

Stenson, Michael, *Class, Race and Colonialism in West Malaysia* (Brisbane: University of Queensland Press, 1980)

Stokes, Eric, *The English Utilitarians and India* (Oxford: Clarendon Press, 1959).

Stoler, Ann L. *Capitalism and Confrontation in Sumatra's Plantation Belt, 1870–1979* (New Haven and London: Yale University Press, 1985).

Straits Settlements, *Annual Departmental Reports* (Singapore: Government Printing Office, various years).

Straits Settlements, *Report of the Commissioners Appointed to Enquire into the State of Labour in the Straits Settlements and Protected Native States* (Singapore: Government Printing Office, 1891).

Straits Settlements, *Proceedings and Report of the Commission appointed to enquire into the cause of the presenting housing difficulties in Singapore, and the steps which should be taken to remedy such difficulties.* Vol I, Instrument of Appointment and Report; Vol II, Evidence and Memoranda (Singapore: Government Printing Office, 1918).

Strang, T. F., *State of Kelantan. Annual Report of the Medical Department for the Year 1936* (Kota Bharu: Cheong Fatt Press, 1936).

Sturrock, A. J., *Annual Report of the British Adviser, Trengganu, for the years A.H.1346 and 1347 (30 June 1927–18 June 1928; 19 June 1928–7 June 1929)* (Singapore: Government Printing Office, 1929).

Sturrock, A. J., *Trengganu. Annual Report for the Year A.H. 1348 (8 June 1929–27 May 1930)* (Singapore: Government Printing Office, 1930).

Suleri, Sara, *The Rhetoric of English India* (Chicago: University of Chicago Press, 1992).

Sullivan, Rodney, Cholera and colonialism in the Philippines, 1899–1903, in Roy MacLeod and Milton Lewis (eds), *Disease, Medicine, and Empire. Perspectives on Western medicine and the experience of European expansion* (London and New York: Routledge, 1988), pp. 284–300.

Szreter, Simon, The importance of social intervention in Britain's mortality decline c. 1850–1914: A re-interpretation of the role of public health, *SHM* 1, 1 (1988): 1–37.

Szreter, Simon, Introduction: The GRO and the Historians. *SHM* 4, 3 (1991): 401–414.

Szreter, Simon, The GRO and the Public Health Movement in Britain, 1837–1914, *SHM* 4, 3 (1991): 443–463.

Tan Chee Khoon, *Memorandum on the Malayanization of the Medical Association of the Federation of Malaya by the Alumni Association of the King Edward VII College of Medicine and Faculty of Medicine, Univerity of Malaya*, 5 December 1955, Rhodes House Library, Colonial Records Project, Mss Indian Ocean S39.

Thomas, Nicholas, Sanitation and seeing: The creation of state power in early colonial Fiji, *Comparative Studies in Social History* 32 (1990): 149–170.

Towers, Bridget A., Health education policy 1916–1926: venereal disease and the prophylaxis dilemma, *MH* 24, 1 (1980): 70–87.

del Tufo, M. V., *Malaya Comprising the Federation of Malaya and the Colony of Singapore. A Report on the 1947 Census of Population* (London: Crown Agents for the Colonies on behalf of the Governments of the Federation of Malaya and the Colony of Singapore, 1949).

Turner, E. B. British Social Hygiene Council notes, *Health and Empire* 1, 4 (1926): 328–329.

Turshen, Meredith, The impact of colonialism on health and health services in Tanzania, *IJHS* 7, 1 (1977): 7–35.

Turshen, Meredith, *The Political Ecology of Disease in Tanzania* (New Brunswick, NJ: Rutgers University Press, 1984).

Twumasi, Patrick A., Colonialism and international health: A study in social change in Ghana, *SSM* 15B (1981): 147–151.

Vaughan, Megan, *Curing their Ills: Colonial power and African illness* (Cambridge: Polity Press, 1991).

Vickers, W. J. and J. H. Strahan, *A Health Survey of the State of Kedah with special reference to rice field malaria, nutrition, and the water supply, 1935–1936* (Kuala Lumpur: Ryle, Palmer, 1936).

Viswanathan, Gauri, *Masks of Conquest. Literary study and British rule in India* (London: Faber and Faber, 1990).

Vlassoff, C. and Eva M. Rathheber, Gender and tropical diseases: New research focus, *SSM* 37, 4 (1993): 513–520.

Vlassoff, Carol and Elssy Bonilla, Gender-related differences in the impact of tropical diseases on women: What do we know? *JBS* 26 (1994): 37–53.

Vlieland, C. A., *British Malaya. A Report on the 1931 Census and certain problems of vital statistics* (London: Crown Agents for the Colonies for the Colony of the Straits Settlements and the Malay States under British Protection, 1932).

Waddington, I., *The Medical Profession in the Industrial Revolution* (Dublin: Gill and Macmillan, 1984).

Warren, James F., *Rickshaw Coolie: A People's History of Singapore* (Singapore: Oxford University Press, 1986).

Warren, James F., *At the Edge of Southeast Asian History: Essays* (Quezon City: New Day Publishers, 1987).

Warren, James F., Prostitution in Singapore society and the *Karayuki-san*, in Peter J. Rimmer and Lisa M. Allen (eds), *The Underside of Malaysian History: Pullers, Prostitutes, Plantation Workers* (Singapore: Singapore University Press, 1990), pp. 161–176.

Warren, James F., *Ah-Ku and Karayuki-san: Prostitution in Singapore, 1870–1940* (Singapore and New York: Oxford University Press, 1993).

Watson, Sir Malcolm, *Some Pages from the History of the Prevention of Malaria.* The Finlayson Memorial Lecture, Glasgow, 29 November 1934 (Glasgow: Alex Macdougall, 1935).

Watson, Sir Malcolm, Malaria and mosquitos: Forty years on. *JRSA* LXXXVII, No. 4505 (1939): 482–502.

Watson, Sir Malcolm, *Some Emergency Anti-malarial Measures* (London: Ross Institute Industrial Advisory Committee, 1942).

Weindling, Paul, The politics of international co-ordination to combat sexually transmitted diseases, 1900–1980s, in Virginia Berridge and Philip Strong (eds), *AIDS in Contemporary History* (Cambridge: Cambridge University Press, forthcoming).

Wellington, A. R., *Hygiene and Sanitation in British Malaya.* Malayan Series No. XVI, British Empire Exhibition, London, 1924 (Singapore: Fraser and Neave, 1923).

Wellington, A. R., *The ways and means adopted by government for the control of malaria in the Federated Malay States.* Paper presented to the Far Eastern Association of Tropical Medicine, Tokyo, October 1925. (Kuala Lumpur: Federated Malay States Government Press, 1925).

White, Douglas, The Straits Settlements Ordinance, October 1930, *Health and Empire* VI, 1 (1931): 18–21.

White, N. J. and D. A. Warrell, The management of severe malaria, in W. H. Wernsdorfer and I. A. McGregor (eds), *Malaria. Principles and Practice of Malariology*, vol.I (Edinburgh: Churchill Livingstone, 1988), pp. 865–888.

Williams, C. D., The life of a Malay child, *JMBMA* 2, 2 (1938): 73–81.

Williams, C. D., Common diseases of children as seen in the General Hospital, Singapore, *JMBMA* 2, 3 (1938): 113–123.

Williams, C. D. and J. W. Scharff, *Preventive Paediatrics. An experiment in health work in Trengganu in 1940–41, with an Appendix containing notes for Dressers and Nurses* (Kuala Lumpur: Department of Public Relations, Federation of Malaya, 1948).

Williams, W., Puerperal mortality, *Transactions of the Epidemiological Society of London* XV (New Series) (1895–1896): 100–133.

Williamson, K. B., The control of rural malaria. *The MAHA Magazine (Official organ of the Malayan Agri-horticultural Association and of the Selangor Gardening Society* 3, 3 (1933–4): 145–150; 3, 4: 201–206; 4, 1: 224–228; 4, 2: 281–291.

Wilson, T., The control of rural malaria in Malaya, 1936. *BIMR* No. 2 (Kuala Lumpur: FMS Government Press, 1939).

Winslow, C. E. A., *The Conquest of Epidemic Disease: A chapter in the history of ideas* (Princeton: Princeton University Press, 1967) (1st pub. 1943).

Winzeler, Robert, Malayan *amok* and *latah* as 'history bound' syndromes, in Peter J. Rimmer and Lisa M. Allen (eds), *The Underside of Malaysian History: Pullers, Prostitutes, Plantation Workers* (Singapore: Singapore University Press, 1990), pp. 214–229.

Woodhull, A. A., *Notes on Congress of Hygiene and Demography, London, 1891* (Trenton, NJ: John L. Murphy, 1892).

Wohl, Anthony S., *Endangered Lives. Public health in Victorian Britain* (London: J. M. Dent, 1983).

Woodham-Smith, Cecil, *Florence Nightingale, 1820–1910* (London: Fontana Books, 1968) (1st pub. 1951).

Woodward, L. M., *Commission of Enquiry into the Conduct of Government Medical Officers, Report* (Kuala Lumpur: Government Printing Office, 1908).

Woolcock, Helen R., 'Our salubrious climate': attitudes to health in colonial Queensland, in Roy MacLeod and Milton Lewis (eds), *Disease, Medicine, and Empire. Perspectives on Western medicine and the experience of European expansion* (London and New York: Routledge, 1988), pp. 176–193.

Worboys, Michael, The emergence of tropical medicine: a study in the establishment of a scientific specialty, in G. Lemain, R. MacLeod, M. Mulkay and P. Weingart (eds), *Perspectives on the Emergence of Scientific Disciplines* (The Hague: Mouton, 1976), pp. 75–98.

Worboys, Michael, Manson, Ross and colonial medical policy: Tropical medicine in London and Liverpool, 1899–1914, in Roy MacLeod and Milton Lewis (eds), *Disease, Medicine, and Empire. Perspectives on Western medicine and the experience of European expansion* (London and New York: Routledge, 1988), pp. 21–37.

Worboys, Michael, The discovery of colonial malnutrition between the wars, in David Arnold (ed.), *Imperial Medicine and Indigenous Societies* (Manchester and New York: Manchester University Press, 1988), pp. 208–225.

Worboys, Michael, British colonial medicine and tropical imperialism: A comparative perspective, in G. M. van Heteren, A. de Knecht-van Eekelen and M. J. D. Poulissen (eds), *Dutch Medicine in the Malay Archipelago, 1816–1942.* Articles presented at a symposium held in honour of Professor Dr D. de Moulin. Nieuwe Nederlandse Bijdragen tot de Gescgiendenis der Geneeskunde en der Natuurwtenschappen No. z35 (Chief editor A. M. Luyendijk-Elshout) (Amsterdam and Atlanta, GA.: Rodopi, 1989), pp. 153–167.

Wylie, E. M. The search for the cause of Beriberi in the Malay Peninsula: The contribution of Dr W. L. Braddon. *JMBRAS* LXI, 2 (1988): 93–122.

Wylie, E. M. Colonial administration and malaria in British Malaya, 1900–1920, Unpublished honours dissertation (Brisbane: Griffith University, 1989).

Wylie, E. M., Economic change and disease in Malaya c.1820–1920: A study in human ecology, unpublished PhD dissertation (Brisbane: Griffith University, 1994).

Yeoh, Brenda, Power and the People: Municipal control and plebeian agency in the control of disease and sanitary conditions in turn-of-the-century Singapore, unpublished paper presented at the Regional Conference of the Asian Studies Association of Australia, Singapore, February 1989.

Archival sources

Arkib Negara Malaysia, Kuala Lumpur
    Federated Malay States
        Files of the Malaria Advisory Board (MAB)
        Files of the Institute of Medical Research (IMR)
        Files of the Selangor Secretariat (Sel. Sec.)
    Kelantan, Files of the British Adviser of Kelantan (BAKel)
    Trengganu, Files of the British Adviser of Trengganu (BATr)
    Kedah, Files of the British Adviser of Kedah (BAK)

Foreign and Commonwealth Office Library, London
    Colonial Reports. Papers relating to Her Majesty's Colonial Possessions, 1873–1891

National Archives of Singapore
    Straits Settlements Records (SSR), 1800–1867
    East India Company Records, 1800–1875

Public Records Office, Kew (London)
    Great Britain, Colonial Office
    Accounts and Papers, ZHCI (ZHCI)
    Files of the Colonial Office, Original Correspondence, Straits Settlements, CO273
    Files of the Colonial Office, Singapore correspondence, CO953
    Files of the Colonial Office, Colonial Development Advisory Committee, CO859
    Files of the Colonial Office, Colonial Medical Research Committee, Papers and Minutes of Meetings, CO913
    Files of the India Office, Factory Records (India Office)
    Files of the British Military Administration (BMA)

Rhodes House, Oxford
    Colonial Records Project
    Individual items listed under author's name (above)

Royal Commonwealth Society, London
    Files of the British Association of Malaya (BAM)

Index

gender, xiv-xv, 16-18, 71; social
  construction of, 71, 212, 228
General Hospital, Malacca, 15; Penang,
  15; purpose of, 36; Singapore
  266 n7
General Register Office, 32
genetic differences, 76, 77
Georgetown Municipality, 124
germ theory, 73
Gerrard, P. N., 145, 233
Gimlette, J. D., 20, 183, 184, 186, 190;
  memorandum on cholera, 49–50
Golomb, L., 20
Grassi, Giovanni, 8

Hailam, Dr Rupert, 197
Hare, G. T., 167, 182, 183
Harrison, M., 7
Hart, D., 20
Haynes, A. S., 90, 132, 145
Headrick, D. R., 7
Health Boards, responsibilities of, 153
health education, for cholera, 48; for
  infant care, 217, 218; for influenza,
  52; for malaria, 154; for use of
  trained midwives, 210; for venereal
  disease, 198, 199
healthy workforce, economic advantage
  of, xiii, 17
Herrmann, E. K., xiii
Hill, Professor Bostock, 198
hill stations, 8, 73, 74
Hill, T. S., 158
historiography, xvii, 3-4, 25–26, 244 n1,
  244 n2, 278 n53
Hobsbawm, E., 4
home visiting, 11, 65, 207, 211, 213,
  215, 222
homelessness, see vagrancy
homicide, 27, 36
homosexual relations, 19, 166, 178, 179
hookworm, 28, 63, 132, 241, 271 n14, 271
  n34; campaign against, 152, 234
Hooper, W. E., 118
hospital returns, Penang, 36; gender
  differences in, 36, 58
hospital use, ethnic differences, 220;
  see also reluctance, delay
hospitals, charges for, 147; conditions of,
  68, 144–47, 257 n5, 273 n79; estate,
  adequacy of, 146–47, 151; ethnic
  differences in use of, 67, 69; fear of,
  67, 263 n109; group hospitals, 145,
  151; stratification in, 232
housing conditions, 83, 113-14, 115; on
  estates, 276 n163; in kampungs, 56,
  84; in Kuala Lumpur, 104

humoral medical theory, 25, 259 n80
hygiene rules of, 74-75

immigrant workers, conditions of
  employment, 80, 270 n4; death
  rates of, 43, 58, 79; exposure to
  disease, 30; recruitment of, 28, 77,
  128, 129; recruitment of women,
  92; repatriation of, 95; risk of
  disease to, 8
immunity, ideas of, 7, 72, 75, 246 n21
India Office, 32, 34
Indian Immigration Enactment, 150
Indian Immigration Fund, 97, 127, 128
Indian Plague Commission, 110, 114
Indochina, labour conditions in, 11
infant feeding, 206, 212, 214–15
infant welfare, policies and programs, 11,
  203; clinics, 65, 215–17, 222;
  changes of staff, 218
infectious disease, decline in, 27
influenza, 51-52, 149; direct deaths from,
  52, 54
injuries, workplace, 81; see also employment
inquiries, into alcohol, 142; into brothel
  clubs, 187, 188; into health on
  estates (1890), 129, 137, 139–40,
  150, for Chinese and Javanese
  labourers (1910), 132, 140, 150,
  among estate labourers (1924), 60,
  134, 147–48, 150, 153, membership
  of, 273–74 n106; into housing
  (1906–07), 114–16, 204; into housing
  (1917), 117, 122; into nutrition in
  the Colonial Empire, 90, 93, 161,
  227; into prostitution and venereal
  disease (1860s), 32, into
  prostitution (1898), 167, 179; on
  tuberculosis (1923), 122
inspection, of houses, 125, 126; see also
  surveillance
Institute of Medical Research, Kuala
  Lumpur, 9, 90, 93, 152, 236
International Labour Organisation, 196
International Sanitary Convention, 51,
  254 n52
isolation, 238; and institutionalisation,
  239; of tuberculosis patients, 122
Ivory Coast, health services, 253 n26

Jackson, J. C., 44
Java, labour conditions on, 11
Javanese, 29
Jelf, A. S., 150
Jenner, E., 8
Johore, deaths from influenza, 52
Johore Bahru, 98